Dying to Care?

Based on major multi-centre research in the UK, *Dying to Care?* aims to identify why work stress is such a problem in healthcare generally, and in HIV healthcare in particular. The similarities and differences between work stress experienced in general healthcare settings and in HIV/AIDS are explored in a state-of-the-art review of international research and experience in the field to date.

Practical in focus, *Dying to Care?* explores ways in which the unique stresses of patient advocacy in HIV/AIDS can be addressed, identifying the best approaches for management. Based on extensive research and clinical experience of the author and the experiences of health workers of all disciplines working in HIV/AIDS and oncology, the book examines the general historical confusion between work stress and burnout, and presents concrete suggestions for burnout prevention. The studies conducted include 'context initiatives' such as:

- ensuring staff vary workloads, enabling expression of work successes
- encouragement for planning non-work periods
- normalising the experience and expression of work stress
- recognising the impact of loss
- incorporating the use of ritual in saying goodbye to dying patients.

This will be a key handbook for managers, physicians, nurses, social workers, health advisers and counsellors working in or alongside healthcare. It will also have practical relevance to similar groups working in the context of other life-threatening diseases.

David Miller is Head of the Department of Psychology and Psychotherapy for HIV/STD at Mortimer Market Centre, London (Camden and Islington NHS Trust), and Honorary Senior Lecturer at Royal Free and University College Medical School, University College London. He is presently the Psychosocial Adviser to UNAIDS, Geneva.

Social Aspects of AIDS

Series editor: Peter Aggleton

Institute of Education, University of London

AIDS is not simply a concern for scientists, doctors and medical researchers, it has important social dimensions as well. These include individual, cultural and media responses to the epidemic, stigmatization and discrimination, counselling, care and health promotion. This series of books brings together work from many disciplines including psychology, sociology, cultural and media studies, anthropology, education and history. The titles will be of interest to the general reader, those involved in education and social research, and scientific researchers who want to examine the social aspects of AIDS.

Dying to Care?
Work, stress and burnout in HIV/AIDS

David Miller

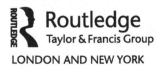

Routledge
Taylor & Francis Group

LONDON AND NEW YORK

First published 2000 by Routledge
2 Park Square, Milton Park, Abingdon, Oxon OX14 4RN
605 Third Avenue, New York, NY 10017

Routledge is an imprint of the Taylor & Francis Group, an informa business

© 2000 David Miller

Typeset in Galliard by
BOOK NOW Ltd

British Library Cataloguing in Publication Data
A catalogue record for this book is available
from the British Library

Library of Congress Cataloging in Publication Data
A catalog record for this book has been requested

ISBN 13: 978-1-85728-820-9 (hbk)
ISBN 13: 978-1-85728-821-6 (pbk)

Social Aspects of AIDS

Series editor: Peter Aggleton

Institute of Education, University of London

This book is dedicated to absent friends and to a new one, Ada P (16.10.98).

Contents

Tables and figures

Series editor's preface

The global epidemics of HIV and AIDS have brought forth both the best and worst in human nature. On the one hand, they have triggered reponses of stigmatisation, ostracisation, discrimination and denial. On the other hand, they have led to constructive and supportive reactions on the part of families, communities and individuals. Key among those who have responded positively to the challenges that AIDS poses are many health care workers and informal sector carers. Without their assistance and support, many people with AIDS would live (or would have lived) much poorer quality lives. Yet providing such care takes its toll and, as David Miller explains, the occupational stresses and 'burnout' associated with this work can be considerable. *Dying to Care?* examines some of these issues in greater depth. It offers an overview of some of the challenges that health care workers and informal sector carers have had to face, and contains recommendations for the better management of occupational stress and burnout. Of relevance to health care workers, social researchers and community and voluntary sector workers in a variety of fields, this book contains over a decade's worth of reflection and contemplation on these important concerns.

Peter Aggleton

Foreword

We are now nearly 20 years in the AIDS epidemic – 20 years of suffering and joy, hard-won victories and deceptions, solidarity and loneliness, exciting discoveries and lost illusions. Recently, much attention has gone to 'long-term survivors' among people infected with HIV, and thanks to the availability of 'highly active anti-retroviral therapy', many people with HIV in high-income countries now live longer and better. However, among the care providers there are also 'long-term survivors' – those who have been working in the field of HIV/AIDS for many years. Many, if not the majority, have gone through phases of burnout, acute stress, and moments of existential doubt as a result of their work.

This book is a timely and – for once – essential addition to the growing and vast literature on AIDS. It uniquely fills a gap by addressing both research and management of HIV/AIDS-related work stress and burnout. It is very much grounded in first-hand experience of the author, and is a reflection of David Miller's sound research methodology, his empathy for people, and his long practical experience on the subject. What I particularly like about this book is the combination of research results and practical lessons on how to prevent and manage burnout. The stories and experience are largely about AIDS, but they are very relevant for basically all health and social professionals. Let us face it: HIV will be with us for a long time, and it is crucial that all of us in this challenging field of HIV/AIDS learn how to cope with the long-term consequences on our own well-being and effectiveness.

This book helps us to recognise, understand and manage better work-related stress and burnout, and is therefore a must for everybody working within the clinical and social HIV area. David Miller is to be congratulated for what will undoubtedly become a classic.

Peter Piot

Preface

It is always important to have a sense of history. This book reflects a decade of contemplation and action in this field of burnout in HIV/AIDS by myself, and by many greatly appreciated colleagues. The initial encouragement and support for working in this area came from Tony Pinching in London, Norman Sartorius in Geneva, and Chris Smith MP. What started as a wistful idea for possible collaboration turned into an especially enjoyable and constructive series of research activities with Pamela Gillies in Nottingham in the 1990s. Much of what follows is a product of our collaboration and her tremendous support. Our colleagues in Nottingham – Alison Broderick, Carol Coupland, Cathy Elliott, Katherine Fielding, Richard Madeley, the late Val Morris, Kerry Nelson, Jim Pearson, Lesley Rushton, Sarah Smith, Mary Stevenson, and Dave Williams – also contributed so graciously their time, their wisdom and skills as the national studies became a reality and bore fruit. The UK studies described in detail in Chapters 7 and 8 owed so much to concerned and committed colleagues in many major sites in the UK: Marilyn Wilson in Leicester; the late Richard Wells and Bob Tindall, Barbara Dicks, Anne Cattell, Anne Fingret, Tony Wingate, William Hartley and Jane Mallett all in London; John Green and Fiona Wallace, Pat Wright, Jane Bruton and Rob Miller, Richard Gilson and John Howson, Jane Anderson, Riva Miller, Derval Murray, Margaret Johnson and Debbie Farmer, Rob George, and Mary Hughes; Tom Snee, Liza Catan, Sandra Williams, Jean Faugier, Ian Hicken, Nick Raisen, and Barbara Salmon; Neil Sherringham, Jonathon Grimshaw, Alan Turkie and Ros Pendlebury; Christopher Eyes, Shirley Magwenzi, Eddie Manning and Seamus Noone; Linda Grant and Marian Lewin; Christopher Spence, Brit Haggar, Hamish MacGregor and Leo Atkins; Nick Partridge, Bill Hendry and Richard Haigh – all and more have their vital contributions reflected in these pages.

It is amazing how work grows. Outstanding work by colleagues in many countries also forms the fabric of much that lies herein – Rachel Baggaley, Marco Bellani, Lydia Bennett, Dieter Kleiber, Lina Maslanka, Mike Ross, Raffaele Visintini, to name a few. Collaborations with them all have been very enjoyable and constructive.

Once the formal research was completed and on the shelf, the impetus to make it more widely presentable and useful was so considerably maintained by John

Cape. Caroline Wintersgill gave constructive suggestions and showed great patience.

We know what we know because vulnerable people inform us of their truths. Extremely busy people gave precious time and vital meaning to the studies and clinical work that has led to the small but growing understanding that now informs so many. As if hard-working health staff and volunteers didn't have enough to do . . .

To all those mentioned and many that are not, most grateful thanks for all the work you did and do for all of those among whom we work.

Finally, this book was written overlooking a springtime Pretorian garden. To Sandra Anderson, my amazed thanks always for this and so much more. And to George and his mates – where now do you weave your sylvan spells . . . ?

David Miller

Part I
Development of the awareness of work stress and burnout

1 Introduction

> It has been claimed that about half the entire working population are unhappy
> in their jobs and as many as 90% may be spending much of their time and
> energy in work that brings them no closer to their goals in life. About 75% of
> those who consult psychiatrists are experiencing problems that can be traced
> to lack of job satisfaction or an inability to relax.
>
> (Levi, 1987)

Imagine . . .

Imagine some mercenary empire-builder, some new corporate re-engineering,
retrenchment-minded money flunkey, hired to make his hospital profitable and
indispensible, named Mr Mercenary[1]. Mr Mercenary decides to impress himself
and others with his ability to manipulate those who work for him in the hospital,
and there is one certain way. For the times are hard. Jobs are hard to come by, and
eagerly enacted. The workforce is getting poorer year on year as salaries reduce in
real terms while overall profits grow, yet the politicians who employ Mr
Mercenary insist that the people have never had it better. Those who grumble are
publicly denounced as not caring about their patients, and as being greedy, so the
public becomes less sympathetic towards them. Soon, many people work harder
to protect what they have. In this setting, Mr Mercenary gets to work. He decides
to design a job specifically with the purpose of making it stressful.

The first thing Mr Mercenary does is to make the tasks of the job vague, for he
knows that a vague job description is both confusing and enables the person who
takes the job – The Candidate – to tread on the toes of many colleagues, making
them suspicious and even hostile towards her. At the same time, Mr Mercenary
makes it clear to all colleagues that the new person is welcome and very necessary.
That way, no-one is clear what The Candidate is supposed to do, or why, or how
much. Because the job is 'important', however, colleagues are intimidated and do
not ask directly what The Candidate is there for. The Candidate doesn't ask either,
because that would show that she *needs* to ask, and make her feel foolish in front of
everyone else. This situation is reinforced by The Candidate not being given a
clear overview of the activities, aims and roles of her organisation, its ethos, and
how her new job fits in to the organisation. What is known is that The Candidate

is a specialist with professional training. However, Mr Mercenary adds another touch – the experience that made The Candidate valuable in the first place is never called upon. In this way, The Candidate is confused, isolated, the object of suspicion *and* de-skilled.

In another scenario, Mr Mercenary might hire The Candidate to fill a specific post, then require her to do something else while staying in the post. In other words, the job stays but the tasks are changed, without negotiation. The demoralised and confused Candidate feels little choice but to comply (jobs are scarce, after all). Before long, all sense of expertise and use are lost, as, in either scenario, The Candidate runs on the spot trying to perform to an agenda that is neither clear nor understandable.

Mr Mercenary then cranks the pressure up by telling The Candidate that she must do more, because the staff is being down-sized. More work! Additionally, The Candidate is informed that she must also attend more meetings, do more paperwork, and see fewer patients. She will be placed on a performance-related pay structure that means she will have salary deducted if she doesn't meet Mr Mercenary's unnegotiated performance targets.

Eventually, The Candidate and her colleagues decide that they have to challenge the situation, and they assemble a list of grievances which are presented to Mr Mercenary. He responds by informing them that they are undermining the welfare of their patients and that their demands are making further redundancies more likely. Indeed, their budget is cut, so they are able to do less with their patients, even when they know they can and should do more. While this is happening, the politicians who hired Mr Mercenary decide that, in order to protect themselves from negative fallout associated with the demands of The Candidate and her colleagues, they will denounce the colleagues in the national media as showing a mercenary spirit, of betraying their sense of vocation, of making the interests of patients secondary to their own financial greed. The charge makes front-page news, and the colleagues feel shocked and betrayed.

The politicians then decide that they will change the nature of the system in which The Candidate and her colleagues work, and Mr Mercenary adds this into his plan. The hospital in which the colleagues all work is turned into a business, where the workers are now called 'providers' and they have to bid for the money and resources to do their job from managers – now known as 'purchasers'. The purchasers have no real experience of the health industry, but are given the power of life and death because they were good at making a profit from selling groceries, cars or coal. In addition, the colleagues are told that they are now in direct competition with their colleagues at neighbouring health facilities. This means that even if they know their colleagues are better at managing specific aspects of health care, they cannot refer their patients on, because that would reduce the basis on which money is allocated to their own hospital.

The colleagues are later told that they will soon have to combine with their competitors to make fewer hospitals because hospitals are so expensive to run. The colleagues are told they must also make the case for being able to keep their jobs. Once that has happened, the colleagues, including The Candidate, are told that their jobs are all being re-graded downwards, and that they must all re-apply for their own jobs that are now broader and busier, and that will in future be paid at a lower rate. Meanwhile, Mr Mercenary is being awarded a pay rise far in excess of those negotiated for the people actually seeing patients, because of his excellent work in reaching performance targets and cutting costs (beds, jobs, resources).

While such job circumstances are being played out cynically by Mr Mercenary on a structural level, major changes are happening at a clinical level also. The colleagues are working with a new disease – one that seems to attack only stigmatised, marginalised social groups, and that causes unpredictable, often catastrophic illnesses that eventually prove fatal. Every time a new drug is identified and employed, it eventually fails. As it is discovered that the disease is caused by a transmissable agent – a virus – the families and loved-ones of The Candidate and her colleagues all beg them to do something else in order to protect their families from possibly 'catching' the newly found bug. Many relationships have been found to crack under the strain. The new disease also means that new knowledge has to be acquired, new procedures learned and adopted, a dramatic expansion of clinical roles, and a rapid broadening of services to meet the needs and demands of previously un-addressed patient groups. There is much negotiation between staff of who should really be doing what, and many staff feel disaffected with the changes to their working arrangements.

It is not all bad news, of course – the media has made stars of some staff and patients, prominent citizens make statements and photo opportunities that work to reduce the stigma and fear surrounding the disease, and more money comes in because the true extent of the infection in the communities becomes clear. Nevertheless, the pressures grow as the patient numbers grow. Colleagues in other areas of health care become resentful and jealous of the new attention and money being given to this new area of work, when they continue to fight for any resources that may be needed.

Soon, staff are calling in sick because they've had too much of death and dying, of not being able to cure, of causing illness with medicines supposedly designed to help, with the disappointment of recurrent failure in their jobs. The Candidate tries so hard to keep up with the rapidly growing and vast knowledge base, to cover for her colleagues, to push the searing disappointment and pain of repeated loss of long-term patients with whom she increasingly identifies, and with Mr Mercenary's constant reminders that she should be doing more with less, for less, and feel lucky that she still has a job to come to, while still trying to find time for life with her family, friends, loved-ones, and for herself. Sleep seems reluctant to visit, so alcohol and drugs are increasingly used fall-backs. Increasingly, those not in the field seem less relevant to the importance of The Candidate's work, and are seen less often. Sheer fatigue makes her feel less communicative, less motivated, less capable of responding to those around her. Yet, whenever she has thought of asking for help from colleagues or Mr Mercenary, she remembers another colleague who once did so, and was told that signs of depression and exhaustion were clear evidence of being unfit to do the work at all, and that colleague was effectively pushed out of his job. What to do but try to work harder, so no-one will notice how low, or tired, and desparate she is . . . ?

It is not hard to see situations like this unfolding across the world, because this is a deliberate expression of a darker side of the extraordinary world of HIV/AIDS care in countries that have many patients, and in formerly socialised medical systems that have, in recent years, moved more directly into privatised medicine and rationalising of current health service structures. Even where the health care systems have been relatively stable, the demands of this health tragedy have had health workers on the back foot from the beginning. And the vehicle of HIV/AIDS has enabled new light to be shed on the issue of workplace stress and morbidity[2], particularly in the field of health care.

Perhaps one of the most important lessons arising from the enriching pain of HIV/AIDS care is that this kind of consequence for health workers does really happen, and that it is entirely legitimate to acknowledge this pain and what it means – for organisations, and for the people who staff and serve them. Indeed, it is entirely necessary to acknowledge it, for if we do not, we risk losing the most vital resource in our global arsenal against the virus: experienced, committed, inspired, caring people. AIDS has also taught us the fatal error of not learning from neighbours, and what lessons there are to reduce HIV spread and the impact of it in communities. When we consider workplace morbidity, we also have lessons to avoid in HIV/AIDS care that have been hard-learned in other theatres of distress.

The costs of ill health at work

The costs of mental-health and occupational stress problems in the general work-force are substantial. The Confederation of British Industry (CBI) has calculated that 360 million working days are lost annually in the UK through sickness, at a cost of STG£8 billion (Sigman, 1992), and the UK Health and Safety Executive estimates that at least half of these lost days are stress-related (Cooper and Cartwright, 1994). These figures and estimates were based only on diagnosed and end-stage illness – absences shorter than 7 days at that time were not medically certified, and therefore not recorded in this calculation. The CBI and Department of Health have also reported that 30 times as many working days are lost through stress and mental illness than through industrial disputes. Other costs of occupational stress and morbidity include: reduced productivity, increased labour turnover, poor timekeeping, lowered staff relations and morale, and increased accidents. In the general work population, Jenkins (1993) noted that mental illness accounts for 14 per cent of certified sickness absence, as well as 14 per cent of National Health Service (NHS) inpatient costs and 23 per cent of NHS pharmaceutical costs. Such high costs are also found in other developed countries. A 1986 commission in the United States found stress-related disorders cost the USA roughly 12 per cent of its Gross National Product (cited by Cooper, 1992). In the 1980s, USA industry lost approximately 550 million working days annually due to absenteeism, and 54 per cent of these lost days were estimated to be stress-related (Elkin and Rosch, 1990).

As such estimates imply, morbidity associated with work is not always easy to identify reliably. Correlate markers of morbidity have therefore been used in some studies. For example, alcohol consumption to excess is often used as an indication of psychosocial morbidity in the workplace. Tissue evidence of alcohol abuse was found in 4.5 per cent of UK aircrew who died in accidents between 1955–79 (Harding and Mills, 1983). Rose, Jenkins and Hurst (1978) found that Boston air-traffic controllers drank alcohol much more heavily than the general population, and a lower proportion than found in the general population remained abstemious. In a toxological study on 1,345 general aviation pilots who had been killed in air accidents in the United States between 1968–74, elevated blood alcohol levels were found in 19.5 per cent; the blood alcohol level was over 0.05 per cent in just under 9 per cent of this population (Rose, Jenkins and Hurst, 1978). In a series of studies of medical staff (Firth-Cozens, 1987; Firth-Cozens and Morrison, 1989) evidence was found of depression in 28 per cent of junior house officers, in whom there was an estimated 50 per cent prevalence of emotional disturbance overall. Heavy drinking and significant drug use for physical illness was also noted in this population, and drinking to excess has also been identified as a coping strategy in recent studies of nurses in Scotland (Plant, Plant and Foster, 1992). A more recent postal survey of hospital consultants, hospital administrative staff, and general practitioners, by Caplan (1994), showed that overall, on the Hospital Anxiety and Depression Scale (HAD), only 46 per cent (n = 178) were free from anxiety, 25 per cent (n = 100) scored as borderline cases, and 29 per cent (n = 111) had clinically measurable symptoms. This same study showed that on the General Health Questionnaire (GHQ), 46 per cent of the consultants, 48 per cent of the GP's, and 46 per cent of the managers scored in the range for 'caseness' (i.e., had marked psychological vulnerability), while only 26.8 per cent of the general population would be expected to score in that range (Caplan, 1994).

Rates of suicide in medical professionals have frequently been demonstrated to be higher than for many other occupational groups. A recent review of morbidity among anaesthetists revealed an excess of deaths by suicide in both British and American anaesthetists compared with all physicians and with life insurance policyholders, especially in those under 55 years of age (Redfern, 1990). Surprisingly, the epidemiology of psychiatric disturbance in the health industry has yet to be comprehensively assessed in the UK. The Caplan (1994) study identified that on postal responses to the HAD, 27 per cent (n = 69) of general practitioners were borderline or clinically depressed, and this group were significantly more likely than hospital consultants to show suicidal thinking.

Birch (1975) showed that 66 per cent of a sample of nursing drop-outs said they left because of the stress of nursing. In more recent years, there has been growing evidence that the threat of job loss – a new phenomenon in the UK health industry – is equivalent in terms of psychological impact to experiences of bereavement and other forms of loss (Whittington, Wilson and Avery, 1993). The most significant increases in GHQ scores in a Swedish study of a plant closure involving 354 workers occurred during initial periods of uncertainty when redundancies were threatened or announced revealed (Arnetz *et al.*, 1988). Similar findings have been found by Warr and Jackson (1985), who noted psychological adjustment following from initial periods of stress in a context of redundancy and job loss.

It is not clear how far work-based factors, as opposed to personality-based factors, influence such levels of morbidity (redundancy excepted). However, a great deal of effort has gone into characterising work-based stressors in an attempt to form a clearer picture of morbidity at work, of how it can be predicted and therefore avoided. Considerable emphasis has also been placed on a relatively recently described and acknowledged phenomenon – burnout in health care workers – particularly in view of the impact it may have on the quality of patient care, and the resulting capacity for and efficiency and effectiveness of health service provision.

Main aims of this book

In many countries of the world, the stress of HIV/AIDS care is no longer avoidable. In a series of training activities in psychosocial management for HIV/ AIDS in many cultures, the same questions have kept arising when the pressures of HIV care are discussed:

- Is there something wrong with me?
- Are other HIV services producing the same problems?
- Why are we all feeling so stressed and exhausted?
- What can we do about it?

This book aims to examine the notion of 'burnout' and occupational morbidity in the context of emotionally stressful fields of health care, especially HIV/AIDS. It seeks to identify how best to deal with work stress and burnout in this occupational setting, in a practical way. There are intrinsic elements of work in this and other health fields that may contribute to health worker stress, such as multiple deaths of patients, uncertainties about treatment effectiveness, the relative youth of many patients, and social stigma associated with having these diseases (Sontag, 1990). And most health care systems have staff who report that they are overworked – overwork almost seems to be a *sine qua non* of health care. In addition, however, the wider context of health care in Britain has been undergoing a period of very considerable change:

- Changes in the structure of health care, including the imposition of purchaser–provider systems introducing competition within different arms of the health care service.
- Changes in means and capacities for resource allocation – including staffing – within NHS Trusts, resulting in the threat of hospital closures and staff redundancies, especially with the merging of major teaching hospitals.
- Changes in the resourcing of specialist areas of health care and research, not

least HIV/AIDS, despite sexual health and prevention of sexually transmitted disease being a priority area in the government statement, 'Health of the Nation'.

This book addresses issues in health worker morbidity that arise in very many cultures, not just those that emerged in the UK. A central tenent of this book is that the phenomenon of health worker stress and burnout is a primary consequence not so much of attributes brought to the workplace by individual health workers, but *mainly* of the structures and processes of health care organisations that so often then rest content to allow staff experiencing the destructive forces of those structures and processes to take responsibility for their appearance and, in some cases, even be pathologised for experiencing them.

Work stress and occupational morbidity have, in the past 15 years, become synonymous with the notion of 'burnout' – a term that has, until recently, had little theoretical substance, and that has been the subject of growing academic debate. This book examines the notion of burnout in the context of occupational stress, and critically examines the degree to which our understanding of the field can be said to have advanced. It will suggest that theories underpinning the development of burnout are not clearly elaborated, and that research is only now coming to the point of providing empirical substance to earlier theories of how burnout develops.

It is tempting to think that understanding of occupational morbidity and burnout is sufficiently advanced to allow for the development of rational, clinically based strategies for intervention, so that with the appropriate allocation of resources such as staff and money, staff stress and burnout can be a thing of the past. This book will, however, demonstrate that there is still a great deal to learn about how work impacts upon the well-being of workers, inside and outside the workplace, and how this can best be managed. Additionally, the book describes in detail two national UK studies that have built upon previous research and methodological lessons. One, the MOMS study, is a large-scale quantitative and qualitative project examining the experiences of work stress and burnout – and preferences for staff support – of 200 health care workers in the fields of HIV/AIDS and oncology. This study also examines independent predictors of workplace stress and burnout in these populations. The second study examines pre-existing models of burnout prevention in four major HIV/AIDS treatment and care facilities, and uses the findings to make suggestions for both generic and targetted staff support programmes.

Perhaps the main aim of this book, however, is to legitimise the experiences of health workers who have recognised the problems of work stress in themselves and in others, yet whose pleas for support from higher authorities have gone unheeded or unrecognised. It is an expected consequence of many health structures that work-related stress should result in further alienation of individual staff. After all, we are not supposed to become emotionally involved in the experiences (especially the care experiences) of our charges. Most health systems convey a double jeopardy for the staff member who is brave enough to acknowledge their own work stress: to do so means admitting a psychological vulnerability and need, which can then be interpreted as due to a lapse in professional detatchment and standards, and even an advertisement of possible future unemployability. Similarly, most employers do not wish to have their structural pathologies revealed or expressed – understandably, they do not wish to advertise themselves as bad employers, not least because that would require that something be done, specifically by investing time and money in staff welfare. Yet for most hospitals or firms, the deliberate ignoring of the psychological welfare of their staff amounts to a studied denial of the realities of health care and its impact on the humans who make it work. Thus, a further agenda in this book is to emphasise the vital importance of investing in carers, by taking forward a new phase of empiricism in testing models of staff support. The need for such investment has never been greater, and the potential benefit for managing the global catastrophe of HIV/ AIDS by supporting staff has also never been so compelling.

Who this book is intended for

The book presents a review of academic research and debate in the areas of work stress and burnout, particularly focusing on the field of HIV/AIDS. As such, it is intended to be read by clinical researchers of all professions, to give background and pointers on future research in this area – what needs to be done, what we need to know, and why. In addition, much of the material is presented as a practical guide to developing strategies for management and prevention of burnout. As such, it is aimed at all health care professionals who might be seeking suggestions for improving workplace conditions, managing crises in colleagues and staff, and wishing to prevent future distress and psychological morbidity in their places of work.

Outline of the book chapters

The book will develop according to the following plan:

Chapter 2: Occupational stress: the background to the development of burnout. This chapter starts with a discussion of what is meant by occupational stress, and what causes stress in the workplace. The roles of factors identified both empirically and conceptually are assessed, together with how these factors led in recent years to the emergence of the concept of burnout.

Chapter 3: Burnout before HIV/AIDS. This chapter considers how burnout happens, the involvement of personality and other factors, and the processes through which burnout progresses. Part of the confusion within this general field has centred on the similarities between burnout and occupational stress generally, so attention is given to why they are similar, and why they may also be different.

Chapter 4: Symptoms and correlates of burnout. The physical, psychological and behavioural symptoms of burnout are reviewed, along with correlative factors associated with its emergence. Empirical symptoms of burnout – and their clinical diagnostic correlates – are described, especially the impact of burnout on personal relationships in and outside the workplace, and the less-well considered but possibly very important factors of gender, age and experience in the workplace.

Chapter 5: Burnout in HIV/AIDS. The significance of burnout for the HIV/AIDS field is examined and empirical evidence to date is reviewed. Examination of staff stresses arising from staffs' fears, issues of association, professional and role issues, and stigma, discrimination and ethical issues then leads to a discussion of known mediators of HIV/AIDS burnout. Using counselling as an example, the power of context is revealed as an impetus to burnout.

Chapter 6: Methodological limitations and issues raised in burnout research to date. The possible biases involved in volunteer-only studies are described, as well as the limitations of questionnaire-only and cross-sectional studies, and difficulties in interpreting burnout measures in relation to other standardised clinical measures. The problems with imposing solutions to management of staffs' reported work stress and burnout are also considered.

Chapter 7: The Multi-centre Occupational Morbidity Study (MOMS): Experiences and independent predictors of workplace stress and burnout. This chapter describes the aims, methodology and results of the first UK multi-centre study on burnout in HIV/AIDS and oncology populations. Associations with – and independently significant predictors of – self-reported and psychometric measures of work-related stress are presented and discussed in relation to key demographic indicators and observations of worker characteristics versus features of the workplace.

Chapter 8: The UK studies on staff preferences for support, and burnout prevention. Results from the MOMS study on stress management and support preferences are presented. Additionally, the two phases of the UK Burnout Prevention Study – and the results – are described. Findings from both studies are then discussed in terms of evidence in favour of targetted staff support, and implications for future staff support designs.

Chapter 9: Volunteers and burnout in HIV/AIDS. The relatively sparse empirical literature on HIV/AIDS volunteer populations is described, with particular emphasis on tensions associated with volunteering – in families, in the breadth and importance of the work done, in motivations, and in and between organisations. The chapter concludes with suggestions for burnout management and prevention.

Chapter 10: Management of occupational stress and burnout. A review of approaches to management of work stress and burnout is presented – an area where the conceptual confusions uncovered earlier in the discussion come to have practical, potentially obstructive significance. The vital distinctions between differing modes of supervision and support are explicated, and benefits and hazards of group approaches are discussed, along with the critical roles of staff management in HIV/AIDS work stress prevention and management. The importance of supervision for addressing boundary issues is described. Finally, possible contractual agendas for staff support, a crisis management algorithm, and critical questions to ask in planning and implementing staff support activities, are suggested.

Chapter 11: Conclusions and recommendations. The essential lessons from research and practice in characterisation and management of HIV/AIDS work stress and burnout are presented, and suggestions for future burnout research and policy are made.

Notes

1   The use of the term 'Mr' is merely a grammatical convention, to make writing easier. There have also been instances of 'Ms' Mercenary, and male Candidates suffering the consequences of their reigns! Throughout, where abstract persons are drawn, they are intended to convey a circumstance, to which female and male genders may equally be appropriately ascribed.

2   The term 'morbidity' is used in the book to mean physical and/or psychological deterioration associated with chronic, unresolved workplace stresses. Morbidity is not assumed to be irreversible – on the contrary, it is assumed in this book that the individual experience of morbidity, and the symptoms and consequences it generates, are manageable with appropriate assessment, diagnosis and intervention.

2 Occupational stress
The background to the development of burnout

Stress models – the springboard for recognition of occupational stress

Early models of stress – whether in or outside the workplace – were unable to capture the human complexity of stress responses. In particular, they failed to incorporate cognitive elements that mediate perception of stresses and subsequent responses to them. These earlier models have been summarised by Cox (1981), and will now be briefly described.

Stimulus-based models of stress

Cox (1981) characterises stimulus-based models of stress as *engineering* models – they posit external stresses giving rise to stress reactions, or 'strains', within the person. All people are held to have some level of built-in resistance to stress, presumably compounded of genetic inheritance, learning and situational resistance, so that stress can be tolerated up to a certain point. Once that point is exceeded, however, serious physical and psychological damage may result. A difficulty with such a model is that it posits stress only associated with high quantity of demand. However, undemanding occupations are often reported as stressful as those with excessive demands. Also, the role of perception of stress – psychological mediation – is not addressed in this formulation. Further, quantifying stress may not be easy in some settings – deciding what makes a situation stressful can be perilously subjective. Additionally, individual differences are not accounted for in models of this type.

Response-based models of stress

Selye (1956) defined stress as '. . . the nonspecific (physiological) response of the body to any demand made upon it'. He held that:

1   The source of the stress does not matter, and the physiological response pattern evoked by the stress represents a universally held defence reaction that is essentially the same for all animals.

2   The stress defence reaction progresses through three stages, together known as the General Adaptation Syndrome (GAS): (a) an alarm reaction and consequent reduction of resistance; (b) increased resistance associated with adaptation to the alarm; then (c) exhaustion which may be terminal, the alarm reaction reappearing as the animal dies.

3   Illness and disease result from prolonged and severe defence responses, illnesses being the cost of exposure to stresses.

Selye's notion of non-specificity has, in recent times, attracted growing criticism, not least because it ignores psychological perceptual processing factors (Cox, 1981). However, his view that coping in the face of stress occurs via adreno-cortical activity and is either adaptive (increased adrenocortical activity [resistance stage]), or maladaptive (adrenocortical exhaustion leading to disease and/or death), helped lay the foundation for contemporary research in psychoneuro-immunology (Miller, Nott and Vedhara, 1994).

Selye's work has been further developed by Kagan and Levi (1971), and Levi (1973, 1974), to incorporate psychological factors as mediators of physical illness. They suggest that most life changes evoke physiological stress responses which prepare the person for coping. If chronic, this physiological response leads to physical decline, which may then lead to illness and even death. In their formu-lation, psychosocial stimuli (life events), interact with genetic factors and with experience (the 'psychobiological programme') to generate the stress response. This process is open to modification by internal and external, mental and physical factors at any time, and these can therefore inform and shape the nature of adaptation.

The weaknesses of these models of stress lie in the label of stressor being applied to any process that elicits a particular stress response. Thus, as Alfred Lord Tennyson's 'bold' Sir Bedivere 'remorsefully regarded thro' his tears' the *morte d'Arthur*, his Selyean stress must be presumed of equivalent impact and potential for illness to that felt by Rupert Brooke's ' . . . wanderers in the middle mist / Who cry for shadows, clutch, and cannot tell / Whether they love at all or, loving, whom'. These models also suffer from the difficulty of distinguishing between stressors and stress responses. Also, the same response may be evoked by different circumstances, for example heart rate may be elevated and sustained by multiple orgasm (Kothari, 1989), or by fear.

What is occupational stress?

Occupational, or work, stress has been defined as

> ' . . . the psychological state that is or represents an imbalance or mismatch between peoples' perceptions of the demands on them (relevant to work) and their ability to cope with those demands'.
>
> (Cox, 1981)

This definition implies that work stress is an individually based, affect-laden experience associated with subjectively perceived stressors (Handy, 1988). As such, it reflects a departure from the earlier stimulus-based and response-based stress models that had given insufficient attention to psychological processes, in particular, the *cognitive mediation* that occurs between the presence of a stressor, and the psychophysiological consequences of it.

It is this focus on cognitive mediation that distinguishes the 'Transactional' model of occupational stress (Cox, 1981; Cox and Mackay, 1981; Cox, Kuk and Leiter, 1993) from the simply *interactional* models of occupational stress, such as that proposed by Cooper and Davidson (1987). This latter model recognises the potential significance and interaction of demands impinging the work arena, including those from outside the work situation, without emphasising the psychological processes of stressor and resource interaction to the extent that the model of Cox does.

As Cox, Kuk and Leiter (1993) note, the psychological appraisal of the transactional model may take into account the resources and supports available to the person for coping, the constraints placed on coping and the person's control of the situation. The demands, resources and constraints may be internal, such as personal needs and expectations of performance and achievement, and individual professional expectations, and/or they may be external to the person, for example, the nature of the work done, the circumstances in which it is done, and performance targets associated with job roles. The way that people perceive and appraise their work situation may drive their coping behaviour, and this, in turn, feeds back in to how they perceive future work situations, including whether the demands of those situations match their (experience-defined) capacities for coping. This process is illustrated in Figure 2.1.

An empirical example illustrating the importance of cognitive mediation in the experience of work stress has been given by Bailey, Steffen and Grout (1980). In one of the largest studies on staff stress in medical settings, these authors applied a 'stress audit' to 1,800 intensive care nurses. Over 80 per cent indicated that the greatest stresses were related to unit management, interpersonal relationships and patient care. However, about 99 per cent indicated that it was patient care, knowledge and skills and interpersonal relationships that were among the elements giving greatest work satisfaction.

Individual perception of work stressors and their meanings was thus shown to be the critical mediator of experienced work stress. It follows that it may be necessary and ultimately most practical or cost-effective to have potentially vulnerable staff define their own stressors at work in development of effective burnout-avoidance programmes. This has rarely been documented as an aspect of intervention programmes.

The 'Transactional' model of occupational stress (Cox and Mackay, 1981; Cox, Kuk and Leiter, 1993) thus integrates findings from research associated with previous occupational stress models, specifically the stimulus-based and response-based models described above. The transactional model of occupational stress has the further advantage that it offers much insight into the links that may be developed between occupational stress and the concept of occupational burnout.

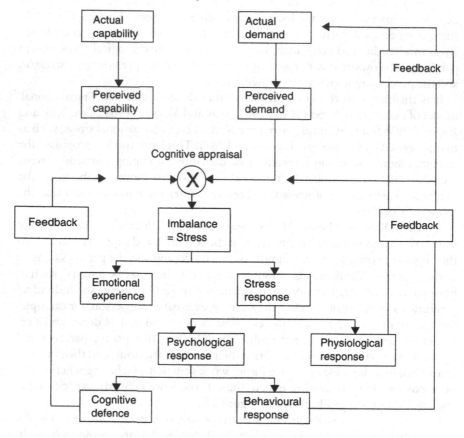

Figure 2.1 Transactional model of stress.
        Source: Cox, Kuk and Leiter, 1993.

Some of the aspects of this analysis, in particular, situational and individual antecedents of stress demands, resources, and supports, will now be considered.

What causes stress at work?

A stressful work situation is one in which coping resources are not well matched to the level of demand placed upon them, where coping has constraints placed upon it, including lack of social support, and where the person has consequent negative emotions which chronically diminish well-being (Cox, Kuk and Leiter, 1993). Attempts at characterising work stress have been made by examining characteristics of the person, of the work situation, and of the non-work situation (Cooper and Davidson, 1987). These areas have varying amounts of empirical evidence from commercial contexts to support their inclusion, although until quite recently only a limited number of studies had been conducted to examine their generalisability to the health industry (Handy, 1988).

Stress in the work arena

One of the earliest attempts to characterise workplace factors that affect production took place during the Second World War. By interviewing 3,000 workers from light and medium engineering firms over a six-month period, Frazer (1947) identified the following factors associated with an increased incidence of 'work neurosis':

- More than 75 hours of industrial work weekly.
- Domestic factors, including inadequate diet, reduced leisure time and restricted social contacts, minimal recreation time and interests, widowhood or separation, problems associated with too much responsibility (e.g., family illness), financial problems, and difficulties with housing and excessive travel;
- Boring and disliked work.
- Work requiring skills above or below the person's competence.
- Very light or sedentary work.
- Work requiring constant vigilance, but with no scope for initiative or the exercise of responsibility.
- Work without variety.
- Tasks for which lighting is unsatisfactory.

The importance of work-based stress for health has been investigated by Theorell (1974), who identified a significantly raised incidence of myocardial infarction in workers experiencing any of the following life events in the 12 months before their illness:

- Change to a new type of work.
- Major change in work schedule.
- Increased or decreased responsibility at work.
- Trouble with their boss and/or with their colleagues.
- Retirement from work.
- Unemployment for more than one month.

Another way of considering the potential for occupational stress is to consider the potential for job satisfaction. Locke (1976) suggests that job satisfaction is the result of appraising one's work in terms of the needs and values one has, and the possibilities for meeting these. Needs may be either physical and bodily, or psychological, and personal growth is a critical aspect of the latter. Locke's characterisation of the most important factors relating to work satisfaction includes:

- Mentally challenging work, which can be successfully managed.
- Personal interest in the work.
- Rewards for the work that fit the person's aspirations.
- Working conditions that enable satisfactory completion of the work, without physical demands.
- High personal self-esteem.
- Basic values which the above do not violate.

Locke suggests that work becomes dissatisfying if some or all of these conditions are not met, with ill health (physical and/or psychological), and negative effects on production, absenteeism, labour relations, and accident rates resulting.

A striking aspect of these and other studies of work and stress is the degree to which the relevance of their findings has endured subsequently, even in new models of work stress. In a review of stress in the workplace, Cooper and Davidson (1987) illustrate a model of occupational stress incorporating categories of work stress characterised earlier by Cooper (1983). This model is useful for: (a) its acknowledgement of the interactional nature of stress elements and thus the stress process (cf. the 'Transactional' model of stress suggested by Cox and Mackay [1981]); and (b) the emphasis the model places on 'extra-organisational' stressors, including the home and social arenas.

Cooper and Davidson's (1987) model identifies five major sources of stress in the work arena:

1 *Factors intrinsic to the job*, including the fit of the person to the job, job satisfaction and use of skills, equipment and training, shiftwork, work overload (quantitative and qualitative), job underload, low task variety, low discretion or opportunity for control over one's work;
2 *Role in organisation*, including role ambiguity and role conflict, responsibility for people and organisational boundaries;
3 *Relationships at work*, including social support in the workplace, and quality of relations with colleagues, supervisors and subordinates;
4 *Career development*, including lack of job security, over-promotion and under-promotion, and satisfaction with pay;
5 *Organisational structure and climate*, including organisational culture (poor communications, lack of team working, office politics, lack of participation), organisational structure (complexity, rigidity, hierarchy, and the role of significant other colleagues), and organisational change (job security, status, power).

These five areas of stress from the work arena combine, in their model, with demands from the home, social, and individual arenas, to generate manifestations of stress when they are unmet by matching coping responses. This process of interaction is illustrated in Figure 2.2.

This model does not make explicit reference to values and professional expectations that may lead to frustration or expression of stress because of reducing professional efficacy (as for Cherniss, 1980). Indeed, many of the aspects of this model have been more fully explicated in the context of research on burnout. However, three of the central aspects can be discussed here.

Factors intrinsic to the job

In his review of physical environmental demand factors found to be associated with work stress, Cox (1981) notes that they have attracted much research

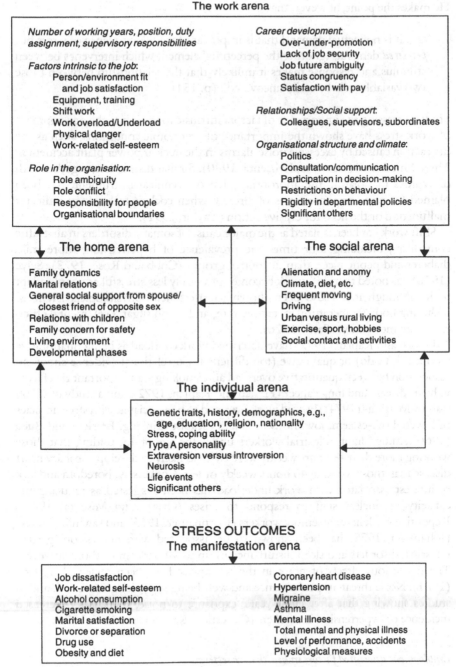

STRESSOR VARIABLES
The work arena

Number of working years, position, duty assignment, supervisory responsibilities

Factors intrinsic to the job:
  Person/environment fit
    and job satisfaction
  Equipment, training
  Shift work
  Work overload/Underload
  Physical danger
  Work-related self-esteem

Role in the organisation:
  Role ambiguity
  Role conflict
  Responsibility for people
  Organisational boundaries

Career development:
  Over-under-promotion
  Lack of job security
  Job future ambiguity
  Status congruency
  Satisfaction with pay

Relationships/Social support:
  Colleagues, supervisors, subordinates

Organisational structure and climate:
  Politics
  Consultation/communication
  Participation in decision-making
  Restrictions on behaviour
  Rigidity in departmental policies
  Significant others

The home arena

Family dynamics
Marital relations
General social support from spouse/
  closest friend of opposite sex
Relations with children
Family concern for safety
Living environment
Developmental phases

The social arena

Alienation and anomy
Climate, diet, etc.
Frequent moving
Driving
Urban versus rural living
Exercise, sport, hobbies
Social contact and activities

The individual arena

Genetic traits, history, demographics, e.g.,
  age, education, religion, nationality
Stress, coping ability
Type A personality
Extraversion versus introversion
Neurosis
Life events
Significant others

STRESS OUTCOMES
The manifestation arena

Job dissatisfaction
Work-related self-esteem
Alcohol consumption
Cigarette smoking
Marital satisfaction
Divorce or separation
Drug use
Obesity and diet

Coronary heart disease
Hypertension
Migraine
Asthma
Mental illness
Total mental and physical illness
Level of performance, accidents
Physiological measures

Figure 2.2 A model of occupational stress.
  Source: Cooper and Davidson, 1987.

attention probably because of the relative ease with which they can be measured. He makes the point, however, that

'. . . it is not actual demand that is important for the occurrence of stress but *perceived* demand. Ignoring the perceptual element which intervenes between stimulus and response makes it unlikely that the relationship between those two variables will be easily uncovered'. (p. 154)

Studies assessing the importance of factors intrinsic to the job in the development of work stress have shown the importance of ergonomic conditions, such as the distraction caused by excessive noise alarms in the nuclear power plant accident at Three Mile Island (Otway and Misenta, 1980). Similar distraction, together with difficulties in isolating the appropriate dial or technical instrument, has been blamed for poor response times of aircrew when cockpit technology indicates malfunction or the need for evasive action (Taylor, 1991).

Shift work has been isolated as the major cause of somatic disorders in air-traffic controllers, including four times the prevalence of hypertension, more mild diabetes and peptic ulcer, than in control groups (Cobb and Rose, 1973). Selye (1976) has noted that shift work becomes physically less stressful as people adapt to it, although it has also been shown to affect neurophysiological rhythms, including body temperature, metabolic rate, and blood sugar level, mental efficiency, and motivation (Selye, 1976).

French and Kaplan (1972) have described work overload as being quantitative (too much to do) or qualitative (too difficult). Correlational evidence shows an association between quantitative overload and smoking – an important risk factor in heart disease and lung cancer (French and Kaplan, 1972), and a study of 1,500 staff by Margolis (1974) showed work overload to be associated with stress indicies of lowered self-esteem, low motivation and escapist drinking. Breslow and Buell (1960) studied light-industrial workers under the age of 45, finding that those working more than 48 hours weekly were twice as likely to develop coronary heart disease than those working 40 hours weekly or less. Conversely, boredom and lack of interest associated with work underload has been suggested as reducing the capacity of nuclear staff to respond to crises (Otway and Misenta, 1980). Repetitive work in car assembly workers (Kornhauser, 1965) and sawmill workers (Johansson, 1975) has been shown to be associated with depression, gastrointestinal disorders and sleep disturbance in up to 40 per cent of those surveyed. The deleterious effects of noise in the workplace have been reviewed by Cox (1981). Noise threatens performance and well-being in the long term, as found in studies showing that after eight years' exposure to noise, there is an increased incidence of hypertension in workers (Carlestam, Karlsson and Levi, 1973).

Employment associated factors in health care settings

Findings from cohorts of oncology staff suggest that specific elements of oncology care, including administration of toxic and illness-inducing chemotherapy, managing the psychosocial needs of dying patients and their families, and unit administration, are major causes of stress. Gray-Toft and Anderson (1980, 1981) examined causes and effects of stress in 122 nurses from hospice, surgery, oncology, cardiovascular and general medical settings. All groups stated that overwork, managing dying patients, and inadequate preparation and training to meet the emotional needs of patients and their families were major causes of stress, although hospice nurses were less prone to such stress than their colleagues in other fields. Trait (i.e., constitutional and/or chronic) anxiety was a good predictor of stress, and correlated significantly with low job satisfaction and with staff turnover.

In structured interviews of 91 nurses and 57 physicians from 13 oncology facilities in Bavaria, Ullrich and FitzGerald (1990) identified variables associated with physical symptoms of work-related stress. They categorised potentially stressful work situations under 11 headings which reflected conflict areas both in the patient–helper relationship and in the helpers' work and home environments. This work was based on the model positing work stress as arising from a misfit between work demands and abilities to cope, and predicting that somatised stress would be predictive of illness.

Ullrich and FitzGerald (1990) found strong associations between specific, situational stressors and reported psychosomatic complaints. For example, in nurses many physical complaints such as irritability and headaches were related to the experience of interpersonal difficulties, both in private lives as a result of the disruption caused by work, and in their dealings with patients. On the other hand, where nurses reported greater identification with the suffering of patients, that is, where they showed what the authors termed 'overcommitment', this was significantly associated with over-tiredness, without other symptoms. Although it was regarded by subjects as a powerful work stress, proximity to dying patients was unrelated to any of the psychosomatic symptoms from which subjects could choose. In physicians, dissatisfaction with the job or with the work environment was associated with malaise. Physicians revealed a general picture of sometimes extreme tiredness associated with the stresses identified in their work. Loss of control was strongly linked to irregular heartbeat, diarrhoea, throat discomfort, dizziness and breathlessness.

Profession, age, sex, hospital size and having trainees emerged as 'life-variable' predictors of stress. Irregular working hours were related to both total level of stress, and total symptom levels. In a comment that appears to reflect the burnout construct of 'depersonalisation' (described in Chapter 3), Ullrich and FitzGerald (1990) noted:

> 'Identification with the patients' suffering, which was linked to tiredness amongst nurses, had effects amongst doctors which suggest an almost physical rejection of the patient'. (p. 1021)

A structured interview study examining work stressors in 600 randomly selected qualified Lothian nurses by Plant, Plant and Foster (1992) employed the

Gray–Toft Nursing Stress Scale, a 34-item standardised instrument divided into seven factors, including death and dying, conflict with doctors, inadequate preparation, lack of support, conflict with other nurses, workload, and uncertainty concerning treatment. Additional structured questions concerned alcohol, tobacco and illicit drug use, AIDS-related attitudes, knowledge and beliefs, general health, and demographics. Using stepwise multiple regression analyses to identify independently significant predictors of stress at work for both male and female nurses, the greatest single predictor of work stress was concern about AIDS. (Indeed, fear of contagion has been a feature of discussions of the impact of HIV/AIDS care on health staff [Horsman and Sheeran, 1995; Barbour, 1994]; this is discussed further in Chapter 5.) For females, other independent significant work stress predictors were administrative workload, and previous week's alcohol consumption. For males, in addition to concern about AIDS, the other reported independent significant predictor of work stress was years of nursing experience (although it was not clear if having fewer or more years of working experience predicted greater stress levels).

A further issue raised in these studies of health worker stress in oncology is the importance of giving health staff adequate preparation and training for management of issues giving rise to stress and anxiety. Working in specific units where expertise and 'insider' understanding can be modelled, and experience at work measured in terms of total months since qualification, has been shown to buffer potentially stressful work circumstances in a study of 64 HIV/AIDS staff (Bennett, Michie and Kippax, 1991).

Role in the organisation

Role conflict and ambiguity are key issues in determining job satisfaction (Kasl, 1978). They can also be major sources of work stress, and have been implicated in the development of coronary heart disease (Shirom *et al.*, 1973). In non-health occupations, management, clerical and professional staff appear more prone to stress associated with role conflict (Cooper and Marshal, 1976). In studies of staff at the Goddard Space Flight Centre, Caplan (1971) found that 60 per cent of staff reported experience of role ambiguity which, in turn, affected job satisfaction, and psychological and physical well-being. Further work at the Kennedy Space Centre by French and Caplan (1972) related role ambiguity to anxiety and depression. In a review of studies of role conflict, Kahn (1974) summarised the emotional costs of role conflict as including increased job tension, lower job satisfaction, reduced confidence in the employing organisation, poor interpersonal relations, and poorer relations with close colleagues.

Job roles involving responsibility for the safety and welfare of others have been shown – in studies of police and of air-traffic controllers – to be major occupational stressors (Kroes, 1976; Crump *et al.*, 1980). There are equivocal reports relating occupational responsibility for others to coronary heary disease (Cox, 1981). However, it may be inferred that care for the lives, including the quality of life and of death, of others may be a significant source of stress in health professionals faced with high levels of direct patient contact. This is to be expected where, for example, both patients and health workers recognise shortfalls in available resources affecting care delivery, and where treatment is associated with administration of toxic regimens of uncertain efficacy.

When considering studies of occupational stress in health care, most prior to HIV/AIDS have been performed on nursing staff, with occasional exceptions, e.g., on physicians (Firth-Cozens, 1987; Ullrich and FitzGerald, 1990), and occupational therapists (Piemme and Bolle, 1990). This fact has important consequences for interpreting many of the results found. For example, in respect of role issues as characterised by Cooper and Davidson (1987), nurses are below physicians on the medical professional heirarchy and, as such, are frequently in clinical positions where they may be spending the greatest amount of time with the patients, but while having the least degree of authority to intervene creatively when crises – or even 'routine' observations – indicate that this might be appropriate. In designing interventions to prevent work stress and burnout, taking issues of seniority and professional group into account is desirable to ensure that preventive and supportive strategies are relevant for all professions and levels of seniority.

In studies of mental health professionals, including family therapists and clinical psychologists, stress has increasingly been found to be a function of denial of the health worker's own emotional needs while continuing to give all care possible to others (e.g., Maynard, 1985; McCarthy, 1989; Walsh, 1990). Perhaps this could be said to reflect the sense of vocation and committment to community service that has traditionally been associated with work in nursing and medicine. It is this sense which, in the context of burnout speculation, has been suggested as a significant source of the 'depersonalisation' experienced by health staff responding defensively to the emotional exhaustion associated with loss of a sense of professional efficacy (Leiter, 1991).

For example, in an anonymous postal survey of 94 clinical psychologists in the UK, Walsh (1990) found that they faced considerable obstacles to admitting and responding to occupational stress. These obstacles included: (a) the 'debilitating nature of professional values' associated with the job, involving the threat of lost credibility, lost equality with non-support-receiving colleagues, and lost job security; and (b) the fear of becoming a client; having needs for emotional support is construed as being unfit to work in the profession. If such results associated with the perception of professional role are generalisable, it is easy to see how personal needs in response to stress at work can be denied, minimised or devalued and may thus lead, if unresolved, to serious personal difficulties. Walsh importantly identified the need to distinguish between receiving professional (case management) support, and receiving emotional (therapeutic) support in this population (see Chapter 10).

Gladding (1991) describes mental health counsellor 'self-abuse' associated with not learning from the past and with not setting proper boundaries for themselves with their clients and colleagues. Gladding suggests anecdotally that burnout can result, along with unethical behaviour and inappropriate countertransference behaviours being manifest. The issue of professional boundaries and burnout is discussed in Chapter 10.

Increasingly, health care is actively multidisciplinary, and this can lead to significant clashes of professional culture resulting in work stress, especially where line management and professional roles and responsibilities become blurred. Bates and Moore (1975) found that stressors such as role conflict and ambiguity, and work overload, were more acutely and more frequently felt by health professionals involved directly with patient care who had a high degree of role responsibility, such as trained nurses and medical interns. Those without such direct and pressing clinical involvements, such as trainee nursing staff and service administrators, were reported to be less stressed.

The trend in occupational stress research in health care has been to survey nurses, and particularly oncology nurses (Miller, 1991). Some early studies did, however, attempt to compare oncology workers with health staff from other fields of care. In a self-report questionnaire-based study of 40 female nurses from four specialty areas of care (oncology, cardiac care, operating room, and intensive care), Stewart *et al.* (1982) found that oncology nurses experienced greater temporary stresses resulting in physical and emotional exhaustion, daily mood swings and difficulties in discussing the conditions of patients than nurses from other health fields. Oncology nurses also experienced significantly more relationship problems, including with patients, than other nurses. A particular stressor for oncology nurses was having the responsibility for administering highly toxic chemotherapies with serious side effects, and the emotional complications and support this entailed.

Constable and Russell (1986) employed a multiple regression analysis of responses to the Maslach Burnout Inventory (MBI) by 310 army nurses to identify major determinants of MBI-defined burnout in this population. The MBI has three main constructs: 'emotional exhaustion'; 'depersonalisation'; and 'reduced sense of personal accomplishment'. The main determinants of burnout were low job enhancement (autonomy, task orientation, clarity, innovation and physical comfort), work pressure, and lack of supervisor support. Thus, they found that nurses are more susceptible to burnout when *not* encouraged to be self-sufficient, when tasks are not clearly understood, when rules and policies are not clearly articulated, where there is a lack of work variety, and when the work environment is unattractive and uncomfortable. Work pressure also correlated positively with MBI emotional exhaustion. Having higher numbers of patients was positively correlated with 'emotional exhaustion' and 'depersonalisation', and not correlated with 'reduced sense of personal accomplishment'. A later study found that having interactions that are more frequent, more direct, longer-lasting or chronic, and with patients who are aggressive, dependent or passive–aggressive, was more likely to induce burnout as defined by MBI-based questionnaire norms (Cordes and Dougherty, 1993).

Cordes and Dougherty (1993) define role *conflict* as the result of disagreement about work expectations communicated to a health worker by their managers. Role *ambiguity*, on the other hand, is associated with the need for certainty and predictability about goals and how to accomplish them. Schwab and Iwanicki (1982) found that role conflict and ambiguity were responsible for significant levels of variance in the 'emotional exhaustion' and 'depersonalisation' components of the MBI in a study of 469 teachers. Also, role ambiguity accounted for a lesser though significant amount of variance in 'personal accomplishment'. In a questionnaire-based study of 248 teachers, Jackson, Schwab and Schuler (1986) found role conflict to be significantly associated with 'emotional exhaustion', but not with the other two MBI-defined burnout dimensions of 'depersonalisation' or 'personal accomplishment'. Role ambiguity, however, was found to be significantly associated with 'reduced sense of personal accomplishment'.

Relationships and support at work

Relationships in the workplace have been one of the main considerations in early burnout research, although this has altered somewhat in recent years. In 1993, Maslach lamented what she saw as the loss or diminution of the earlier focus given to 'social interaction between the provider and the recipient'. By giving extra attention to job factors, industrial/organisational theories and variables, and methodologies,

'... it may have shifted the focus away from the interpersonal, relational roots of burnout to the view that burnout is just another job phenomenon'. (p. 31)

Role ambiguity has been cited as a major reason for poor work relationships, and consequent work stress (French and Kaplan, 1972). Given what Smail (1993) describes as the coarsening of social and community spirit in the UK associated with political and commercial trends in the 1980s and 1990s, relationships in the health care workplace may be expected to be further driven by competitiveness, fears of redundancy, and an emergent attitude of individual, rather than communal, priority.

On the other hand, social support among colleagues has been suggested as a potential buffer and reliever of job stress, in the 'social buffering hypothesis' of stress coping (House, 1981). This hypothesis states that social support does not necessarily lower levels of work stress experienced by the employee, but instead helps them to cope with stressful parts of their work. Empirical results concerning this hypothesis have been inconsistent. Constable and Russell (1986) examined the impact (beneficial or otherwise) of social support on the effects of perceived work stress by administering the MBI, the Work Environment Scale (Moos and Insel, 1974), and a social support measure by House and Wells (1978), to 310 qualified US Army nurses (they had a questionnaire return rate of 79 per cent, suggesting that participation was not compulsory). Multiple regression analyses were performed to assess the effects of social support on burnout, and whether social support had a buffering effect on the negative aspects of the work environment and burnout. They found that the major predictors of high scoring (i.e., being a 'case') on the MBI subscale variables were job enhancement, work pressure, and supervisor support. As they expected from the buffering hypothesis of social support, their results suggested that as supervisory support increased, emotional exhaustion decreased – indeed supervisor support interacted with job enhancement to predict reduced 'emotional exhaustion'. However, Constable and Russell (1986) found that there was no significant relationship between *burnout* and support from colleagues, spouses, and/or family and friends. A similar result has been found in a study of factory workers by House (1981), which revealed that support from supervisors – and not from co-workers – was the most significant source of buffering and reducing the effects of work stress on workers' health.

A study by Leiter and Maslach (1988) examined the effects of different sources of interpersonal contact on MBI-subscale scores of staff in mental health settings. In making a distinction between pleasant and unpleasant co-worker and supervisor contacts in a group of nurses, they found that unpleasant supervisor contact was related to 'emotional exhaustion', whereas pleasant supervisor contact was negatively related to 'depersonalisation', and pleasant co-worker contact was positively related to 'personal accomplishment'. In other words, a pleasant boss reduces work stress and negativity, and pleasant colleagues foster a sense of achievement. It is not clear from this and other studies what this result might mean for work productivity, although the inference must be that in health care at least, less stress, negativity, and enhanced self-esteem would correlate with higher standards of work, not least because less staff morbidity would be associated with greater staff continuity and work satisfaction.

Many research studies considering the buffering effects of support on burnout have been performed by Leiter (1988, 1990, 1991). Leiter worked with Maslach and Jackson to develop the validation of the MBI, and his related work on social support and burnout with populations of mental health workers is significant for its empirical distinction between personal (i.e., having family resources), informal and professional support. Leiter (1988) identified that having *informal* contacts and support mechanisms was significantly related to higher levels of MBI-measured 'personal accomplishment', while professional support was related to higher levels of 'personal accomplishment' *and* 'emotional exhaustion'. In other words, professional support coming from the *wrong* quarter may actually *increase* 'emotional exhaustion'! In a later report, Leiter (1990) further defined organisational support as the opportunity constructively to implement and develop work skills, and found negative correlations between personal support and 'emotional exhaustion' and 'depersonalisation', and organisational support was negatively related to 'depersonalisation' and 'reduced sense of personal accomplishment'. In other words, having personal support was significantly associated with *not* being emotionally exhausted or detatched from the needs and concerns of patients. Having support *from the workplace* resulted in a relative absence of detatchment and cynicism about patients' needs, and being able to recognise one's professional accomplishments. A third report (Leiter, 1991) found that co-worker support was positively related to a sense of 'personal accomplishment', and that support by supervisors was not significantly related to any of the MBI subscales – in contrast to the findings by Constable and Russell (1986).

A second major approach to the study of the social buffering hypothesis has involved examining the consequences and correlates of occupational stress on non-work relationships, particularly family life. Relevant empirical data comes mainly from the field of research on burnout, and this is considered in detail in subsequent chapters.

To summarise, stress at work has been significantly associated with factors intrinsic to jobs, such as giving toxic drugs, anxieties about contagion (e.g., from HIV infection), situational and environmental stressors, and organisational and professional roles. Role is based on, among other things, staffs' perceptions of their vocational commitments, and it is such commitment that can have negative consequences for the individual worker. Further, heirarchy in professional contexts has not been clearly addressed in studies of role-related stress, and this may confound the generalisability of earlier studies. Relationships in the workplace are also central to much reported workplace stress – supervisor support has been identified as a critical buffer of work stress.

Can we confidently generalise from these other fields of care to HIV/AIDS? As with research findings for issues relating to professional roles, the influence of associated factors of gender, age, professional group, seniority, and length of professional experience also needs clarification in the context of HIV management. HIV/AIDS has been an important vehicle for furthering our understanding of burnout. The emergence of burnout in health care workers, and the roles of these other factors, will be considered in the next chapter. The significance of burnout in the specific field of HIV/AIDS will be discussed in Chapter 5.

3 Burnout before HIV/AIDS

Aside from the limitations of the traditional theories of stress and hence occupational stress, that were identified by Cox (1981), another conspicuous early feature of the occupational stress literature was the relative absence of reports on health workers. Much of the understanding about work stress and its impact on health workers has come from the burgeoning literature on burnout, perhaps mainly because health care has been seen from the beginning of the burnout movement as a rightful domain of such work (Maslach and Schaufeli, 1993). Also, the term 'burnout' was coined following observations of stressed staff in a community health clinic (Freudenberger, 1974).

Maslach (1993) has described three 'phases' of burnout research. The first phase concerned the characterising of burnout, giving it a definition and identifying the scope and symptoms of burnout in a series of anecdotal and correlational studies. Second, Maslach describes the 'empirical' phase, in which further correlational evidence married organisational and some individual characteristics to subscale scores on the Maslach Burnout Inventory (MBI). This measurement of burnout constructs in relation to defined stressors and their modifiers is the hallmark of the second phase. The third phase is presently evolving, and concerns the attempt to marry empirical information to a theoretical structure which, until very recently, had been lacking in this field. The expression of theoretical development is most refined in the process models of burnout described below.

Leiter (1991) makes the additional point that the critical 'added value' of the burnout research enterprise lies in its having focused attention on the role of the *meaning* of work in development of work stress, and in its amelioration. To appreciate the importance of such research, however, we should first examine what burnout is, where it comes from, how it works, and where it is going. Accordingly, this chapter will examine work on the process of burnout, and how it has been distinguished from formulations of work stress.

What is burnout?

Definitions and models of burnout

Burnout has been described predominantly as an extreme expression of work stress – the *end stage* of a chronic process of deterioration and frustration in the individual worker. Models suggesting how people get to the point of burnout will be described below, but the elements common to most definitions of burnout have been distilled by Maslach and Schaufeli (1993):

1 A predominance of dysphoric symptoms such as mental or emotional exhaustion, fatigue, and depression.
2 An emphasis on mental and behavioural symptoms rather than on major physical symptoms.
3 Symptoms are work-related.
4 Symptoms appear in people without prior histories of psychopathological disturbance.
5 Decreased effectiveness and work performance occur because of negative attitudes and behaviours.

The primary emphasis on exhaustion, or 'a general state of severe fatigue', also features in the subjective and objective diagnostic criteria for burnout proposed by Bibeau *et al.* (1989). This principal *subjective indicator* of exhaustion is accompanied by:

• Loss of self-esteem arising from a feeling of professional incompetence and job dissatisfaction.
• Multiple physical symptoms of distress without identifiable organic illness.
• Problems in concentration, irritability, and negativism.

The principal *objective indicator* of burnout is significantly reduced work performance over several months, which is observable in relation to:

• Service recipients – patients and clients receive poorer quality services.
• Supervisors – they see increasing absenteeism and reduced work effectiveness.
• Colleagues – they observe a general loss of interest in work-related issues.

These authors also include three exclusion criteria to enable a diagnosis of burnout to be differentiated from, say, depression, by suggesting that these subjective and objective indicators should *not* be the result of:

1 Sheer incompetence (there must have been a prior stable period of good performance).
2 Major psychopathology.
3 Family-related problems.

Finally, Bibeau *et al.* (1989) also exclude severe fatigue as a result of monotonous work or overwork, as this is not necessarily accompanied by lowered productivity or by a feeling of incompetence.

Burnout was first discussed as a clinical entity in the literature by Freudenberger (1974), who identified a state of fatigue and frustration arising from excessive demands on personal resources in staff working in free clinics in the United States of America. In these settings work was characterised by long hours, low pay, emotionally demanding encounters with clients and colleagues, and meagre resources, all of which were obviated by staff dedication and camaraderie. He suggested that the worker, in attempting to achieve unrealistic expectations imposed socially or internally, becomes exhausted, physically and mentally. Freudenberger (1977) thus proposed the 'depletion' model of burnout, in which organisational conditions – including role ambiguity and resource shortages – lead to depleted personal capacity. Other researchers and reviewers (e.g., Lyall, 1989; Selder and Paustian, 1989) have also suggested that burnout is a direct consequence of aiming too high, or of failing to live up to personal or professional ideals. Management demands also play their part in this:

'The way people manage [others] is all about punishment. [Yet] we are all looking for rewards from people in senior positions' (Lyall, 1989).

Other models have also developed the notion of *organisational* respnsibility for burnout, including the 'crisis of competence' model proposed by Cherniss (1980), and by Meier (1983), in which burnout is composed significantly of the diminished confidence associated with lack of expected job recognition and reward. This model has been substantially explicated in work by Leiter (e.g., 1991, 1993). The 'alienation' model of Karger (1981) and Berkeley Planning Associates (1977) suggests that organisational factors, again, conspire to reduce committment as jobs become split and novelty is lost over time.

Wallace and Brinkerhoff (1991) describe burnout as referring to individual workers' inability to respond adequately to perceived demands, and to their accompanying anticipation of negative consequences for such inadequate responses. Field, McCabe and Schneiderman (1985) describe an 'expected lowering of self-esteem' where performance at work has a public professional scrutiny.

Perlman and Hartman (1982) reviewed research from the decade prior to their review and, in order to clarify the common themes from the 48 separate definitions they found at that time, they developed a 'synthetic' definition, describing burnout as a response to chronic emotional stress with three major components:

1   Emotional and/or physical exhaustion.
2   Lowered job productivity.
3   Overdepersonalisation.

The Perlman and Hartman (1982) definition was very similar to that generated in the most influential work to date on the subject. The 'attributional/environmental' model of Maslach and Jackson has gained ascenancy particularly because: (a) they developed a conceptual and empirical base that has been the starting point for much subsequent research activity; and (b) the development of the burnout concept subsequently has been closely linked with its assessment, and one of the earliest standardised measures of burnout was developed by Maslach and Jackson.

In their model, Maslach and Jackson (1982) identify 'burnout' as a multi-dimensional process with three central constructs (what Maslach and Ozer [1995] refer to as an 'operational definition'):

- *Emotional exhaustion* – having no capacity left to offer psychological suport to others.
- *Depersonalisation* – a negative and callous attitude to colleagues and patients.
- *Reduced sense of personal accomplishment* – playing down or disregarding positive job performance and past achievements.

As these constructs imply, burnout is seen by Maslach as a state that attaches especially to people working in jobs involving much personal interaction, and jobs with a potential for a high emotional content, such as working with patients, clients, or service recipients (Maslach and Ozer, 1995). Shinn *et al.* (1984) state that human service work is the area most appropriate for study of burnout because

'. . . workers must use themselves as the technology for meeting the needs of clients, who, in turn, do not always express gratitude or appreciation'. (p. 865)

Maslach (1993) characterises emotional exhaustion as an expected correlate of working with difficult or unpleasant patients, breaking bad news, dealing with patient deaths, and conflict with co-workers and/or supervisors. Depersonalisation is seen as an extension of 'detatched concern', where the health worker distances themselves psychologically, avoids over-involvement with patients, sees the patient as a symptom cluster, and derogates patients and their views. Reduced sense of personal accomplishment involves feeling unprofessional, experiencing emotional turmoil, negative self-evaluations and finding a lack of satisfaction or existential meaning from working. The job factors critical in the development of burnout are those that increase the level of emotional stress in the health worker, that produce negative perceptions of care recipients, and reduce the worker's sense of efficacy.

These three constructs form the subscales of the most widely accepted and used burnout measurement instrument, the MBI (Maslach and Jackson, 1982).

How does burnout happen?

The importance of timing

'Thus the whirligig of time begins in his revenges.'

(Shakespeare, *Twelfth Night*, V1)

The importance of *timing* in the individual experience of burnout has been largely unexamined, yet in burnout, as in good comedy, timing is of central importance. While differing routes to burnout have been suggested, most writers concur that burnout is an *end-state of a chronic process*, and that chronicity is a diagnostic discriminant of burnout as opposed to, say, reactive depression or an acute anxiety state (Leiter, 1993).

Additionally, while descriptions of symptoms of burnout have been offered by many authors (e.g., Maslach and Jackson, 1982; McElroy 1982; Greer and Mor, 1986; Keinan and Melamed, 1987; Ullrich and FitzGerald, 1990 – summarised in Chapter 4), such symptom clusters have typically been characterised only in the context of short-term analyses, never as long-term sequalae to occupational trauma (Davidson and Jackson, 1985). Indeed, timing (as opposed to the process) of burnout has not been explored empirically in interactions between individual and organisational characteristics, particularly the critical periods in careers for increasing self-efficacy (Roth, 1995).

We also need to know how long burnout takes to appear as different to – or as the end-stage of – work stress, and how long it takes to disappear once circumstances change. The main consequence of the lack of information on timing – as opposed to the sequences – of burnout is that no theoretical models for this have yet been tested. Further, approaches to recovery from burnout do not usually acknowledge that the full recovery process may be protracted (as it would be for correlate clinical disorders, such as chronic depression and anxiety states), and much effort has gone instead into the 'weekend get-well seminar' approach for staff at risk (Reynolds and Briner, 1994).

In a rare study truly examining burnout from a longitudinal perspective (i.e., beyond three to six months), Cherniss (1992) reported on the relationship between early career burnout and subsequent adaptation over a 12-year period. A small sample of 25 lawyers, high-school teachers, public health nurses and mental health professionals were interviewed twice in their first year of full-time professional practice, then again subsequently 12 years later. At the follow-up interview, subjects were also asked to complete the MBI; their original interviews were post-rated on five different dimensions relating to the three MBI subscales – occupational satisfaction, internal work motivation, feelings about clients, trust in clients, and emotional detatchment. Confidants of the participants were also asked to complete short rating scales as a validation exercise, following subject interviews. Cherniss found that people who had experienced burnout early in their careers (in the first year) were significantly less likely to change careers in the next decade, and were seen as more flexible by confidantes 10 years later. In explaining the results, Cherniss suggested that early career experience may simply lose its impact over time. A further point is that in the health services, career change is different to job change – there may be many job changes within a career. Cherniss noted that research by Kahn *et al.* (1964) demonstrated flexible subjects as having more role conflict and ambiguity than rigid personalities, so it may have been that personal flexibility contributed to career burnout early on. Burned out staff may have felt disinclined to change career because they feared burning out again in a new field, while those doing well would have had the confidence to try new fields. Or perhaps, having survived early burnout, they felt a greater commitment to their career field.

Overall, the importance of this exploratory study lies in demonstrating that for this small sample at least, early burnout appeared to have no long-term adverse consequences for the individuals involved – conversely, they were more likely to stay in their careers and became more flexible as their experience grew. This study also alludes to the possible importance of recognising *personality* factors in the context of occupational stress and burnout – another surprisingly neglected area of burnout research given the apparent readiness in burnout management to tie the responsibility for constructive change to individuals, rather than to the organisational forces that conspire to generate burnout in individuals (Leiter, 1991).

Thus, it becomes increasingly clear that more factors need to be admitted to the examination of burnout processes. To paraphrase Handy (1988), many studies have used too similar ranges of mechanistically conceptualised characteristics to arrive at similar conclusions. A useful way out of this conceptual rut would be to ask staff to identify their own stressors in burnout research, rather than only imposing limited choices of stressors from which responses are correlated to MBI subscales. Also, a clearer view of Cherniss's (1992) outcome might be gained by asking health staff how they cope with stresses, and by examining how work stresses impact on life outside work, particularly non-work relationships (see Chapter 4).

A criticism of approaches to burnout conceived and employed during the empirical phase, was that of applying 'various presumptive elements using predetermined categories' (Handy, 1988). It was argued that imposing a choice of stressors then inferring the experience of respondent stress did not explain why particular *patterns* of burnout had developed, or the ways they may be maintained in work environments. This is the context against which the third phase of burnout research – the theoretical – has started to grow, and its noblest blooms are the process models of burnout.

Process models of burnout

Models examining the *process* of burnout have been developed only latterly in the conceptual development phase of burnout research (Maslach and Schaufeli, 1993). Thus, in their 1982 review of burnout research in the preceding decade, Perlman and Hartman developed a 'perceptual-feedback stress paradigm' containing four principal aspects:

1 The degree to which a situation is conducive to stress, because of an inadequate fit between the person and the job.
2 The degree to which a person perceives the situation as stressful.
3 The physiological, cognitive/affective and behavioural responses to stress.
4 Burnout – a multifaceted experience of chronic emotional stress.

This formulation saw burnout as an expression primarily of emotional exhaustion, but was important also for its emphasis on burnout as a process.

In keeping with a process orientation centering on emotional exhaustion as the focus of burnout, Edelwich and Brodsky (1980) have described burnout developing in four stages:

1   *Enthusiasm* – 'a tendency to be overly available and to overidentify with clients, and to have unrealistic expectations of the job' (cf. Cherniss, 1980; Leiter, 1991).
2   *Stagnation* – 'expectations shrink to normal proportions and personal discontent begins to surface (i.e., the fact that the job will not make up for whatever is missing elsewhere in life)'.
3   *Frustration* – difficulties seem to multiply, the helper questions their own competence, becomes bored, less tolerant, less sympathetic, and starts coping by avoiding and withdrawing from relationships.
4   *Apathy* – characterised by depression and listlessness in response to chronic frustrations – this stage represents the embodiment of the burnout experience.

The Edelwich and Brodsky model was adopted as the basis for an exploratory questionnaire study of 152 health workers from Rome and Milan by di Giann-antonio *et al.* (1993). Demographic and professional characteristics were found to be unrelated to each of these stages. However, statistically significant associations with growing stagnation were found with contextual issues (described as career development issues in the Cooper and Davidson [1987] model), such as low salary and perceived lack of choice for job change. Growing frustration was significantly related to interpersonal relations and issues coming under the organisational structure and climate category in Figure 2.2, such as communication avoidance with colleagues, and the sense that better organisation of care could help sicker patients more. Stage four – apathy – was related in this study to blaming patients for their disease, fatigue, overwork, and anxiety about becoming infected at work – issues more conventionally associated with Maslach's concept of depersonalisation.

   To understand the way burnout works requires recognition of the process by which it develops, and this requires a capacity to measure burnout. The use of the MBI has been very important in this respect, as it is the most reliable, valid and employed instrument in the field (Schaufeli, Enzmann and Girault, 1993). While an increasing body of work employs the MBI in correlational studies examining workplace phenomena in order to identify stressful work situations, the MBI has also been used to identify how burnout unfolds, particularly by examining the interrelationships of the three MBI subscale constructs. In examining some of the process models of burnout, we will focus on three recent characterisations, each of which have similar elements and each of which enables a development of theoretical consensus.

Leiter's developmental process model of burnout

Leiter (1991) has described a process model of burnout based on two general hypotheses:

1   The three MBI-defined components of burnout influence one another as they develop over time.

2   Each of the three components has distinct relations with environmental conditions and individual factors.

Leiter has employed structural equation modelling to explore this process model, as it allows an exploration of relations between the three MBI subscales, and of organisational predictors of burnout. His developmental process model is illustrated in Figure 3.1.

Relations among the MBI subscales

In Leiter's model, *emotional exhaustion* is a primary and central reaction to occupational stressors. This, in turn, mediates the impact of occupational stressors on outcomes including *depersonalisation*, while the presence of resources, including social support, and opportunities for skill enhancement, influences *personal accomplishment*. For the most part, these aspects of burnout have distinct predictors, although some conditions, such as coping styles, appear to contribute to both exhaustion and diminished accomplishment. The model predicts that problemmatic occupational consequences – reduced committment, health problems, absenteeism, etc. – arise with emotional exhaustion. Reduced personal accomplishment is a further consequence of emotional exhaustion and depersonalisation. Leiter (1993) notes that in his own and others' research on the

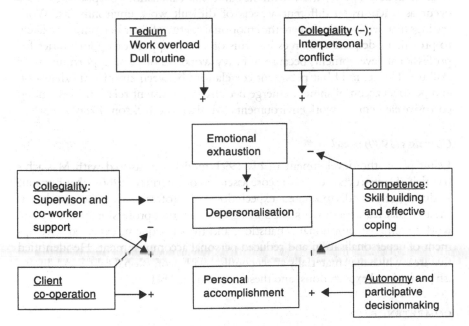

Figure 3.1 Process model of burnout.
    Source: Leiter, 1991.

interrelations of the MBI subscales, correlations of personal accomplishment to the other two subscales are always weaker than between emotional exhaustion and depersonalisation. He suggests these latter two have closer associations with supportive aspects of the workplace, although in a longitudinal (12-month) study of the impact of family and organisational resources on the development of burnout, reduced personal accomplishment was found to come before emotional exhaustion. This result indicates the need to give a more central role to how organisational roles are possibly impeding or supporting the expectations of self-efficacy of professional staff.

In considering organisational *predictors* of burnout, Leiter (1991) gives a central role to the conflict between personal aspirations and organisational limitations. In the illustration of his process model of burnout (Figure 3.1), the main stressors are work overload and conflicts with people at work, both of which are held by Leiter to have a distinct relation to emotional exhaustion. There are, of course, many other stressors that may influence the development of emotional exhaustion. Wherever they emerge, stressors affect committment and depersonalisation to the extent that they have an impact on emotional exhaustion. The level of emotional exhaustion generated in response to work stressors is partially a function of supportive resources, as strong social and supportive networks (e.g., with supervisors) are associated with reduced levels of burnout and higher levels of staff retention (see also Chapters 2, 4 and 5).

Leiter's model proposes that the reduced personal accomplishment component of burnout develops in parallel with the emotional exhaustion component, as they occur as reactions to different aspects of difficult work environments. Work settings that persistently deplete the emotional energy of their personnel are likely to provide inadequate resources in terms of social support or opportunities for professional development, because of heavy workload or poor opportunities for skill use. Hence, mild but persistent correlations between emotional exhaustion and personal accomplishment emerge because of consistent relationships among corrosive elements of work environments (Maslach and Jackson, 1986).

Cherniss's (1980) model

Leiter places the development of his 1991 model – measured with Maslach's tryptich of constructs – upon the core assertion of Cherniss (1980), that burnout is due largely to disappointed expectations of professionals. Cherniss hypothesised that features of work supporting or generating professional efficacy will work to diminish emotional exhaustion, and the subsequent, expected development of depersonalisation and reduced personal accomplishment. He identified five areas which may materially affect conflicts with professional values and diminish professional expectations, and these are examined below.

COMPETENCE

The capacity to use skills developed in training and/or with experience is critical in determining professional self-efficacy. For example, studies comparing mental health nurses with those in intensive care, emergency and neonatal settings, revealed that high skill use was negatively associated with burnout, while low skill use was associated with very low levels of personal accomplishment (Leiter, 1988). In subsequent studies looking at the impact of coping style and skill use on problem-solving in health workers, staff employing *control coping* – using skills and strategies to confront problems – were less likely to score as burned out on the MBI than those using *escape coping* – avoiding or ignoring difficult situations.

Control coping is likely to support expectations of personal efficacy by increasing the probability of workers developing work environments conducive to their expectations, and by enhancing the sense of self-efficacy through successfully solving work problems. Escape coping, however, helps maintain problems by fostering and maintaining defeatist approaches and avoidance, although of course where management is unresponsive, workers may have no other coping options. Finally, Leiter (1991) draws attention to the importance of a supportive working atmosphere in the development of control coping:

> 'People are more likely to address problems actively when embedded in collegial relationships, than in an atmosphere of suspicion and mistrust'.
> (p. 552)

AUTONOMY AND CONTROL

Perhaps the clearest professional dilemma involving autonomy and control in health staff is seen in the context of nursing, where nurses frequently have major responsibility for the care of patients, but often without sufficient authority to make acute critical decisions about clinical management. An example of this concerned the recent case of a senior nursing Sister in the UK, sacked after copying a continuing care drugs sheet for a terminally ill patient which a physician then forgot to sign. Following five months of organised protest, and after being cleared of gross professional misconduct by the UKCC, she was reinstated at her previous post, grade, salary and job title (*Nursing Times*, 19 October, 1994, Vol. 90, No. 42). There was no record of the physician being disciplined.

Paradoxically, multidisciplinary management of patients may further compromise professional autonomy, since the actions of one team member may have distinct repercussons for other team members. The normal accommodation of such processes can be obstructed when administrative structures give more power to one professional group (e.g., physicians) than others (e.g., nurses). Similarly, the unilateral decision-making of administrators, perhaps responding to political imperatives (Smail, 1993; Halton, 1995), may direct and limit professional autonomy, thus leading to resentment and alienation, e.g., regarding funding reductions, role re-allocations, unit closures, and so on.

One of the paradoxes of multidisciplinary team-working, where job roles and even responsibilities may be overlapping, is that such approaches help staff to achieve what they want – more decision-making latitude (Shinn *et al.*, 1984). In medical and mental health staff, participation and involvement in organisational decisions has been consistently related to lower MBI scores (Leiter, 1989), and can powerfully enhance commitment to organisational goals, but only where the staff involved felt that their participation was meaningful, i.e., not an expression of tokenism. On the other hand, as Leiter (1991) has indicated, it is the very overlap of roles, of decision-making responsibility and all the hassles and uncertainty that this may entail across professions and administrative structures that has been associated with increasing MBI-defined emotional exhaustion, and psychological morbidity in medical staff (e.g., BMA, 1992).

ROUTINE AND TEDIUM

Paperwork obstructing clinical care and the application of clinical skills can undermine the motivation of clinical workers, because it can distance the practitioner from skill use, and from a sense of constructive professional autonomy. Rugg *et al.* (1989) have documented how monotony and routine – even in as intensive a context as HIV pre-test counselling – can lead to burnout in HIV/AIDS counsellors.

PROBLEMS IN COLLEGIALITY

Leiter's (1991) model includes collegiate relations in two ways. First, conflict among colleagues directly contributes to emotional exhaustion, just as excessive, tedious work does. In a study of 110 hospital nurses, when asked the open-ended question, 'What causes you stress in your job?', only 12 per cent of replies referred to patients – the remainder referred to difficulties with colleagues, other professionals or administrators. Second, having good relations with colleagues reduces the impact of emotional exhaustion, depersonalisation, and reduced personal accomplishment. Evidence to support this view comes from social buffering research (see also Chapter 2).

Leiter (1991) argues that aside from personal differences that give rise to conflict among colleagues, aspects of organisational design and management also encourage it, especially performance appraisals which focus on individuals, rather than their work setting and milieu which is more often the critical unit of performance. Leiter suggests appraisals be based instead on group processes and organisational behaviour.

CLIENT CO-OPERATION

In Leiter's (1991) analysis, adequacy of agency resources in the light of expectations for client services becomes the focus, rather than the demands of specific client problems. This is reminiscent of Freudenberger's assessment of the Free Clinic movement that spawned the burnout movement, where he identified how the conditions of work in such surroundings were setting-up the professionals for failure. Important agency resources include the provision of in-service training to extend skills (including the skills to identify and analyse organisational problems), having adequate equipment for the work, and support personnel – and the resource of time in which to use them.

In summary, Leiter's analysis is that whether people tend towards increased professional efficacy or towards burnout is a function of their reactions to persistent elements in their work environment. The relations between the three burnout constructs reflect organisational consistencies, and personal processes. Leiter's process model based on the concepts of Cherniss helps to fill the gap concerning the role of psychological and interpersonal processes that had been neglected in earlier models of occupational stress until the transactional model of Cox, and the interactive schema of Cooper and Davidson (1987). In later work, Leiter was to join forces with Cox in reconciling the transactional model of occupational stress to the professional expectancy and process models of burnout. Finally, this model is consistent with other research and models giving a central role to emotional exhaustion as an expression of burnout.

Roth's (1995) model of 'mutual influence'

The transactional model of occupational stress has recently been extended in the context of burnout by Roth (1995). Her position essentially states that burnout research offers an opportunity for a more acute focus on psychological issues that mediate individual behaviour and responses, and organisational processes and demands, that precede the appearance of burnout. She argues that an analysis of burnout must necessarily take account of the broader societal structures in which human and occupational discourse take place. While agreeing that self-efficacy is important (following from the concepts of Cherniss), Roth also argues that as a concept it does not fully address the range of individual, organisational and societal features that might interact to create burnout.

Roth's position is very similar in scope and domain to that of Handy (1988). In a review of theoretical and methodological problems in burnout research, Handy argued that it is necessary to view burnout and occupational stress – which she regards as essentially similar – in the context of societal constructions which impinge on individual experience. Handy suggests that limitations in the burnout and work stress literatures arise from the neglect of the relations between higher order organisational and societal issues, and the subjective experiences of employees. These limitations could, however, be overcome by supplementing the current models with salient concepts from sociological literature. Roth (1995) has, accordingly, obliged and begins from research citing two primary causes of burnout:

1   The worker's inability to do what they aim for (e.g., heal the sick).
2   Work overload and lack of resources.

The first is attributed by Roth to individual factors, the second to organisational factors (Leiter would disagree, saying both were more likely to be a function of organisational deficiencies). The antecedents for *individual* factors are subdivided into: (a) demographic issues – gender, age, tenure in the job, and tenure in the profession; and (b) psychological characteristics, including self-efficacy. Antecedents for *organisational* factors include: (a) the organisational structure, including role ambiguity and conflict; and (b) features associated with the selection, attraction and maintenance of employees.

This model suggests that work organisations are one type of social activity system that is continually (re)structured through the interaction of individual, institutional and social forces, each of which may be either acknowledged or unacknowledged by the persons involved. Other relevant social activity systems include family, educational, political and religious systems. For example, an acknowledged individual force is cognition – how individuals psychologically classify an issue. Such classifications may be socially constructed (like race, or sexuality), but some people can change their classifications through interaction, and compounding individual experience. Unacknowledged individual forces are described as psychological, and those psychological forces associated with burnout include lack of self-efficacy, anxiety and depression. Acknowledged organisational forces may include organisational structure, and staff selection and recruitment practices, while unacknowledged forces may include organisational culture – 'how things are done'. These (together with social forces) all influence human behaviour, and human behaviour influences them all – they are mutually influencing.

Roth does not dismiss the findings or constructs of earlier models. Critically, this model posits 'mutual influence' as central in the maintenance of organisational culture and expressions of organisational decline, including burnout of staff members. She hypothesises that burnout is a process structured during interactions between the worker and the workplace – including the interactions between a provider and a client. Roth sees such interactions being constrained by workplace resources, but the interactions may also facilitate more effective client/provider interactions. She suggests that her model offers many advantages and overcomes many of the limitations associated with current models. For example, her model:

- Encourages longitudinal research designs.
- Focuses on relations between individual and organisational factors.
- Focuses on provider-client (power) relationships.
- Places communication – between individuals, organisational and societal forces – at the centre of the analysis.
- Overcomes an emphasis on either individual or organisational factors by focusing on an interaction of the two – burnout becomes a construct of the *system* rather than being assigned to any individual or organisation.

The process model of Cordes and Dougherty (1993)

Just as Perlman and Hartman (1982) performed a review of literature in an attempt to streamline the understanding of burnout to that point, in 1993 Cordes and Dougherty attempted a review and integration of research on job burnout in order to establish the generalisability of the concept to industries other than human service settings. In particular, they adopted the three-component model of Maslach and Jackson (1982), and aimed to clarify the interrelations between the three components of emotional exhaustion, depersonalisation and reduced personal accomplishment. Their process model is illustrated in Figure 3.2.

Using the jargon of the 'engineering' approach to stress, Cordes and Dougherty suggest that people experience the strongest responses ('strains') to work demands and constraints when they perceive *uncertainty* about their ability to handle them, and when the consequences of coping or not are important. They see burnout as a response to demand stressors (such as workload) and say it can be distinguished from other forms of stress,

'. . . because it represents a set of responses to a high level of chronic work demands, entailing very important interpersonal obligations and responses'. (p. 640)

Because of the high arousal generated in the face of such important demands, repeated exposure to them leads to emotional exhaustion, and depersonalisation towards clients follows as a coping strategy. A reduced sense of personal accomplishment follows as the work environment provides less and less feedback, and fewer rewards in the light of emotional exhaustion and of depersonalisation.

The key issue in burnout is emotional exhaustion, and the main determinants of emotional exhaustion in Cordes and Dougherty's model reflect organisational and personal demands placed on employees – such as work overload, and unrealistic standards of personal performance. Job demands contributing to burnout are also seen in role conflict, individual demands are seen in expectations for the organisation, and in personal expectations for achievement and the nature of interpersonal interactions with others, for example, clients.

Cordes and Dougherty describe depersonalisation (cynical, dehumanising and negative attitudes towards clients) as a stress response unique to burnout – it is not characterised or examined elsewhere in the occupational stress literature. They characterise depersonalisation as a defensive coping response to emotional exhaustion: 'an expedient alternative for dealing with emotional exhaustion when other coping resources are not available' (p. 644). Leiter (1991) has also suggested that unrealistic professional expectations are a function of professional socialisation and the cultural context of human service work. The use of depersonalisation may be partly due to professional socialisation – in professional training, health professionals are told to maintain clinical detatchment and a highly professional demeanour. It would not be surprising for depersonalisation to be the recourse when client–provider interactions become difficult or characterised by intense, negative emotions, for example, during anticipatory bereavement. The authors suggest that gender may also influence propensity to depersonalisation – research by Maslach and Jackson (1985) revealed sex-role socialisation resulted in women emphasising caring, nurturing, and showing

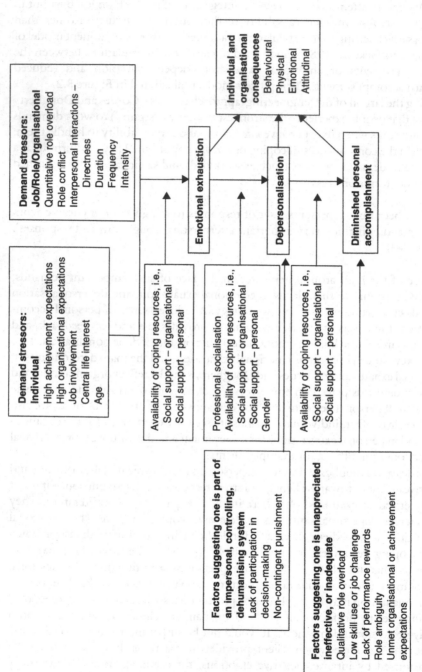

Figure 3.2 A conceptual framework for burnout.
Source: Cordes and Dougherty, 1993.

concern for others, whereas men appeared more decisive and callous in inter-personal behaviour. Further contributors to depersonalisation may include lack of workplace control (Cherniss, 1980), and lack of participation in decision-making (Savicki and Cooley, 1983). Research in learned helplessness has demonstrated how perceived control is a major mediator of stress. Where the possibilities for control or participation in decision-making are missing, individuals will mechan-ise or depersonalise their relations with colleagues, clients or the organisation in order to cope (Cordes and Dougherty, 1993).

Reduced personal accomplishment follows mainly from depersonalisation, and from factors suggesting one is ineffective, incompetent, or unappreciated, according to this model. Thus, the construct of perceived self-efficacy is central. Particularly relevant factors include qualitative work overload, role ambiguity, lack of performance-contingent rewards (i.e., absence of feedback about work performance), and unmet organisational and personal achievement expectations.

Finally, Cordes and Dougherty (1993) suggest the burnout process is moder-ated at three different points by availability of coping resources. First, between the appearance of stressors and emotional exhaustion, second between emotional exhaustion and depersonalisation, and third, between depersonalisation and reduced personal accomplishment. Two common coping resources are organi-sational social support and personal social support. In organisational contexts, social support may give the confidence that one can cope, and redefine the potential for harm (and reduce the threat from aspects of work). Leiter (1991) has argued that being able to use skills at work instead of having skill use obstructed is a form of organisational social support and is positively related to increased sense of personal accomplishment. Coping can also be enhanced by personal social support. For example, a spouse may act as a buffer for work stress, and help to enforce a balanced perspective that work is not everything in life – marriage has been significantly associated with lower levels of emotional exhaustion. Staff with families also have lower emotional exhaustion levels. Why? Perhaps family-based staff are more mature, and therefore more emotionally stable. Or perhaps they are more used to dealing with emotional conflicts and emotional problems, and become less immediately reactive or stresses when new potential stresses arise.

Consensus across process models of burnout

To summarise, there is a growing consensus regarding the processes of burnout. The three process models discussed here agree that emotional exhaustion is the central aspect of burnout. Further, they all agree that key organisational features involve work overload and role conflict. Individual factors held in common in relation to emotional exhaustion centre around disappointed professional expec-tations – for personal performance, for organisational standards, for relations with colleagues and patients. Roth has extended the consensus, however, by suggesting a broader 'societal' focus on issues behind individual aims and expec-tations, such as gender, race, psychological characteristics (including propensity towards affective disturbance), and tenure.

Further, the models of Leiter (1991) and of Cordes and Dougherty (1993) share an emphasis on the importance of available coping resources in relation to each component of burnout, and the possible gender and professional social-isation processes described in Cordes and Dougherty (1993) also fit the analyses of both Leiter (1991) and Roth (1995). The explication of demands leading to emotional exhaustion in Leiter's analysis are grouped under organisational features only for Cordes and Dougherty, although Leiter would not object to this, given the role of individual perception and *meaning* that mediates all demand stressors. It is interesting to see that Cordes and Dougherty's individual demand stressors match many of those identified as within the individual arena in the occupational stress model of Cooper and Davidson (1987).

Contrasts across models are seen in the depersonalisation factors of Cordes and Dougherty's model being accorded to the development of personal accomplish-ment by Leiter (i.e., lack of participation in decision-making, and autonomy). Also, the factors suggested by Cordes and Dougherty as directly associated with reduced personal accomplishment, such as role overload, and lack of skill usage, feed directly into emotional exhaustion in Leiter's model, although parallel develop-ment of these constructs has subsequently been acknowledged by Leiter (1993).

The main point, however, is the substantial agreement that burnout is a process that requires time and interaction between individual and organisational elements (and Roth would add societal elements also) to enable it to happen. None of these analyses has an empirical basis in the context of HIV/AIDS, and they have given little emphasis to additional personal factors, such as length of professional experience, and experience in the job. The role of gender, age, and professional occupation needs further elaboration in respect of burnout constructs, and especially in the context of HIV/AIDS care for, while there may be similarities between this and other health care fields (such as oncology), this cannot be presumed. These analyses would also affirm that burnout is a distinct process to that of general occupational stress, although the nature of the relationship between burnout and occupational stress requires clarification.

Distinguishing burnout from stress, and from occupational stress

Popular and historical conclusion

Much of the confusion over the specificity of burnout, and over the relationship of burnout to occupational stress, arises from its linkage with common discourse and – at the same time – with scientific definition and measurement (Cox, Kuk and Leiter, 1993). Burnout is a 'buzzword' – as Maslach and Schaufeli (1993) note:

> '. . . at various times burnout has been equated with tedium, (job) stress, (job) dissatisfaction, (reactive or professional) depression, alienation, low morale, anxiety, (job) strain, tension, feeling 'worn out', experiencing 'flame-out', ten-sion, conflict, pressure, 'nerves', boredom, (chronic or emotional) fatigue, poor mental health, crisis, helplessness, vital exhaustion, and hopelessness'. (p. 9)

These same authors make the additional comment that '. . . a concept that has been expanded to mean everything ends up meaning nothing at all' (p. 4).

As if that were not enough, concepts with which burnout is closely associated are also susceptible to populist confusion – concepts like stress and depression. Some of the confusion can also be attributed to the way the concept of burnout has been adopted and fostered by overlapping but also distinctive disciplines related to organisational psychology. For example, Freudenberger (1974) coined the term from the perspective of the psychiatric clinician, following observations of staff under stress working in free clinics. However, the next phase of burnout research development was the empirical phase, most notably characterised by the development of measurement instruments enabling further quantification of the syndrome Freudenberger described. That this phase took place mainly in the context of social psychology has had at least two consequences that are relevant today:

- The crossover between social and clinical (and organisational) psychology in burnout research has generated different emphases in interpretation – the social psychological approach has led to suggestions for intervention based on the social and organisational work environments, while the clinical approach has focussed on individuals' responses (Cox, Kuk, and Leiter, 1993).
- Burnout has continued in many studies to be conceptualised in operational terms implied and reinforced by the measurement instruments, such as the MBI, leading to a narrowing of the conceptual debate and a presumptive approach to staff burnout identification and intervention (Miller, 1992; Maslach and Schaufeli, 1993).

A further difficulty in drawing legitimate comparisons between the domains of burnout and occupational stress lies in the relatively rapid evolution of burnout research through its phases of clinical enquiry and characterisation, empirical verification and, more recently, theoretical development. For example, before the articulation of the transactional model of occupational stress, a major difference suggested between conceptions of burnout and of occupational stress was with burnout having its conceptual base within an explicitly stated cognitive process concerning the *meaning* of work for the human service professional (Leiter, 1991). This view is not shared universally. Payne (1984) concluded that in comparing the two fields, the burnout literature up to 1984 was merely an inferior and sensationalist version of the stress literature, rediscovering the same concepts and perpetuating poorly designed empirical research – a view with which many subsequent commentators have agreed, at least with respect to the *quality* of burnout research (Schaufeli, Maslach and Marek, 1993). Handy (1988) has suggested the definitions of burnout she surveyed – which did not, surprisingly, include the three constructs articulated by Maslach and Jackson (1982) which have formed the platform for most research since the mid-1980s – were simply more extreme versions of the definitions of job stress then current (the interactionist models), illustrating '. . . the somewhat sensationalist character of much of the burnout research' (p. 353).

Indeed, recent critiques by Briner (1998) and Barley and Knight (1992) suggest that sensationalism has been extremely useful in bringing work stress into the context of political rhetoric with the aim of improving work conditions, garnering public sympathy with collective industrial action, and de-individualising stress discourse, thus avoiding individual pathologising of workers reporting work stress.

In addition, Handy (1988) has criticised burnout research for merely re-tracing the research agenda of occupational stress. Maslach and Schaufeli (1993), in their review of the historical development of burnout, acknowledge that there are no sharp boundaries, and they offer the somewhat capitulatory view that burnout can be distinguished from occupational stress only 'in a relative way'. They do suggest, however, that two relative distinctions can be drawn between burnout and stress with respect to time, and between burnout and both depression and satisfaction with respect to domain.

Citing the work of the pioneer stress researcher, Selye, who postulated the 'general adaptation syndrome' in response to stressors (consisting of the phases of alarm, resistance and exhaustion), Maslach and Schaufeli suggest that stress and burnout cannot be distinguished on the basis of symptoms, but only on the basis of the *process* – of the time it takes burnout to appear. They regard burnout as a consequence of a breakdown in adaptation to chronic stress accompanied by chronic malfunctioning – exhaustion may be reached before the individual is aware of the earlier Seylean phases. The time element is thus a critical discriminant.

Other writing on the subject also relates burnout to occupational stress in ways reflecting the stimulus- and response-based models of work stress described earlier. For example, a postal survey by Shinn *et al.* (1984) explicitly employed the engineering analogy in examining methods and effects of coping with burnout in 141 group therapists. In an attempt to link research on burnout with previous work on job stress, strain and coping, they conceptualised burnout as psychological strain resulting from the stress of human service work. For these authors, stress was composed of negative work features, strain was the psychological and physiological responses, and coping was the effort to reduce stress and strain.

Attempts to draw a distinction between burnout and occupational stress as research foci has further, perhaps unexpected, aspects that are revealed when one considers why the concept of burnout has gained such popularity. As Cox, Kuk and Leiter (1993) suggest, unlike other related concepts such as work stress and depression, burnout does not necessarily stigmatize the individual worker. Instead, the person is assigned a more passive role in theories of burnout that emphasise the social context and determination of the condition, than in theories of stress which emphasise the interaction between person and environment. These authors argue that conceptions of burnout, by assigning responsibility less to the individuals concerned, are more amenable to diagnosis and interventions, presumably because they allow interventions to be posited within the broader domains of occupational environmental initiatives. A second and equally important reason suggested by Cox, Kuk and Leiter (1993), and endorsed by

Barley and Knight (1992) and Briner (1998), for the popular appeal of burnout is its provision for social and health services of an explanation of why their members are so adversely affected during a time of budgetary stringency and increasing public expectations of what they can offer. They suggest it has been useful for health and human services staff to have a notion of their own occupational distress that was both socially and scientifically acceptable, that pointed to the causes of their distress, yet without blaming the staffs involved for their conditions.

Contemporary views of the differences between burnout and occupational stress

In their review of research on burnout, Cordes and Dougherty (1993) consider that the distinction between burnout and stress is not clearly delineated – they suggest that burnout is a kind of stress, '. . . a chronic affective response pattern to stressful work conditions that features (sic) high levels of interpersonal contact' (p. 625). They add that there had been little definitional or operational agreement among job stress conceptualisations until the work of Schuler (1980) who identified stress as a dynamic condition in which the individual faces demands or constraints on what one is wanting to do and for which resolution is perceived to have uncertainty but which will lead to important outcomes. Cordes and Dougherty suggest that such a definition subsumes burnout: Burnout starts as a pattern of response – as a result of demands including interpersonal stressors – and, as such, represents a type of job stress with its own pattern of emotional exhaustion, depersonalisation and reduced personal accomplishment. They suggest further that the concepts of uncertainty and importance of outcomes is as important in burnout as in other kinds of stress response generated by constraints and demands.

Ullrich and FitzGerald (1990) state, 'The syndrome [of burnout] is now best seen as a subcategory of stress effects' (p. 1013). In their research on the impact of cancer care on physicians and nurses, Ullrich and Fitzgerald characterise stress as resulting '. . . from an imbalance between the demands of the workplace and the individual's ability to cope', and its effects as primarily somatic in the form of physical complaints. Perhaps the clearest (and also simplest) characterisation is that given by Maslach and Ozer (1995), when they state 'Burnout is a type of prolonged response to chronic emotional and interpersonal stressors on the job'. As such, this formulation posits stress and its sequalae as a function of the individual and of the organisation, but it does no more. No theoretical framework is explicated to account explicitly for the process of burnout development. In particular, processes of psychological mediation are not admitted explicitly, despite evidence (e.g., Bailey, Steffen and Grout, 1980; Treiber, Shaw and Malcolm, 1987) indicating the importance of doing so.

In his review of burnout as a developmental process, Leiter (1993) notes that while the three-dimensional quality of burnout increases the potential for burnout to make a distinct contribution to organisational psychology, the empirical focus on emotional exhaustion lessens the contrast between burnout research and work on general occupational stress, as well as the particular relevance of burnout for the human service professions. In a similar vein, Maslach (1993) has suggested that of the three components of burnout, emotional exhaustion is the closest to an orthodox stress variable – factors hypothesised to relate to emotional exhaustion are very similar to those in the general literature on stress, so similar findings are not unexpected. On the other hand, the dimensions of depersonalisation and personal accomplishment do encourage a focus on theraputic relationships with service users and the development of professional efficacy.

Are the differences between occupational stress and burnout a problem?: reconciling the differences

Cox, Kuk and Leiter (1993) consider that theories of burnout and work stress can be reconciled by examining the conceptual and empirical comonalities between the dominant models of burnout (i.e., that of Maslach and Jackson, 1982 – and subsequently modified by Leiter, 1991), and of work stress (i.e., the transactional models of Cox, 1981, and of Cooper and Davidson, 1987). They define work stress as involving a process of appraisal – of work demands and of personal capabilities to meet those demands – these complex cognitive and perceptual processes underpin the interactions described in the Cooper and Davidson model. The appraisal process takes into account resources and supports for coping, along with constraints and personal control that mediate the processes of coping. Each of these elements may be mapped on to by what they describe as a 'deconstructed' analysis of the components of burnout, although the authors add the caveat that burnout is probably only something that applies in this sense to human service workers, and thus is only a particular phenomenon within the (work) stress process. Thus, they concur that emotional exhaustion is, along with depersonalisation, a response to stressors affecting human service workers. Emotional exhaustion is a general response, encompassing notions of emotion and wellbeing, and which seems to give rise to a coping response (depersonalisation). Reduced sense of personal accomplishment is based more on appraisal outcome, reflecting Cherniss's (1980) conception of the meaning of work, and frustrated professional expectation. Accordingly, these authors argue that from the context of the transactional model of occupational stress, burnout '. . . can be seen to be a particular slice across the stress process that is a relatively common occurrence in human service workers' (Cox, Kuk and Leiter, 1993, p. 188).

Leiter (1991) has based his empirical examinations of the aetiology and antecedents of burnout on the model of frustrated professional expectations, first described by Cherniss (1980). In recalling the emphasis placed on the cognitive and perceptual discriminants of burnout as opposed to work stress generally, Leiter (1991) notes,

> '. . . the emphasis of the [burnout] syndrome on the *meaning* of professional work makes a distinct contribution [to that of the study of occupational stress] to organisational and clinical psychology'. (p. 554)

In concluding this section on relating burnout to occupational stress in general, it is pertinent to consider Leiter's (1993) suggestion that the name of this research field be changed from that of burnout to something else – he suggests 'professional efficacy' or 'career crisis' as appropriate alternatives that focus attention not just on one negative end of a continuum of work experience, and will also encourage consideration of the middle ranges of the MBI subscales. Such renaming may also aid the clinical specificity attached to the field and its constructs. In reality, it is probably too late to do so, but Leiter's points are well made – we need to dig deeper and broader in our consideration of burnout processes and their management.

The next chapter will consider symptoms of burnout, and some more of the issues affecting the experience of burnout. Chapter 5 will also extend the clinical and empirical developments in burnout research to the field of HIV/AIDS.

4   Symptoms and correlates of burnout

Symptoms of burnout

Aside from research initiatives that have explored the burnout experience in a quantitative fashion, qualitative clinical reports have described an often spectacular phenomenology associated with burnout in its most extreme presentations. For example, McElroy (1982) portrays a cumulative, chronic process in which, as emotional and physical exhaustion are unresolved, and illness and proneness to disease become more pronounced, behavioural and social symptoms appear and relationships with others (including colleagues and patients) become less important. Cognitive and intellectual signs then increasingly appear, including difficulties in decision-making, impaired problem-solving and decreased listening. Attitudinal changes occur, alongside quickness to anger, difficulty in holding in feelings, and a sense of omnipotence. Next comes detatchment, with overlaying cynicism, intellectual rigidity, stubbornness and obstructiveness. Longer hours are spent with less being accomplished and pervasive feelings of boredom at work and at home. The final phase of this process sees the anger and destructiveness turned inwards, resulting in depression and an overwhelming sense of personal failure.

While such descriptions are compelling, it is unusual to observe clinically the full spectrum of described features knit together in a destructive welter. Rather, it seems that most health workers subjected to stressful (particularly clinical) working circumstances will identify some symptoms that recur and come to characterise their perceptions of health work. In most circumstances, these are manageable to the extent that their most conspicuous features can be contained, although not necessarily cured. Commonly reported symptoms of staff stress, and those frequently reported in the literature in association with staff burnout, have been summarised by Miller (1991), and are listed in Table 4.1.

In a review of symptoms of burnout published in 1988, Kahill suggested that the profusion of symptoms currently identified in the literature (84 had been identified prior to her review) may be a consequence the general imprecision and lack of conceptual clarity of the burnout field. Kahill (1988) also notes that such symptom profusion may result from burnout being

'. . . a generalized psychological distress reaction that is necessarily experienced somewhat differently by each individual, . . . thus hav[ing] no clearly delineated symptomatology' (p. 285).

Table 4.1 Reported symptoms of staff stress and burnout

Physical
- Physical exhaustion
- Lingering minor illnesses
- Headaches and back pain
- Sleeplessness
- Gastrointestinal disturbances
- Malaise

Behavioural
- Readiness to be irritated
- Proneness to anger
- Increased alcohol and drug use
- Marital and relationship problems
- Inflexibility in problem-solving
- Impulsivity and acting-out
- Self-righteousness
- Withdrawal from non-colleagues

Cognitive/affective
- Emotional numbness
- Emotional hypersensitivity
- Over-identification with patients
- Grief and sadness
- Pessimism and hopelessness
- Boredom and cynicism
- Indecision and inattention
- Depression

Source: Miller (1991), based on data in Greer and Mor (1986), Keinan and Melamed (1987), Ullrich and FitzGerald (1990), McElroy (1982), Maslach and Jackson (1982).

She groups symptoms 'for convenience' into five major categories: physical, emotional, behavioural, interpersonal, and attitudinal.

Physical symptoms of burnout

In the literature, it is difficult to find hard evidence linking empirically measured burnout (defined as an elevated score on MBI subscales of emotional exhaustion, depersonalisation, and reduced sense of personal accomplishment) with diagnosed symptoms of physical disease. There may be a number of reasons for this:

- Burnout may be a construct that is too extreme to be reliably measured in 'normal' samples or populations of health workers.
- There may be few serious physical illnesses that link reliably and directly with measurable burnout.
- Measures of burnout that have been used may be too soft – they may be measures of initial phases of burnout-associated morbidity only.
- Symptoms of illness may appear long after the stress that led to their development has occurred and been dealt with.

Although at least one report (Schneider, 1984) has suggested that MBI-measured and/or self-reported burnout may lead eventually to physical disease, including heart attack, cancer or suicide, evidence linking burnout with physical disease is not nearly as compelling as might be expected. In Kahill's review, while there is some evidence relating burnout to declining physical health (see Table 4.1), only a few major physical illnesses (e.g., gallbladder and cardiovascular disorders, ulcers and kidney disorders) have been linked to MBI-measured burnout, and these have been done so inconsistently – by the same researchers! It is also pertinent to remember Maslach and Schaufeli's (1993) list of common elements in burnout definitions – one of the common elements cited was an emphasis on 'mental and behavioural symptoms rather than physical symptoms' (p. 15). Relatively minor somatic disorders are generally the most often reported correlates of high MBI burnout scores and self-reported burnout, and formed the foundation of a stress study in oncology physicians and nurses by Ullrich and FitzGerald (1990). It has recently been suggested that low correlations between burnout as measured on the MBI and physical symptoms in cross-sectional studies may also be explained by the expected latency of 6–12 months between negative life-events and physical symptoms, as in life-events research (Bennett, Miller and Ross, 1995).

Emotional symptoms

The empirical link with affective disorders, in particular depression, is much firmer, although evidence of associations with other emotional symptoms can surprisingly only best be described as 'suggestive [yet] insufficient to permit firm conclusions at this time' (Kahill, 1988, p. 288). There is clearly a need to link burnout measures, such as the MBI, to reliable and valid clinical scales in order to help clarify the nature of the link between burnout and clinical affective states.

Clinical correlates of burnout

An evident tension in the burnout literature has concerned reconciling the proposed state of burnout to an identifiable clinical process. Indeed, one of the pitfalls of early discussion and searches for definition in this field (see reviews by Pearlman and Hartman [1982]; Kahill [1988]; Miller [1991]), has been the tendency to refer to burnout as an end-stage entity, something arrived at, not a process (Bennett [1992b]; Price and Murphy [1984]). Clinically, this makes little sense: clinical phenomena associated with burnout reports are typically consequences of chronic processes (see Table 4.1). Ignoring this puts grave restrictions on the potential for meaningful observation and intervention.

Maslach and Schaufeli (1993) are concerned to differentiate burnout from affective states of depression and job dissatisfaction. Freudenberger (1981) cites clinical evidence to suggest that symptoms of burnout are, at least initially, job-related and situation-specific, rather than generalised as for clinical depression. The same position is taken by Warr (1987), although it could be argued –

particularly in the light of the necessary time periods to be passed before depression becomes formally diagnostic – that in the early stages of burnout, depression may be focal and the two would therefore be difficult to tell apart.

While Maslach and Schaufeli (1993) see a conceptual agreement that burnout is more job-related than depression, evidence from empirical studies suggests that the emotional exhaustion component of MBI-measured burnout is substantively related to depression. For example, Meier (1984) used a multi-trait–multi-method approach in an MBI-based survey of 320 faculty members to conclude that there was considerable overlap between the MBI and several depression measures. The difficulty with this study was that Meier scored the MBI by summing the responses from all items, rather than summing subscale items only – his results cannot therefore be interpreted or generalised. A more interpretable study by Firth *et al.* (1986) compared MBI scores with those of 200 nurses on the Beck Depression Inventory (BDI), finding that the emotional exhaustion subscale was significantly related to BDI depression. Relationships with the MBI subscales of depersonalisation and reduced personal accomplishment were much less significant statistically.

In terms of formal psychiatric classifications, burnout is not specified in the major nosologies. However, it comes best under the DSM-IV sub-categorisation of Adjustment Disorder 'with significant impairment in social or occupational (academic) functioning' (American Psychiatric Association, 1994). Adjustment disorders are a residual category used to describe clinical presentations that are a response to identifiable stressors and that do not meet crtieria for other specific Axis I disorders, such as a Major Depressive Episode. They can, however, be diagnosed in addition to another Axis I disorder, and may be coded formally according to subtypes that best characterise the predominant symptoms, such as depressed mood or anxiety. Adjustment disorders can be either acute (less than six months but more than three months' duration), or chronic (more than six months' duration). Burnout comes under the same categorisation in the ICD-10 codes developed by the World Health Organization.

A study of unpaid volunteer HIV/AIDS staff by Claxton, Burgess and Catalan (1993) aimed to identify factors associated with burnout and psychosocial distress in order to refine recruitment and training procedures for volunteer workers at the London-based Terrence Higgins Trust. Claxton administered the MBI and the HAD depression scale to 267 registered 'Buddies' (volunteer befrienders and domestic helpers of people with HIV disease). Some 26 per cent overall scored above the cut-off levels for probable cases of burnout on one or more of the MBI subscales, although they scored lower overall than other, comparison groups of HIV health workers. Multiple regression analyses revealed only small amounts of variance associated with anxiety, depression and burnout, although poor outcome from volunteering was significantly associated with wanting to feel 'needed', and 'wanting to help others'.

In reviewing studies attempting to link MBI scores to job satisfaction, Schaufeli, Enzmann and Girault (1993) suggest that there are consistent findings indicating MBI-measured emotional exhaustion has moderately negative correlations with job satisfaction (coefficients ranging from 0.35 to 0.45), and while depersonalisation is only slightly negatively correlated (coefficients between 0.25 and 0.35), personal accomplishment is positively but insignificantly related to job satisfaction. This is in spite of the MBI Users's Manual reporting only weak and insignificant relationships with job satisfaction.

Behavioural symptoms

Behavioural symptoms have more reliably been shown to have statistically significant associations with reported burnout, particularly in relation to work-related behaviours. Staff turnover, whether actual or desired, has been strongly linked in the pioneering studies of burnout by Berkeley Planning Associates (1977), and links have also been made between burnout and neglect of duties, making mistakes, and lowered discipline in a study of burned-out nurses (Jones, 1981). Findings for absenteeism are 'mixed' – for example, although a relationship is reported between burnout and absenteeism by Jones (1981), no details are given. Maslach and Jackson (1981), however, report a correlation of 0.30 between absenteeism rated by co-workers and the scores on the depersonalisation subscale of the MBI in mental health workers. Piecemeal findings from other industrial and commercial settings are equally equivocal for absenteeism, and suggest that in future studies, this area (important for helping to determine the cost-effectiveness of burnout prevention interventions) needs closer attention.

Consumption behaviours (alcohol, caffeine and drug use) have been shown to have variably strong statistically significant links with burnout in a number of studies of health care and social services workers (Kahill, 1988). Jones (1981) reported a positive and reliable correlation between irrational beliefs, violence, use of alcohol on the job and staff burnout scores (replicated by Jackson and Maslach, 1982, and Maslach and Jackson, 1978). There has also been an interaction noted between burnout and theft of drugs in nurses (Jones, 1981).

Finally, in considering reports of research on behavioural correlates of burnout, Johns (1991) observes that such studies are invariably disappointing because work behaviours are substantially constrained in their variance by organisational, social and individual factors, such as those discussed above.

Symptoms associated with interpersonal relations

Roth (1995) states that '. . . a model of burnout may be incomplete unless it accommodates societal influences beyond the individual and the workplace on burnout' (p. 14). Roth is making a clear request for extending the realm of empirical examination of burnout to relationships between the worker and non-work meaningful others, something that has received relatively little attention to date. There are at least two main strands of consideration in this context: (a) examining the consequences of occupational stress on non-work relationships, particularly family life; and (b) examining the ameliorative effects of strategies such as social support on experienced occupational stress and burnout. As with all aspects of burnout research, findings in these areas are still best described as preliminary and, in a recent review, Cordes and Dougherty (1993) were moved to conclude that

'A better understanding of the intricacies of the work-nonwork interface, and the implications that this interface has for personal sources of support, is an important and timely concern' (p. 635).

Non-work relationships

With respect to the impact of work stress on non-work relationships, studies of teachers by Rottier, Kelly and Tomhave (1983) revealed that 31 per cent felt that work had interfered negatively with their family life. In a study of language pathologists, Miller and Potter (1982) found that 78 per cent of burned out subjects felt their personal lives had been negatively affected by work, compared with 21 per cent of those with moderate burnout and none of non-burned-out subjects.

A ground-breaking study using the MBI was undertaken in populations of police personnel and their spouses in the United States. Jackson and Maslach (1982) studied 142 couples where one spouse was a police officer, applying the MBI in an interview of each party. Those scoring as having MBI-defined burnout had significantly lower levels of social activity, with correlations of 0.18 to 0.32 on each of the MBI subscales, compared to those with no burnout. Correlations with avoiding people and being solitary, with the MBI subscale scores for 'caseness' on emotional exhaustion and depersonalisation, were 0.21 and 0.42 respectively. Burnout has been associated with overall quality of family life among police ($r = 0.52$) and the burnt-out police officers' ratings of marital satisfaction ($r = 0.52$ for depersonalisation and reduced personal accomplishment). It was noted anecdotally by spouses that the police staff behaved towards their own children as they would towards those they encountered in their professional roles.

Spouses of MBI-defined burned-out police were described as anxious, irritable and isolated, and were more likely to express anger towards spouse and family ($r = 0.26$ with emotional exhaustion, and $r = 0.28$ with depersonalisation). Wives of burned-out policemen were more likely to describe themselves as being depressed, to feel their husband did not care as much about them ($r = 0.17$ with depersonalisation), and that he did not share her friends ($r = 0.24$ with depersonalisation). Depersonalisation was also the subscale showing significant negative associations with involvement in family matters ($r = -0.18$) in those who were burnt out. Burnt-out police staff were twice as likely as non-burned-out staff to believe their wives failed to understand the pressures associated with the job, and the higher their MBI scores, the less likely their work was considered a source of pride and prestige to their family ($r = -0.22$ and -0.26 with emotional exhaustion).

These results seem to affirm that emotional exhaustion and depersonalisation in the human service worker can affect family as much as clients or 'recipients' of such staff, and that much more work is necessary to assess the true nature of non-work impact of work stress and burnout. It may be, for example, that police staff suffer exceptionally because of the dangers associated with their work, and that health staff have less negative consequences of work on their home lives because of the different, often more predictable, circumstances in which they work.

Burke, Shearer and Deszca (1984) examined the impact of police officers' jobs and demands associated with them on aspects of home, personal and family life, and derived a single measure of work–non-work conflict based on the combined findings. Those staff reporting higher levels of burnout-related effects also reported a correspondingly greater deleterious impact of work on personal, home and family lives. This study suffers, however, from its use of non-standardised instruments.

A further study of 169 police staff and support personnel, based on MBI responses, by Gaines and Jermier (1983) found no relation between marital status and any of the MBI subscale scores. A similar finding was made in a study of 469 school teachers given the MBI by Schwab and Iwanicki (1982) – there was no significant relation found between marital status and any of the burnout components. This is in contrast to another cross-sectional MBI-based survey on 462 teachers conducted by Gold (1985), finding that single teachers experienced significantly greater emotional exhaustion and depersonalisation. Similarly, a study of MBI responses of 316 teachers by Russell, Altmaier and Van Velzen (1987) showed that married teaching staff have significantly higher levels of personal accomplishment. These latter findings fit those from Maslach and Jackson's (1981) MBI validation study based on 1,025 human service personnel, and a further (1985) study based on 845 telephone company staff: they found that married staff experience significantly less emotional exhaustion, and depersonalisation, and greater levels of personal accomplishment. Conversely, staff with children experienced significantly less MBI-measured emotional exhaustion and depersonalisation, and more personal accomplishment (Maslach and Jackson, 1985).

van Servellen and Leake (1993) administered the MBI to a convenience sample of 237 nurses from 18 units in seven hospitals, including special care units managing people with AIDS, cancer, medical intensive care, and general medical diseases. Regression analyses for the emotional exhaustion and personal accomplishment subscales showed that marital status, and number of dependent children had no significant relation to MBI subscale scores.

Leiter (1990) hypothesised that family coping resources would take some time to appear as influences on the experience of burnout, and in a study of 122 hospital workers, conducted over two time points six months apart, found that family resources complement professionally based resources to alleviate burnout or prevent its development. Leiter found that family coping resources were largely independent to work-related coping resources, and extended the individual's capacity for coping with work stress – people with more resources for coping with family problems were more able to overcome work-related exhaustion, either by not having family issues adding to work stress, and/or by having family supports adding to actions to reduce work stress. Family coping resources were not related to diminished personal accomplishment in this study.

A non-MBI-based survey of 91 nurses and 57 physicians from 13 oncology institutions in Bavaria attempted to examine the relation between work situational stressors (such as interpersonal difficulties, dealing with patients, dying and death, therapy decisions) and psychosomatic complaints (Ullrich and FitzGerald, 1990). As expected, they found abundant links between stress and physical symptoms. For nurses in particular, private life stress (mainly as a result of the disruption their work caused) had product–moment correlations of more than 0.35 with headaches/pressure in the head, tiredness, tendency to cry, loss of appetite, irritability and neck/shoulder pain. Ullrich and FitzGerald (1990) suggested that somatization is likely if life outside work fails to relieve stress generated in the job.

A rare study examining the impact of HIV/AIDS work on non-work relationships was conducted by Ancona *et al.* (1991) employing a non-standardised self-report multiple-choice questionnaire with 67 health care workers in Italy. The authors found a surprisingly high number of persons with difficulties in their domestic lives (35–56 per cent), and many staff also reporting feeling 'destroyed' following routine daily activities in caring for people with HIV. This qualitative study suffers for having no standardised referents, for having no report of measures used, and for the impressionistic nature of the study.

An interview survey of 103 HIV/AIDS and 100 oncology staff by Miller and Gillies (1996) found that most reported spending considerable amounts of time discussing work with domestic partners, and work-related subjects caused significant conflict for just under half the total sample. Thirty-nine per cent reported that their partners complained regularly about their committment to work, and one-quarter overall reported that their relationship had seriously suffered as a result of their work in HIV or oncology – mainly by separation or divorce. There were few statistically significant differences between HIV/AIDS and oncology, although friends of HIV staff were more likely to be supportive of their working in such a field, and HIV staff were less likely to avoid discussing their work socially than oncology staff. On the other hand, families of oncology staff were more supportive of their work than were families of HIV/AIDS staff.

One study has been conducted examining the impact of HIV on the *roles* within discordant couples (i.e., one with HIV, one without) by Church, Kocsis and Green (1988). This semi-structured interview study of care-giving partners of people with HIV revealed that 25 per cent of those surveyed reported they were more anxious and depressed than those they were caring for, and 57 per cent reported having high levels of stress. Most reported that their work, social life, recreation and sexual relations had been greatly affected by living indirectly with HIV. Those carers who perceived themselves as having higher social support than the person with HIV were found to have low stress levels, whereas when the person with HIV received higher levels of social support, the carer had higher levels of stress.

An increasing amount of anecdotal and survey literature is presently identifying the impact of HIV/AIDS on the home lives of families in developing countries (e.g., Ankrah, 1991). Reports such as this are serving to remind that in so many parts of the world where the HIV epidemic rages silently, it is the families, spouses, children and parents who are the health workers for those with disease. It is revealing that in low-resource settings, emotional, psychological and spiritual needs of HIV-caring family members have been subsumed under directly pressing (and stressing) burdens of economic need associated with prohibitive costs of medicines, special foods, and funerals. At the same time, families face a declining ability to earn money because they struggle with chronic debilitating illness, and the deaths of income-generating family members (Ankrah, Lubega and Nkumbi, 1989; Ankrah, 1991).

A study examining the impact of HIV counselling on the non-work behaviours of 101 counsellors in Zambia has highlighted the particular tensions that may arise between the messages that health workers give others, and those that they take home and are able to use themselves, especially in relation to HIV and sexual behaviour (Baggaley *et al.*, 1996). Of those surveyed, 70 had a relative who had died of AIDS, but only a few had been able to discuss HIV with them and, while the same proportion worried about their HIV status, only 24 had been tested for HIV (53 did not want to know their status). A little over half those interviewed were female, and many of the women worried because of their partners' sexual behaviour, yet few could discuss this with them. Indeed, while promotion of condom use was an important part of their work, only 27 had ever used one. Baggaley *et al.* (1996) suggest the tensions evident in such findings may be due in part to the social context of HIV management – characterised in Zambia at that time by stigma and discrimination against those with HIV, traditional barriers to condom use, and to sexual negotiation by women, barriers to public sexual discussion, and the high background HIV seroprevalence. The need to address such issues in counsellor training is particularly clear.

The social support buffering hypothesis

Social support has been considered as a potential buffer of work stress and burnout. The buffering hypothesis states that social support does not necessarily lower the stress experienced by the worker, but acts as an aid to coping with work stress. Empirical results concerning this hypothesis have been inconsistent, however. Constable and Russell (1986) examined the impact (beneficial or other-wise) of social support on the effects of perceived work stress by administering the MBI, the Work Environment Scale (Moos and Insel, 1974), and a social support measure by House and Wells (1978), to 310 US Army nurses. Multiple regression analyses were performed to assess the effects of social support on burnout, and whether social support had a buffering effect on the negative aspects of the work environment and burnout. They found that the major predictors of the MBI subscale variables were job enhancement, work pressure and supervisor support. As they expected from the buffering hypothesis of social support, their results suggested that as supervisory support increased, emotional exhaustion decreased – indeed supervisor support interacted with job enhancement to predict emotional exhaustion. However, Constable and Russell (1986) found that there was no significant relationship between burnout and support from colleagues, spouses, and/or family and friends. A similar result has been found in a study of factory workers by House (1981), which revealed that support from supervisors – and not from co-workers – was the most significant source of support in buffering and reducing the effects of stress on workers' health.

A study by Leiter and Maslach (1988) examined the effects of different sources of interpersonal contact on MBI subscale scores in mental health settings. In making a distinction between pleasant and unpleasant co-worker and supervisor contacts in a group of nurses, they found that unpleasant supervisor contact was related to emotional exhaustion, whereas pleasant supervisor contact was negatively related to depersonalisation, and pleasant co-worker contact was positively related to personal accomplishment.

In a study of 266 volunteers who had been working at Gay Mens' Health Crisis in New York City for six months or more, Maslanka (1992) employed path analyses to assess the role of social support in influencing the degree of stress experienced as a volunteer. She found that formal staff support was more important than peer support in reducing negative outcomes of volunteering. Maslanka found that staff support (emotional support through listening, being helpful and reliable) directly decreased levels of (MBI-defined) burnout and indirectly increased the levels of reward experienced by volunteers. However, she also found that the characteristics volunteers themselves brought to their work – such as the need for companionship or for a new career – played a major role in the development of experienced burnout. Further, those volunteers with high levels of reward from their volunteer work were also those experiencing high levels of burnout, especially if they were younger. Intensity of work and of work committment may be important here – studies have shown that it is the intensity, not the chronicity, of patient contact that can lead to burnout (Horstman and McKusick, 1986). Having said this, Maslanka found that overall MBI burnout levels for volunteers after six months were generally low, and rewards felt were generally high.

Some of the most significant research studies considering the buffering effects of support on burnout have been performed by Leiter (1988, 1990, 1991), and these have been described in Chapter 2. These studies revealed that professional support coming from the *wrong* quarter (i.e., a negatively-regarded supervisor) may actually *increase* 'emotional exhaustion'. Additionally, having personal support was significantly associated with *not* being emotionally exhausted or detached from the needs and concerns of patients. Having support *from the workplace* resulted in a relative absence of detatchment and cynicism about patients' needs, and being able to recognise one's professional accomplishments.

To summarise, it appears that support coming from different sources has different effects as measured on the MBI subscales, but social and organisational support may also have negative effects or no effects at all. Perhaps the most reliable general conclusion to be drawn is that professional and personal sources and experiences of support are indeed different and may have independent effects. It also appears possible that marriage may be recommendable for burnout prevention! The availability of social and/or staff support should, however – on the basis of evidence to date – result in increased levels of personal accomplishment. It is certainly the case that more research is required to establish the true extent of work-stress impact on family lives, the degree to which work-based social support carries over into non-work socialisation, and whether strategies for coping with work stress require active participation of family members and, if so, in what way. Furthermore, it may well be the case that admission of non-work relationship issues is appropriate in work-based staff support programmes if substantial effects are found (Miller and Gillies, 1996).

Other issues affecting the experience of burnout

Burnout research has seen increasing reference in recent years to specific issues that, in addition to organisational and interpersonal constraints, may materially affect susceptibility to experiences of emotional exhaustion, depersonalisation and personal accomplishment. By focusing on individual-based issues such as gender, age and seniority, a greater understanding of how interactional processes are driven and confounded, or modified, can be gained.

Gender issues and burnout

Burnout research has given low emphasis to gender issues, although gender is a standard demographic variable in many burnout studies. As with studies attempting to examine deterministic relations between MBI subscales and demographic issues such as age, marital status and experience in work, the relations found between MBI subscale scores and gender in cross-sectional studies to date are equivocal (Pretty, McCarthy and Catano, 1992), despite females usually showing higher levels of burnout effects than males in studies across cultures (Golembiewski, Scherb and Boudreau, 1993).

For example, in a study of 67 GPs, Lemkau *et al.* (1987) found no relation between any of the MBI subscale scores and gender. In a study of Australian nurses, Bennett, Michie and Kippax (1991) found the same result. However, other studies have identified aparrently gender-specific significant relations with MBI subscales. For example, emotional exhaustion has been identified as being experienced more by females in a study of 169 police staff by Gaines and Jermier (1983), and in a study of 1,025 health professionals by Maslach and Jackson (1985). Confusingly, the same authors found that there was no relation between gender and MBI emotional exhaustion subscale scores in a survey of 845 telephone company staff.

In a population of 433 telecommunication workers, Pretty, McCarthy and Catano (1992) found that there were no differences according to gender in levels of emotional exhaustion, depersonalisation or personal accomplishment, until job levels were taken into account. Women reported more emotional exhaustion and depersonalisation if they were *non-managers*, i.e., if they were dealing face-to-face (or ear-to-mouth) with the public. Men, on the other hand, experienced more emotional exhaustion and depersonalisation if they were managers. In looking at what the authors call the 'psychological environment' of work according to individual MBI subscale scores, emotional exhaustion was related to work pressure for both men and women; however, female managers were more sensitive to staff interactions, while males were more sensitive to the demands of their bosses. For depersonalisation, men were more vulnerable to issues of control, while women were more vulnerable to work relationship issues and peer cohesion. For personal accomplishment, the experiences of female managers were related to oppor- tunities for creative skill use and work variety, while the perceptions of male managers related to peer involvement. For both sexes, personal accomplishment was positively related to control exerted by upper management.

This study also made significant findings with respect to 'sense of community' – akin to the social support notion empirically tested by, e.g., Constable and Russell (1986), and Leiter (1992), and to organisational committment (Cooper and Davidson, 1987). All groups experienced significantly more emotional exhaustion and depersonalisation when they experienced a lower sense of community at work. And all groups except female non-managers experienced higher personal accomplishment when also experiencing a greater sense of community. These authors conclude overall that womens' burnout experiences were more sensitive to work climate factors than those reported by men. Such issues form an important backdrop to issues of organisational and clinical ethos emerging in the context of management of possibly marginalised patient populations, such as is the case with HIV/AIDS care (see Chapter 5).

No relation between gender and emotional exhaustion or personal accom- plishment was found in MBI-based surveys of teachers by Russell, Altmaier and Van Velzen (1987) and Schwab and Iwanicki (1982), although both these studies, and that by Maslach and Jackson, 1985, on telephone workers, and on health professionals, identified males as experiencing greater levels of depersonalisation. In their comparison study of nurses in four nursing settings, van Servellen and Leake (1993) found that male nurses were more likely than females to report higher levels of MBI depersonalisation. Finally, a survey of 462 teachers by Gold (1985) showed that females experience less depersonalisation and more personal accomplishment than males.

A cross-sectional survey of 600 medical, surgical and psychiatric nurses in non- HIV/AIDS workplaces in Scotland by Plant, Plant and Foster (1992) suggested that workplace variables best predicted stress in female nurses. Multivariate analyses revealed that concerns about HIV/AIDS – in these non-HIV/AIDS settings – were the most significant predictors of stress, followed by proportions of time spent in administration, alcohol and coffee consumption for females. For males, a significant predictor of work stress in addition to HIV/AIDS concern was number of years of nursing experience. A difficulty in this study was the lack of psychometric data regarding the structure and reliability of their 14-item scale measuring AIDS concerns.

Roth (1995) suggests that gender differences on MBI subscale scores may be consequences of features of the larger society. For example, she cites studies showing that women are expected to do the housework and childcare, regardless of whether or not they also have paid employment outside the home (Hochschild, 1989). The weight of such extra burdens may explain higher female scores on the MBI emotional exhaustion subscale. Roth (1995) also cites studies suggesting that self-perception is different between men and women, with women seeing themselves in relation to others, while men see themselves according to notions of separateness and difference from those around them, a perception that would logically manifest in higher levels of depersonalisation in intimate work settings. In view of these issues, and differing work experiences associated with sexual discrimination, pay inequality, and career handicaps especially at higher levels, it is surprising that more consistent gender differences in burnout measures are not found (Pretty, McCarthy and Catano, 1992).

In summary, the evidence to date suggests that MBI subscales differentiate the experience of work stress according to gender, though not consistently, and they do so differently for different populations. It is conceivable that gender differences may emerge more clearly than they have done to date if job seniority is clarified in multivariate analyses, as the lack of consideration of this variable may have confounded interpretations of earlier studies (Pretty, McCarthy and Catano, 1992).

Age and experience and burnout

The age of health workers has consistently been implicated in studies looking for vulnerabilities in respect of occupational stress and morbidity. In human service industries, especially health care settings where chronic, life-threatening disease in age peers is the working norm, one might intuitively expect young age and inexperience to be associated with special vulnerability, perhaps because coping skills have yet to be learned, roles within an organisation have yet to be fully identified, and the confidence and psychological armour that comes only with years of experience has yet to grow.

Indeed, it can be argued that the field of HIV/AIDS is itself young, and therefore practitioners of all ages in this field, facing the de-skilling challenges of a new virus and its seemingly burgeoning complications with relatively few proven approaches to management, prophylaxis, prevention and cure, may be especially susceptible to occupational morbidity on that basis alone. The same sense of clinical impotence may have been a part of approaching any new disease, or even an old, proven killer like cancer, and may have its residual echoes in the alacrity with which new managements, or even approaches to management (e.g., antibody testing) are seized upon as though they may offer a breakthrough in care (Shilts, 1987; Miller, 1995a).

In a study of occupational stress in psychiatric nurses that employed burnout-based interpretations of time-sampling, diaries, participant observation and interviews, Handy (1987) identified *how* relative youth and inexperience may impact on the modification of work behaviours. She found that many of the younger nurses were aware of, and troubled by, the discrepancies between their therapeutic ideals and the content and conduct of their daily ward routines (cf. Cherniss, 1980). Sometimes this awareness would lead to *ad hoc* attempts to develop more theraputically oriented relations with individuals in their care, although such attempts often failed because of their inexperience, and because of the 'control-oriented structure' within which they were working. When such attempts failed repeatedly, feelings of intense insecurity and rejection would be triggered in staff, leading, Handy says, to defensive reactions in which patients were blamed for being unmotivated to change. In consequence, staff became more routine-oriented and aloof – an attitude encouraged by more experienced colleagues as it made ward life easier to organise, and also shielded the younger staff from future disappointments in their dealings with their patients.

While not employing the typical constructs of burnout research, Handy's (1988) study can be described in those terms, such that the assault on the younger staffs' professional ideals leads to increased innovative activity (making closer relationships with patients), then a heightened sense of failure, resulting in depersonalisation (blaming patients for the difficulties experienced) which is professionally reinforced.

In their study linking occupational stress situations with somatic sequelae in oncology physicians and nurses, Ullrich and FitzGerald (1990) found that age, sex, profession (i.e., being a nurse or a physician) and hospital size were the 'life-variables' predicting self-reported stress. They found that stress reduced as staff aged, and that younger physicians were the most fatigued. (Additionally, they found that staff working in smaller units experienced more stress because of having greater identification with a smaller number of patients, and nurses had more physical complaints associated with physical exertion in their work.)

In their review of studies associating MBI-measured burnout with age and amount of professional experience, Cordes and Dougherty (1993) describe the pattern and complexity of gender relations to each of the MBI subscales as 'mixed'. What is decipherable is the finding that younger people consistently report higher scores than older staff on the three MBI subscales. For example, this has been found in studies of teachers by Russell, Altmaier and Van Velzen (1987), Zabel and Zabel (1982), and Anderson and Iwanicki (1984). Two other studies in groups of teachers (Schwab and Iwanicki, 1982; Gold, 1985) confirmed this finding, and found also that younger staff also had elevated depersonalisation subscale scores. Maslach and Jackson (1981) found the same in their MBI validation study of 1025 health service professionals.

Bennett, Kelaher and Ross (1994), in a longitudinal study of HIV/AIDS nurses, physicians and social workers based in two hospitals in Sydney, found age to be one of the variables that was significantly predictive of higher MBI subscale scores, along with a reliance on external coping mechanisms, and patient-related stress. Younger age has also predicted HIV/AIDS-related MBI-measured burnout in populations of social workers and paramedical staff (Egan, 1993).

van Servellen and Leake (1993), in comparing nurses working with AIDS, oncology, general medical and intensive care patients, found low but significant associations between nurses MBI subscale scores and age, years of nursing practice, and years of practice in their current units. These authors reported that older nurses with more practice time had significantly lower emotional exhaustion scores, and that those with more practice and unit experience were significantly more likely to have low personal accomplishment subscale scores – i.e., a lower sense of personal accomplishment. It is noteworthy that nurses working in AIDS special care units were significantly more likely to report exhaustion than nurses on other units. van Servellen and Leake (1993) concluded that the lower personal accomplishment subscale scores indicate that whereas practice experience may guard against emotional exhaustion, there may also be a blunting effect on sense of accomplishment that comes with experience and age. Is it that experience generates a greater realism about the eventual outcome of management in chronic, life-threatening illness? Experience may produce a longer-term view that deflects attention away from short-term clinical and therapeutic gains to longer-term outcomes, putting more immediate successes in the context of final treatment failure.

It is important to examine the issue of age and seniority further in the context of health care, not least because of the costs of specialist training mean that the potential loss of youthful staff is very expensive, and the potential loss of experienced staff places higher work burdens on less experienced – and more vulnerable – staff. In seeking to design strategies for managing and preventing occupational stress and burnout, it seems likely that not accounting for age, experience, seniority and gender could result in approaches that have less direct relevance or impact.

Burnout and personality

'More . . . prospective studies are needed to assess personality characteristics . . . But . . . I am afraid that use of conventional research paradigms for another 20 years will result in more data but not much more knowledge. Even more sophisticated investigations of burnout etiology resemble an attempt to predict the outcome of a football match on the basis of the teams' average height and weight on the one hand, and from the prevailing wind direction and speed on the other. What is more, outcome in terms of scores is probably not the most interesting part of the game.'

(Burisch, 1993, p. 88)

One of the few published studies that extends beyond a mere cataloguing of stressors in medical environments concerns the possibility of a 'burnout-prone personality' (Keinan and Melamed, 1987). To 79 male hospital physicians in Israel, these authors administered:

- A 'burnout inventory' (Pines, Aronson and Kafry, 1981), together with scales measuring.

- Repression–sensitisation – the tendency to deal with threatening situations by avoidance strategies such as denial and rationalisation, and to show extreme vigilance to all aspects of stressful circumstances.
- Emotional reactivity – experiencing intrusive or repetitive thoughts following emotional events, lack of control over emotional arousal, experiencing anticipatory emotional arousal, and emotional reactions of excessive magnitude and duration.
- Self control.
- 'Type A' behaviour (insistent, pushy, ambitious, overachieving, behaviourally rigid, impulsive and agressive).
- Hostility.

They found that burnout correlated positively with a tendency to deal with threatening situations by avoidance, denial, rationalisation and showing extreme vigilance. Emotional reactivity was also positively correlated with burnout. On the other hand, learned resourcefulness – the habit of constructive and successful problem-solving – was found to be negatively correlated with burnout and lowered the likelihood of chronic occupational morbidity. A problem with this study was that burnout and work stress were not self-reported – stress was inferred by the researchers from the nature of the physicians' tasks. Yet the study by Bailey, Steffen and Grout (1980) on the role of perception in appreciation of work stressors and rewards (see Chapter 2) affirmed how necessary it is for respondents of such surveys to be able to nominate their own stressors.

A more recent Italian study of 194 HIV/AIDS staff examined personality factors in psychometrically measured burnout. Bellani *et al.*, (1996) administered the 16PF, IPAT, anxiety and depression scales, the AIDS Impact Scale (Bennett, Kelaher and Ross, 1994) and the MBI, to 139 nurses and 55 physicians. They found that burnout was predicted by 'ego weakness', and reduced personal accomplishment was predicted by 'shyness'. In practical terms, this result suggetst that predictors for burnout include not being able to manage others, or to manage group situations, thus giving substance to the appropriateness of burnout prevention through careful staff selection (Bellani *et al.*, 1996; Visintini *et al.*, 1996).

Other personal characteristics that may influence the construct of personality, such as gender, age and interprsonal relationships, are discussed as correlates of burnout in more detail in subsequent chapters.

Conclusions

To conclude, this chapter has examined qualitative and quantitative symptoms of reported burnout emerging from mainly correlational studies and some health-worker phenomenological surveys. It does not present the complete picture, however. For example, the context of HIV/AIDS care involves working with marginalised populations in the context of a feared disease. Therefore, issues of stigma and discrimination, perceived dangers and fears, levels of training and felt competence, support of families and loved-ones, and identification with populations at risk, all matter as possible vectors for health worker stress and burnout. Also, HIV is a new disease that has seen a dramatic evolution of new modalities of health care. For example, there are new professional roles and responsibilities, such as that of HIV/AIDS counselling. And there are new contexts of structured staff involvement, such as volunteering, and the development of the 'buddy' system.

Thus, while HIV has, in its bewildering growth, given a new window on the forms and impacts of HIV-related work stress and burnout, it has also been a very useful vehicle for driving forward our understanding of work stress and burnout, and how to address it. The UK studies described in Chapters 7 and 8 extend this understanding by further examining cognitive, behavioural and emotional correlates of self-reported and psychometrically measured burnout in the context of HIV/AIDS. The literature in this field forms the focus of Chapter 5.

Part II
Burnout in the context of HIV/AIDS

5   Burnout in HIV/AIDS

Are the stresses, and the possibilities for burnout, faced by health workers in the field of HIV/AIDS really different to those of health workers managing other health problems? If so, how different are they, and what makes them so?

There seems always to have been some controversy over whether HIV/AIDS carers experienced unique stresses (e.g., Miller, 1991; Kleiber et al., 1992; Van Dis and Van Dongen, 1993). Van Dis and Van Dongen (1993) suggest that unique characteristics of HIV/AIDS care include:

- The secondary stigmatisation of working with a stigmatising disease.
- The identification with, and emotional involvement with, clients who may have the carers' own sexual orientation and experiences, or substance use difficulties.
- The absence of a cure for HIV disease and a universally fatal outcome.
- The intensity of the epidemic and the high numbers of those infected.
- Fears of HIV infection in the course of occupational exposure.
- Exposure to death and dying.

Other reports suggested that although the burdens faced by HIV/AIDS health care workers were not yet proven to be unique (Kleiber et al., 1992), the recognition accorded the potential for staff stress in this context by media, by patients, and health staff groups probably was. From the outset of the HIV pandemic, clinical and social stresses in HIV/AIDS work were compounded by the high profile and often contradictory media emphases that the pandemic attracted, due in part at least to public stigma and fear associated with myths about homosexuality (Pinching, 1986; Green and Miller, 1987). Yet a criticism often laid at the door of HIV/AIDS burnout research has been the relative absence of studies correlating HIV/AIDS work stress with stresses measured from other fields. Where this has been done, it has usually been with colleagues in oncology (e.g., van Servellen and Leake, 1993; Miller, 1995c), and psychogeriatrics (e.g., Kleiber, Enzmann and Gusy, 1995). Further, in her review of the impact of working with people with HIV, Barbour (1994) noted an additional challenge to representativeness:

'Research appears to have been built up serendipitously rather than systematically, with many researchers opportunistically confining their investigations to the hospital or medical centre where they happened to be based'. (p. 223)

Table 5.1 Health worker impact of HIV/AIDS care

1. Staff fears
- Anxiety over staff safety (e.g., Gordin *et al.*, 1987; Trieber *et al.*, 1987; Davidson and Gillies, 1993)
- Fears of HIV contagion (e.g., Bennett, 1992; Horsman and Sheeran, 1995)

2. Issues of association
- Intense, long-term relationships with patients (e.g., Morin and Batchelor, 1984; Miller, 1987, 1995a; Ross and Seeger, 1988; Bennett, Michie and Kippax, 1991)
- Self-identification with people with HIV (e.g., Horstman and McKusick, 1986)
- Managing distressed relatives and loved-ones of patients (e.g., Miller, Gillies and Elliott, 1996)
- Bereavement overload (e.g., Bolle, 1988; Piemme and Bolle, 1990)
- Grief (e.g., Pasacreta and Jacobsen, 1989; Nesbitt *et al.*, 1996)
- Motivations to work in this field (e.g., Paradis *et al.*, 1987; Barbour, 1994; Maslanka, 1996; Miller and Gillies, 1996)
- Boundary problems between staff and patients (e.g., Williams, 1988; Gessler *et al.*, 1996)

3. Professional and role issues
- The context of care (e.g., Barbour, 1994, 1995; Miller, 1995a)
- Professional role expansion (e.g., taking on counselling) (e.g., Pearlin, Semple and Turner, 1988; Miller and Brown, 1988; Coyle and Soodin, 1992; Barbour, 1995; Miller *et al.*, 1999)
- Intensity of HIV/AIDS work (e.g., Bennett *et al.*, 1992; Bennett, Miller and Ross, 1995; Bellani *et al.*, 1996)
- Discomfort in addressing issues of patient sexuality (e.g., Eakin and Taylor, 1990; Baggaley *et al.*, 1996)
- Neurological management difficulties (e.g., Ross and Seeger, 1988; Sorensen *et al.*, 1989)
- Professional inadequacy (e.g., Burisch, 1989; Miller, 1991, 1995)
- Role ambiguity (e.g., Miller, 1995a; Miller, Gillies and Elliott, 1996)
- Professional rewards (e.g., Ross and Seeger, 1988; Barbour, 1995)
- Newness of HIV/AIDS and of professional responses (e.g., Pinching, 1986; Barbour, 1995; Lloyd, 1995)
- Inadequate training (e.g., Brimlow, 1995; Horsman and Sheeran, 1995)
- Absence of a cure (e.g., Morin and Batchelor, 1984; Bennett, Miller and Ross, 1995)
- Staff working with uncertainty (e.g., over new treatment impacts) while encouraging patients to hope (e.g., Miller, 1996; Bennett and Kelaher, 1993)
- Pressures associated with volunteer work (e.g., Maslanka, 1995; Nesbitt *et al.*, 1996)

4. Stigma, discrimination and ethical issues
- Social contagion (e.g., Munodawafa, Bower and Webb, 1993; Blumenfield *et al.*, 1987)
- Homophobia (and prejudice against IDUs) (e.g., O'Donnell *et al.*, 1987; Pomerance and Shields, 1989; Eakin and Taylor, 1990)
- Ethical dilemmas (e.g., Gilmore and Somerville, 1995; Barbour, 1995)
- Poor social support (e.g., Miller, 1991; Bennett and Kelaher, 1993; Maslach and Ozer, 1995)

In the context of HIV/AIDS health worker stress and burnout, most of the issues of relevance that have received empirical, acecdotal and speculative attention can be identified under the following headings (Table 5.1):

- Staff fears.
- Issues of association.
- Professional and role issues.
- Stigma, discrimination and ethical issues.

While the list in Table 5.1 is not exhaustive, it conveys the substantial interest in health worker impact that has been generated by the HIV pandemic. This chapter will consider the issues under each heading below.

Staff fears

In a review of carers' responses to working with HIV/AIDS patients, Eakin and Taylor (1990) identified fear of contagion, along with social contamination, discomfort with the sexual dimensions of AIDS, the sense of professional inadequacy, and reward and challenge, as the most identifiable themes character-ising health workers' psychosocial responses to working in this field. Evidence of the impact of staff fears on their professional perspectives and conduct has come from a number of studies. For example, early reports concerning the possibility of patients being refused care by health personnel highlighted concerns about the illness being transmitted to staff (e.g., Nicholls, 1986). In an often-quoted study, Trieber, Shaw and Malcom (1987) examined the psychological impact on eight nurses and four physicians of caring for a person with AIDS, compared to working with a person with a non-AIDS illness but with closely matched demographic and disease characteristics – they applied three standardised self-report measures of psychological distress following their treatment of both. These researchers found that care of the person with AIDS produced greater levels of anxiety and general psychological distress in staff than care of the patient with identical treatment requirements, and that the patient with AIDS was perceived by all staff to be 'much more difficult to manage', despite both patients having identical treatment requirements. In the workplace, staff had more anxiety and more negative perceptions of the behaviour of the person with AIDS during routine medical procedures. Outside the workplace, staff had ruminations about contracting HIV from the patient, and nursing staff were more adversely affected.

It seems that the growth in understanding about HIV transmission and infection control procedures has had at best a variable impact on staff responses (Parsons, 1995), particularly where the seroprevalence of the community remains lower than in treatment epicentres. In a postal survey of 1,530 hospital staff from Nottingham (response rate of 63 per cent; N = 958), Davidson and Gillies (1993) found that 62 per cent of staff overall (593/958), including 38 per cent of physicians (36/94), and 52 per cent of nurses (67/128) thought that patients should be routinely tested for HIV on admission, and 17 per cent of physicians and 19 per cent of nurses felt that HIV patients should be isolated in hospital.

While this survey took place in a low-prevalence area of the United Kingdom, the results suggest that the need for active dissemination of information and guidance on an on-going basis is necessary to quell fears of contagion in all hospital staff.

Fear of contagion has also been identified as an issue for health staff in studies by Amchin and Polan (1986), in which 55 per cent of subjects reported spending less time dealing with a person with AIDS than with other patients. Additionally, only 16 per cent said they would volunteer to work in an AIDS unit. Horsman and Sheeran (1995) drew a distinction between perceptions of *physical* contagion, and perceptions of *social* contagion, in which the staff member is perceived as being negatively altered by their association with HIV/AIDS care (this latter aspect is discussed on pages 83–85 of this chapter ('Stigma, discrimination and ethical issues'). They identified 33 studies up to 1993 in which staff identified serious fears of occupational infection out of proportion to the actual risk.

These authors make the point, emerging from the literature on risk-taking, that decisions about risk behaviour in the context of very low probabilities will be either ignored or grossly over-weighted – the aversiveness of small chances of severe negative outcomes will thus be amplified. This has been borne out in studies of health workers' estimates of HIV risk involving both physicians and nurses, and they further note that reassurances about low risk and virus fragility in the context of 'extraordinary, inconvenient and expensive infection control measures' (Gerbert *et al.*, 1988) may seem to trivialise staffs' fears by appearing to ignore the risks involved in this work (Horsman and Sheeran, 1995). In view of these findings, it is interesting to consider Miller's (1995a) finding that HIV/AIDS staff reporting a personal history of potential exposure to HIV since 1980, compared with those not reporting such potential exposure, were over seven times more likely to report that they currently experienced stress associated with their work.

Contrasted to the difficulties associated with risk perceptions is the often equivocal adherence to suggested infection control measures. Indeed, *knowledge* of prevention of occupational risk is by no means related to prevention *behaviour* (just as with cohorts of sexually active people in the 'external' communities!) (Gruber *et al.*, 1989; Smyser *et al.*, 1990; McNabb and Kelter, 1991; Baggaley *et al.*, 1996). This is highlighted in the scenario concerning the impact on ward nurses of caring for a colleague acquiring HIV occupationally, below.

Issues of association

HIV/AIDS staff are required to cope with the stress of identifying with patients from their own age and peer groups, with the grieving of patients and of their loved-ones and families, and with concerns about HIV in a social context of potential stigma and ostracism (Green and Miller, 1987). Indeed, the MOMS study (Miller, 1995c; Miller and Gillies, 1996) identified that involvements of health staff with patients' families/loved-ones was a major source of stress for both HIV/AIDS and oncology staff. In a related study (see Chapters 7 and 8), Miller, Gillies and Elliott (1996) found that 40 per cent of HIV/AIDS staff working across four main treatment sites cited the management of distressed relatives as their major work stress.

Case scenario: Too close for comfort?

Nurse AB was admitted to the ward with a lymphoma on a morning in February. She was well known to the staff because she had visited friends who had been ill on the ward before, and she had also attended regularly for her own check-ups. The staff knew she was previously a nurse on an infectious diseases ward, working with people with HIV and AIDS, and had acquired HIV at work. She was seriously ill, though awake and alert. She was calm, though confided that she knew the end was close.

The call to the psychology and psychotherapy services came after AB had been on the ward for one week. Junior staff particularly were finding that, although she was responding well to treatment, her familiarity with their procedures, with the 'routine' difficulties of managing patients and their families, and her age and similarity to them, was increasingly upsetting. When she had talked to her 'special' (i.e., personal) nurse about how she had acquired her HIV infection, and this was shared at a staff meeting, a few of the nursing staff became very anxious and some asked if they could be excused from her care.

The psychologist involved spoke with the nursing team in two shifts (to cover all those with whom AB might have contact). At each meeting, staff were asked how they felt at the present time about having AB on the ward, and how they had noticed their feelings changing over the duration of her stay. Four main issues emerged:

1 She was 'just like them' as a person – the same age, aspirations, life history, personal and work experiences, attitudes and anxieties.
2 She had acquired her HIV infection by doing exactly what they did every day. This included pushing used needles and syringes down into the sharps tin when it was getting too full, having splashes and cuts when gloves and glasses were not worn, and not reporting them every time they occurred.
3 She was well known to the staff for a number of years, because her 'case' of occupational infection through a deep needle-stick involving fluids from a known infected patient had made the national media, and was a high-profile case in the nursing journals – and now she was getting seriously sick for the first time.
4 Staff were feeling guilty that their views of AB were altering, and that she may recognise that they were 'backing away' from her.

Subsequent discussions focussed on the inconsistency between preventive knowledge and practice, and why this inconsistency existed. Ward procedures and expectations that may contribute to risk behaviour were reviewed, and a plan for improving infection control and accident observance

was devised. Further discussion focussed on personal emotional responses to AB's admission, and how identification with peers of any kind was
expected. The ways in which this might affect AB's care were also
rehearsed, without suggesting blame or professional inappropriateness. It
was discussed that AB might be feeling such things also, and that this might
become a topic for specific discussion with those she had closest contact
with, including her counsellor.

In addition, intense relationships have been reported to develop between carers and people with HIV, and the organisations representing them (e.g., Morin and Batchelor, 1984; Moreland and Legg, 1991). This finding has become so common that a recent research report suggested confidently that the health worker is 'inclined to get involved in the relationship with the patient to compensate for his therapeutic limits' (Visintini *et al.*, 1995).

A number of studies have suggested that such issues, and the pressures arising from them, can have adverse effects on HIV/AIDS health workers. An early example was by Horstman and McKusick (1986), who described a self-report questionnaire study in San Fransisco of 82 physicians. Some 56 per cent of those surveyed reported more stress, 46 per cent reported a greater fear of death, and 44 per cent reported increased anxiety since they had started working in the field of AIDS care. Unfortunately, none of the measures of morbidity was specifically described. Self-reported morbidity was significantly higher in those identifying themselves as gay or lesbian (65 per cent), than in non-identifiers or hetero-sexuals. Subsequent interviews revealed that such increases were associated with self-identification of possible risk for HIV disease, and with gay patients for whom they could not offer a cure. Morbidity in the form of self-reported stress anxiety or depression was associated with the *intensity*, not the chronicity, of patient contact, indicating that as patient cohorts become sicker, stress on staff will increase. Also, 40 per cent of those surveyed reported greater intellectual stimulation since working with AIDS (a factor discussed on pages 76–83 of this chapter, Professional and role issues).

The notion of bereavement overload is one borrowed from oncology (Delvaux, Razaki and Farvacques, 1988), and which has been identified as important for HIV care. In their early qualitative survey, Ross and Seeger (1988) identified this issue as contributing to stress for HIV health professionals. Studies by Bolle (1988), and Piemme and Bolle (1990) confirm this finding. In a study comparing equal groups of oncology and HIV/AIDS health workers, Miller (1995a) found that patient deaths were significantly more likely to be reported as a work stress by junior staff of all professions than senior staff, and that junior staff experienced work stress significantly more than senior staff in response to the perceived danger of their occupation in the field of HIV/AIDS.

Of course, an expected response to bereavement is *grief* – a consequence reported for HIV/AIDS staff, especially in the earlier phases of the pandemic when anti-retroviral regimes were less accessible and less effective. Although studies are starting to suggest that emotional consequences for health staff can be managed by regulating exposure to patient morbidity, as well as the topography of job tasks (see Chapter 10), grief appears to be inevitable where prevalence is high. Also, staff become very attached to their patients over the longer term, and the impact of bereavement should come as no surprise to the enlightened manager, professionalism and professional discipline notwithstanding. The issue of bereavement overload (Pasacreta and Jacobsen, 1989) has already been mentioned. However, one of the few studies directly addressing grief found no direct relationship between grief and burnout in volunteer health worker populations (Nesbitt *et al.*, 1996). This study of 174 religious volunteers did find that the best predictors of grief in volunteers were time spent volunteering per week (more hours weekly meant less grief was experienced), and levels of available emotional support to volunteers (more available support meant less grief).

An issue of importance from a clinical psychological perspective which has received relatively little scrutiny is that of *motivation* for being involved in HIV/AIDS care, and how this relates to work stress and burnout. In her review of HIV/AIDS health worker impact, Barbour (1994) identified that assessment of motivations for HIV/AIDS work was critical in enabling answers to why people become stressed. In particular, she argues, previous work experience, and knowledge of whether staff opted in – or were simply deployed in – to HIV/AIDS care might help explain different staffs' reactions to work stresses. Miller and Gillies (1996) found in their survey of HIV/AIDS and oncology staff that 47 per cent of respondents had close family workers who had also been a health worker, and 77 per cent of HIV/AIDS staff had experienced chronic life-threatening illness in a close family member. However, less than 30 per cent overall said these issues influenced their choice of career field. On the other hand, HIV/AIDS workers were found to be significantly more likely than oncology staff to be motivated for their work by gay/peer concern, by interest in closely related elements of work, or wider sociopolitical issues, and less likely to be motivated by career potential ($P = 0.005$) (Miller and Gillies, 1996).

Maslanka's (1996) study of volunteers at Gay Men's Health Crisis in New York revealed that specific motivations (including 'joining the AIDS cause', 'personal growth', 'social contact', 'helping the gay family', and 'career enhancement') can lead to an increased sense of reward, but may also leave individuals vulnerable to negative psychological outcomes – something that staff support may only partly mediate.

Where motivations such as these may be unrecognised or not specifically addressed in staff orientation, training and supervision programmes (see Chapter 10), boundary problems may appear (Pasacreta and Jacobsen, 1989; Maslanka, 1996). Although this issue will be discussed in Chapter 10, it is pertinent to note Gessler, Alcorn and Miller's (1996) point that encouragement to violate boundaries may come as much or more from environmental, structural factors – i.e., the manner in which the context of HIV/AIDS care is provided – as from any proven individual factors, such as personality issues or lapses in professionalism.

Professional and role issues

As shown in Table 5.1, professional and role issues may contribute to HIV/AIDS health worker burnout in numerous and varied ways. They range from the structural, contextual elements that define the environment of work – both organisational and broader, political elements – to the individual aspects that involve the health worker's perception of their adequacy, their role, and the confdence with which they can fulfill it.

For example, an Australian study by Ross and Seeger (1988) found that 33 per cent and 43 per cent respectively of 108 health professionals working with AIDS reported stress and overwork resulting from AIDS-related work. Some 22 per cent of the sample reported experiencing a 'lot' of stress associated with the youth of the patients seen, clinical neurological difficulties in patients, and having patients dying. The reported areas of HIV work found most difficult included a sense of futility in treating people with AIDS, coping with patients' emotional traumas, and the uncertainty of disease progression. They concluded that 'the emotional needs of patients and inability to deal with them may be a more useful area in which to provide information and support to reduce burnout in staff . . .'. They also noted that there were no significant correlations found between self-reported burnout and personality, suggesting that it is the ambient stresses of patient management that result in burnout, or perhaps that burnout is not something that would appear until staff had had much more experience with such work pressures as were described. The lack of any information on sample selection, response rate, the lack of validity and reliability information on the unspecified scales used, and the use of 'open-ended questions about coping' which were not specified leads to an inability to interpret or replicate these findings, or to place firm conclusions upon them.

However, Ross and Seeger (1988) also found that 55 per cent of their sample reported intellectual *stimulation* from their work – similar to the finding from Horstman and McKusick (1986). This was described as a 'compensation' for the stresses described above, as were the feelings identified by Bennett *et al.* (1994) of working in a challenging and stimulating new field, the social recognition and reward of working in a personally relevant area, the gratitude of clients and patients, and a sense of achievement in making psychosocial progress with patients. Indeed, reward may come in many ways in HIV/AIDS work. Guinan *et al.* (1991) identified reward categories of personal effectiveness, emotional support, social support, and empathy/self-knowing in HIV/AIDS staff. A study of Scottish HIV/AIDS health workers by Barbour (1995), involving detailed qualitative interviews, revealed that despite high levels of concern about burnout,

'. . . interviewees were unanimous in describing some aspects of AIDS work as particularly rewarding, either in terms of providing confirmation of the strength posessed by individuals to weather personal tragedy, allowing staff to contribute to partial or temporary improvement in patients despite a terminal prognosis, or offering intellectual, clinical, and/or professional challenges. Of those considering making a move, the reason most commonly given related to general career moves rather than a desire to get out of AIDS work' (p. 527).

Bennett (1992a) described a sense of new-found freedom from prejudice and secrecy felt by gay male nurses working in this field, where their closer affiliation with those in their care may even make them *more* desirable as colleagues and carers than they may have experienced previously. Studies of HIV/AIDS volunteer workers reveal a sense of reward arising from belonging to the 'AIDS cause' and enhancing the sense of community (Maslanka, 1996), and having a greater sense of efficacy in doing something about the HIV threat (particularly with 'Buddy' work). More recent studies involving a cohort of religious volunteers in Houston, Texas, suggest that social support reward is an important factor in balancing the impact of grief and emotional response to the stress of HIV/AIDS care (Nesbitt *et al.*, 1996). This is not surprising given the presumed common bond in this cohort being a religiously inspired ethos of collaborative support for the vulnerable, just as studies of gay health workers also show that community identification and bonding is a major impetus and reward. And, as described earlier in this book, social support can be a critical mediator of stress in the workplace.

Thus, identification can be exultant or exhausting. The studies by Nesbitt *et al.* (1996) and Maslanka (1996), along with an analysis of data from the same cohort by Bennett *et al.* (1996), do draw attention, however, to the importance of nurturing such bonding and constructive potential by ensuring appropriate mechanisms are put in place for addressing the impact of this stressful work – including appropriate support activities (see Chapter 10).

The notion of rewards counterbalancing the negative aspects of work that manifest as burnout has been investigated and developed psychometrically, based on work by Bennett and her colleagues. Bennett, Kelaher and Ross (1994) describe The AIDS Impact Scale (AIS) based on a longitudial study of HIV/AIDS health workers in Australia. The AIS has 24 items derived from qualitative staff inter-views, designed to measure positive and negative aspects of work. Items are ranked on a 5-point Likert scale, and correspond to five subscales: Recognition/Reward, Grief/Powerlessness, Gay affiliation, Identification/Responsibility, and Stigma/Discrimination. The Recognition/Reward factor was found to be related to relationship stability and satisfaction, and negatively related to homophobia and social withdrawal. Subsequent research revealed that those with low burnout scores on the MBI had higher scores on social recognition and reward (Bennett *et al.*, 1994). Grief/Powerlessness was positively associated with social withdrawal and external coping strategies, and negatively related to negative coping strate-gies; Gay affiliation was negatively related to homophobia, and the MBI subscale constructs of lack of personal accomplishment, and depersonalisation; the Identification/Responsibility (i.e., identification with and responsibility for people living with HIV) factor was positively related to external coping and negatively related to social withdrawal and choice of work arena; Stigma/Discrimination was negatively related to scores on social withdrawal and internal coping (Bennett *et al.*, 1994; Kelaher and Ross, 1995). A subsequent validation study of the AIS in 410 Italian HIV/AIDS nurses by Visintini *et al.* (1996) revealed that the AIS 'social reward' (Recognition/Reward) factor positively predicts personal accomplishment, and negatively predicts emotional exhaustion and depersonalisation.

On a cautionary note, Bennett, Ross and Sutherland (1996) state that while the recognition and reward factor was a clearly discernible one,

> '. . . items on this scale are very specific to AIDS care as opposed to items in other scales measuring the general rewards of care-giving. The rewards of AIDS care-giving and the recognition received may be different to that experienced in other carer roles' (p. 146).

In an attempt to address directly which issues of care gave the greatest stress for HIV/AIDS health workers, Barbour (1995) asked 152 Scottish health staff from a variety of fields of care (injecting drug use, heterosexual and homosexual sex risk) whether HIV/AIDS care made *unique* demands – 71 per cent said yes overall, and 81 per cent of those working with IDU particularly agreed it does. Overall, the most demanding aspect reported of their work was working with families of people with HIV, and providing psychological support – these accounted for 38.5 per cent of responses. Other aspects of work described as the most demanding included inter-agency involvement, deaths of patients, dealing with drug users, the scale and complexity of clients' social problems, multi-disciplinary team working, and the youth of clients. Unfortunately, these issues were about the most demanding aspects of work – not what, in the eyes of respondents, made HIV care unique.

A study by Miller, Gillies and Elliott (1996) (reported more fully in Chapter 8) also asked HIV health workers about their stresses (and not about what made HIV unique), this time by rating the stressfulness of their work on a 0 (no stress) to 10 (high stress) scale. Overall, 65 per cent reported 'moderate to high' workplace stress. When asked what caused their jobs to be stressful, four principal ongoing stresses were identified:

1   HIV-specific issues, such as coping with distressed relatives, as well as deadlines, increasing workloads, and having insufficient time or resources for task completion.
2   Staff issues and relationships, including staff conflicts, problems of communication, staff shortages, supporting stressed colleagues, and problems with staff management.
3   Patient issues, including observing decline in deaths of people known for a long time, maintaining staff–patient boundaries, and managing difficult or aggressive patients (particularly for those working in relative isolation).
4   Management issues, including poor decision-making, restructuring and redundancies, and lack of acknowledgement of staff stress.

Another study by Miller (1995a; see Chapters 7 and 8) found that for HIV/AIDS staff, independently significant predictors for finding HIV work stressful included having colleagues experiencing burnout, and having difficulty with patient deaths.

So far, then, it seems that while HIV/AIDS care has specific characteristics mentioned by a number of commentators and researchers, the things that make work stressful do not appear to be those that make HIV unique as a health care issue. Perhaps the 'newness' of the HIV/AIDS phenomenon has contributed to the sense that the stresses it poses for staff are unique. This has been suggested by Barbour (1995), not least because the complexity of the HIV/AIDS matrix of danger from behaviour, social context and preventive/care challenges demands a breadth of professional engagement previously unseen by most professionals (e.g., as seen in the issue of counselling, pp. 89–91). This notion of newness leading to a confusion of imperatives and professional responses, the very experience of which is stressful, has been seen in the context of commentaries about HIV management from a variety of professional perspectives, e.g., psychiatric management of people with HIV (Pinching, 1986), and social work challenges with people with HIV (Lloyd, 1995).

The professional challenge of 'newness' is demonstrated also in the difficulties described concerning discomfort about embracing sexuality as a professional focus (Milne and Keen, 1988), especially when it cannot be embraced on a personal, individual level by those staff (Baggaley *et al.*, 1996), growing worries about professional inadequacy (Burisch, 1989; Miller, 1991), and concerns about adequacy of professional training (Brimlow, 1995). Additional pressures come from the tensions of expansion of professional roles (Miller and Brown, 1988), and the ambiguities that can emerge in such a circumstance (Raphael *et al.*, 1990; Coyle and Soodin, 1992; Miller, Gillies and Elliott, 1996).

Professional adequacy may be challenged in a variety of ways. Anxiety about both professional and systemic adequacy for managing manifestations of HIV was described in stress reports from staff facing neurological effects of HIV disease in their patients for the first time (Ross and Seeger, 1988; Barbour, 1995). Burisch (1989) gave a warning in the era of anti-retroviral monotherapy about the 'inevitable disappointments' of caring for AIDS patients, giving examples of staff suffering recurrent stress, disturbed dreams and exhaustion, with the most enthusiastic staff being the most affected. Burisch noted that because the symptoms of staff may appear minor in relation to the symptoms and the prognoses of their patients, senior staff may overlook or discount them. Other challenges may come from perceived conflict between traditional health work goals, and the consequences they cause for some patients, particularly when new treatment opportunities arise and are clamoured for by an increasingly anxious population, only to then fail or make patients more sick. For many health staff, the gnawing cycles of hope, uncertainty and despair they mediate for patients they gradually come to know as people beyond the symptoms becomes a question of whether they are prolonging life or prolonging death. This process is central to the case scenario on p. 81 ('How can I keep doing this?').

Bulkin *et al.* (1988) highlighted dilemmas associated with giving aggressive acute care to young people with terminal illness – hospice workers have had to adapt their skills to increasingly heterogeneous patient groups, including patients of a much younger average age than previously. Martin and Julian (1987) describe the difficulty of general practitioners handing care of their patients over to teams of in-patient specialists who they may not know or whose processes and ethos they may not be familiar with, and feeling that by doing so they are admitting they have failed and are giving up. What happens when infection control practices clash with a clinical ethos of overcoming isolation, loneliness and fear? And for health workers striving to entertain notions of hanging on for the hope of a cure or a breakthrough, when is it the best time to suggest writing final letters, putting affairs in order, saying goodbye?

On top of such circumstances, some staff have had the additional burdens of feeling responsible for the illnesses they have come to treat, in addition to the chronic health burdens in their patient cohorts. As Miller *et al.* (1989) describe:

> 'Initially many staff in Haemophilia Centres experienced a 'role change'. They had felt optimistic and helpful, giving Factor VIII and IX treatment and after the discovery of HIV reported feeling 'useless' and 'helpless'. . . Some staff can feel 'guilty' because they infused the Factor VIII that was contaminated [with HIV] and may not be able to take the view that they acted in good faith at that time' (p. 61).

Other studies have illustrated stresses associated with health worker impact that might be expected from the findings discussed from the earlier work stress literature, and that are consistent with the themes in HIV/AIDS work stress already described. For example, a small study by Sherr and George (1989) found that 33 per cent of HIV staff working in a hospital setting found work 'very stressful', and 57 per cent found it more stressful than other areas of health care. However, the stressors cited most frequently included death of a patient, staff shortages, demanding clinical situations, not being appreciated, and having to follow policies one did not agree with. Rugg *et al.* (1989) examined stresses faced by HIV pre-test counsellors in a variety of HIV alternative counselling and testing sites in California. They found that, for those working more than 20 hours per week in the task of pre-test counselling, the relative lack of choice over alternative work options to this led to significantly elevated levels of self-reported stress.

In one of the first studies of occupational stress and 'burnout' in HIV/AIDS staff that employed standardised instruments measuring burnout (i.e., the MBI), Bennett, Michie and Kippax (1991) performed a qualitative and quantitative survey of 32 HIV nurses and 32 oncology nurses in Sydney. They found that the staff–patient ratios and constancy of care with individual patients may directly affect MBI-measured emotional exhaustion in each group. As with the study by Horstman and McKusick (1986), intensity rather than chronicity of HIV patient care appeared to contribute to self-reported morbidity in HIV staff. Inexperience of staff was also found to contribute to the likelihood of self-reported burnout.

Case scenario: How can I keep doing this?

CD was referred by a senior colleague with whom she was doing a training placement. She was 29 years old, a junior medical officer on a clinical training rotation that meant she would be in her current job for about two years. However, after five months CD had gone to her boss and burst into tears, asking 'How can I keep doing this?'. This was the second time she had 'broken down' emotionally in two weeks.

CD had worked previously in the context of chronic disease as a junior member of medical staff. She was known for working hard, being completely professional, being an advocate for her patients and also for junior medical colleagues on hospital and professional committees. She was terrified that if she took time away from work, she would get even further behind in her inherited research activity, and would be adding to the stress of her medical colleagues who would have to cover her absences.

She described feeling increasingly emotional on her current placement, when a number of her patients had started a new drug trial amid high – and publicly announced – hopes for a breakthrough in treatment. From the beginning, some of her patients had been unable to tolerate the drug, and two had experienced temporarily crippling side effects that required immediate cessation and hospitalisation. With other patients, she was bombarded with requests for information, with dilemmas about whether they should start the treatment even though they felt perfectly healthy, and had lifestyles that would be significantly disrupted by undertaking the new regime of therapy. While all this was happening, some of the patients whose care she had taken over became acutely ill and died.

At the time of her interview with the clinical psychologist, CD described bingeing on alcohol and drugs, experiencing major mood swings in a context of underlying depression and agitation. She described feeling like a failure professionally and emotionally, having also separated from her boyfriend of four years some months previously. She also felt that by reacting in the current way she was disappointing her parents who had worked so hard to support her (she was the first member of her family to attend university). In particular, she felt she was unable to answer her patients' questions with any certainty, while at the same time encouraging many to take part in a new programme of intervention that she felt would poison a significant proportion of them. In addition to the pressures she was facing at the time of her referral, she was also questioning whether the constant stress of academic, clinical and other professional burdens was really what she wanted to do.

Over a period of six weekly sessions with the psychologist, CD reviewed her life decisions and career aspirations. She made immediate arrangements to have a work break of two weeks so she could start planning her future in a less reactive manner. She agreed to a short course of antidepressants to assist with her depression, and identified a programme of long-term individual support to help with her decisions about the future. At her last session she reported feeling much better, more stable, and clearer about why she was doing what she did. In particular, she felt that talking to an outsider gave her some distance with which to consider her reactions to her work, and the stress and rewards that went with it.

Van Servellen and Leake (1993) reported that numbers of AIDS patients seen in the previous six months were significantly predictive of MBI-measured emotional exhaustion, and both numbers of patients seen and increases in workload or responsibility were positively related to distress in nurses surveyed.

In a longitudinal study involving a total of 708 health staff from the fields of HIV/AIDS, oncology, and geriatrics, Kleiber *et al.* (1995) examined responses to survey questionnaires incorporating the three subscales of the MBI, and questions relating to social support and coping, at three 11-month intervals. In examining for differential group effects on the MBI subscale scores, *no* effects for occupational groups could be found, although workers in the AIDS field showed significantly *lower* mean scores for emotional exhaustion than workers in the non-AIDS fields. Psychosocial staff in the AIDS field showed relatively higher levels of emotional exhaustion and depersonalisation than those in medical and nursing occupations, while the opposite was found in the fields of cancer care and geriatrics. Workers in the AIDS field were found to experience less time pressure in their work than workers in the other fields, and they also reported greater latitude and autonomy in decision-making – particularly psychosocial as opposed to medical and nursing workers – than oncology and geriatric care staff. Curiously, confrontation with death and dying occurred significantly more often in the fields of geriatrics and cancer care than in the field of AIDS. Certainly the introduction of anti-retroviral regimes involving protease inhibitors and combination therapies has seen drammatic reductions in mortality in some Western cohorts. However, as the case scenario above illustrates, increased stress may be expected in health staff if and when new regimes fail, or side effects and toxicities appear leading to loss of health, or of hope, and/or of confidence and trust in those facilitating access to such regimes (a consistent finding in the context of cancer care) (WHO/UNAIDS meeting on ARV, 1997).

Further, in the study by Kleiber *et al.* (1995), AIDS staff overall reported significantly fewer problems when interacting with clients than workers in the other fields, possibly reflecting closer staff-patient peer identification in long-term cohorts. It is noteworthy that cohorts of staff from developing countries describe increased problems of interacting with patients in social settings of high HIV prevalence, denial, stigma and discrimination (e.g., Kaleeba, Ray and Willmore, 1991; Kalibala, 1995, Baggaley *et al.*, 1996).

In examining the effects of stressors and their mediators/moderators on AIDS and non-AIDS fields, and specifically on interactions with burnout components, Kleiber and colleagues used structural equation modelling techniques contrasting scores over two time periods to identify temporal effects. In HIV/AIDS staff, emotional exhaustion at time 2 was determined by time-1 variables of 'time pressure', 'lack of decision latitude/autonomy', 'problems in interacting with clients', and 'confrontation with death and dying'. Emotional exhaustion thus appeared to be the component of burnout most sensitive to changes. Depersonalisation was found to be caused mainly by 'problems in interacting with clients', while reduced personal accomplishment was best explained by 'knowledge of results' (of medical tests/interventions). Each of these are the findings one might expect given the nature of the MBI constructs, and findings from other, earlier studies in other fields of care (see Chapters 3 and 4).

When contrasting these AIDS-field results with those from the other fields of care, while AIDS staff were confronted with death and dying significantly less often, this appeared to have a stronger impact on emotional exhaustion in them than in staff from the other fields. Further, while problems in interacting with clients led to a significant increase in feelings of personal accomplishment in AIDS staff, it had the opposite effect in geriatric and oncology staff (as one would conventionally expect). The authors concluded that AIDS care problems actually appear to promote a sense of professional identity (AIDS care is considered to be a particularly difficult area of work), by confirming professional identities and esteem.

Stigma, discrimination and ethical issues

One of the features of HIV/AIDS work impact most frequently addressed has been that of social contagion. The threat of HIV transmission, no matter how mis-perceived, and the association of HIV/AIDS care with marginalised and stigmatised social groups, appear to determine the manner in which such work – and the workers doing it – are seen by those around them, occupationally, domestically and recreationally.

In the earliest phase of the HIV pandemic, Reed *et al.* (1984) found that the willingness of nurses to work with AIDS patients was influenced considerably by the level of concern shown by their partners, and in physicians, Bresolin *et al.* (1990) found that 66 per cent of primary care physicians said their family would become concerned if they were to (knowingly) treat more people with HIV. Barbour (1995) found that 41 per cent of HIV health staff in her survey had received negative comments about their HIV-related work – 25 per cent from their families, 12.5 per cent from their own professional peer group, and 9 per cent from friends. The level of adverse comment was even greater if the staff member had opted in to HIV care. Such circumstances have led to nurses denying their work with HIV to those outside the workplace (Blumenfield *et al.*, 1987).

In the UK MOMS study, Miller and Gillies (1996) found that although 53 per cent of their respondents described families' reactions to their work as 'supportive/positive', 19 per cent were 'equivocal/fearful', 15 per cent said their families were 'intolerant' or 'against' their work, and for 13 per cent, the matter was so contentious it could not be discussed with families. Families of HIV/AIDS workers were significantly more likely than those of oncology staff to be 'equivocal/fearful'. Interestingly, HIV/AIDS staff were significantly less likely than oncology staff to avoid discussing their work socially – because they appeared to be significantly more likely to socialise with colleagues. The ethos of HIV/AIDS care, and the apparent reaction to stigmatisation about their work, seemed to lead to a greater staff social cohesion outside the workplace, although this was not necessarily associated with greater trust among colleagues within the workplace (Miller, 1995a).

Negative attitudes may also come from colleagues. Bennett (1992a) described how HIV/AIDS nurses in Sydney experienced negative remarks and discrimination as a result of their work involvement, and Bennett, Michie and Kippax (1991) identified stigma as one of the stress-producing factors of their HIV work. These findings support results found in earlier reports by Pasacreta and Jacobsen (1989), and Fernandez *et al.* (1989).

Social contagion is also seen in the concern of health staff for the impact of known HIV/AIDS work on their own clinical practice. For example, Taylor *et al.* (1990) found that 38 per cent of physicians felt having HIV patients may affect perceptions of their own sexuality, and one-third were concerned about the stigmatising impact of having HIV patients in their practice. A study of physicians by Bredfeldt *et al.* (1991) revealed that 40 per cent were convinced they would lose patients or have problems attracting them, if their work with people with AIDS was known. The notion of presumption about sexuality or even morality following work with people with AIDS has been seen in a comparative study of nursing students in the United States and Zimbabwe (Munodawafa, Bower and Webb, 1993). Some 30 per cent of the US nurses were concerned that people would think they were gay if they acquired HIV/AIDS, while 74 per cent of the Zimbabwean students were worried that people would think they were prostitutes. This correlates with findings from Uganda, where people with AIDS have reportedly been considered 'immoral' because they have AIDS (Ankrah, 1993).

While many such reports are based in evident concern about transmission of HIV through occupational association, reports also suggest that social contagion is also based on prejudice against gay men, sex workers and injecting drug users. Studies of health workers themselves (e.g., Marks *et al.*, 1988; van Servellen, Lewis and Leake, 1988; Hunter and Ross, 1991) reveal significant associations between homophobia and attitudes to people with HIV. The review by Horsman and Sheeran (1995) revealed instances of health staff having homophobic attitudes and an unwillingness to care for people with HIV, a situation shared by injecting drug users. Care refusal rates were found to be highest for IDUs in a national US survey (e.g., Hayward and Shapiro, 1991), and IDUs were ranked 'as bad as prostitutes' in another survey (Breault and Polifroni, 1992), because of their behaviour which was described as 'non-compliant, uncooperative, manipulative and difficult'. Discomfort with management of IDUs has been shown in a recent survey of Italian HIV/AIDS staff (Bellani *et al.*, 1996). The uncritical or naive transfer of care regimes into the HIV sphere from outside it has reportedly led to some agencies having unrealistic expectations (and correspondingly, disappointments and possibly a hardening of attitudes) of change involving IDUs with HIV (Brettle *et al.*, 1994).

The ethical issues raised in the light of such findings are both significant and often directly related to quality of care provided (Gilmore and Somerville, 1995). Is it acceptable that health staff should be able to refuse care to those in need on the basis of their perceptions of self-inflicted maladies, or attitudes and beliefs about lifestyle and sexuality? While examination of these issues is beyond the remit of this book, it is important to recognise the pressures that ethical considerations like this may raise (quite apart from dilemmas about access to restricted treatments, access to toxic regimes, and decisions about when to stop treatment). Reviews by Barbour (1994), Horsman and Sheeran (1995) and Gilmore and Somerville (1995) have raised many instances of health staff being clear in their views that it is not unethical to refuse treatment to people with HIV/AIDS. The bases of such beliefs have led to possible distortions in public health arguments and responses, not least because of political views about the nature of sexuality, and homosexuality in particular, being represented in prevention programmes for school-aged children and young sexually active people. Similar concerns have led to major difficulties in establishment of needle-exchange and related HIV-prevention services for IDUs in the UK and the USA, and to HIV testing regimes that have questionable bases in public health and individual clinical health (Gilmore and Somerville, 1995). In all such instances, the frustrations for HIV/AIDS health staff, and the additional pressure of stigma and discrimination and requirements for justification associated with their work, must be presumed to increase the stress and tension – and propensities towards burnout – in HIV/AIDS workers. For example, Martin (1990) found that 35 per cent of nurses surveyed said they would experience feelings of high stress, and 46 per cent would have feelings of moderate stress, in response to presented ethical scenarios concerning terminally ill patients.

Mediators of HIV/AIDS burnout

Given the fact of stresses associated with HIV/AIDS work, the question then becomes one of why workers respond to them in the ways they do – what is it that makes one worker's stress another worker's satisfaction? Studies examining this issue have done so largely on the basis of cross-sectional surveys that fail to give a clear picture of the *evolution* of staff stress development. However, aside from the issues discussed already that relate to the process and content of HIV/AIDS care, many clues have emerged in relation to gender, age and seniority, and more recently personality. There is also growing recognition of the importance of *context of care* and the *development of new roles* and expectations that go with them, which will be discussed in more detail below.

The critical role of age and experience has already been identified in the context of burnout studies prior to HIV/AIDS (Chapter 4). Youth and inexperience is seen as conferring greater vulnerability in many studies, although not in all: Barbour (1995) found that those health workers with less post-qualification experience were significantly more likely to describe deaths of patients as their most important stressor. Visintini *et al.* (1996), on the other hand, found no association between burnout and age, and only a weak association was found with 'length of work with HIV-infected patients'. Miller, Gillies and Elliott (1996) found no significant association between professional seniority (presumed to increase with age) and self-reported or psychometrically measured stress measures, although the relatively small numbers may have contributed to this finding. The MOMS study (Miller, 1995a – reported more fully in Chapters 7 and 8) found that for health workers in both HIV and oncology, at the 1 per cent level, people *over 30 years of age were more likely* to identify proneness to anger and prejudice in themselves as symptoms of work-related stress, to over-identify with patients' needs, and to know colleagues who had burned out. Those with greater seniority in their professions were more likely to do 11 hours or more overtime per week, to rate their work atmosphere highly, and to feel a higher sense of MBI-measured personal accomplishment. *Junior staff*, on the other hand, were more likely (at the 1 per cent level) to report emotional numbness/indifference as a stress symptom, to find the involvement of patients' loved-ones stressful, to find close relationships with patients problematic, to have problems breaking bad news, to find death and dying stressful, to have difficulty in showing distress about work-related issues, and to have a lower sense of MBI-measured personal accomplishment (see Chapter 7). In a study of Italian HIV/AIDS nurses, Bellani *et al.* (1996) found that younger staff were significantly more burned out on the basis of their MBI scores, but also had higher personal accomplishment.

And the reasons? Bellani *et al.* (1996) have suggested the following:

> '. . . younger workers, because of lack of experience, are more prone than older ones to an excessive job involvement, leading them to 'burnout'. But to be young also entails feeling a greater enthusiasm for one's work, leading to higher job satisfaction'.

Other commentators would also draw attention to younger and less experienced staff having significantly less control over their jobs and the topography of their work tasks (e.g., Maslach and Ozer, 1995). In health care contexts of increasing financial stringency, many health organisations in the UK are requiring staff to go through retrenchment processes that have them re-applying for their present jobs at a lower grade and level of pay. As might be expected, many experienced staff prefer to leave work, and the assault to their vocational committment that such initiatives represent, leaving younger, less experienced staff performing a greater quantity of work at relatively higher levels of complexity and responsibility than might have previously been the case. In addition, the broader health system has been through a process of radical transition, leaving staff of all grades often negotiating new collaborative arrangements as the terminology and topography of their financial and structural arrangements change around them, without their active involvement or assent. The pressures of such a transitional time have been dramatically captured by Halton (1995), whose description of the challenge to skills and to coping strategies perhaps enables a normalisation of the resulting bewilderment that should come as no surprise, as well as the morbidity such madness encourages:

> 'As a result of introducing market forces within the organisation through the purchaser–provider split, professionals are forced into market conflict with each other in relationships dominated by survival-anxiety [that is, self-interest and fear] . . . Whatever the feelings of individual staff, the new structures propel competition forward. Whole institutions compete with each other for survival; clinicians compete with service managers over resources and patient safety; units within hospitals compete; staff compete with each other for their former jobs . . . Clinicians are forced into management functions and budget-holding. Managers are appointed from outside, who have never worked in the disciplines they are organising . . . [However] it is not just the inefficient unit that is closed by market pressure. Successful units, which have engaged fully with the new system, may just as suddenly find themselves surplus to requirement, located in the wrong zone or on the wrong side of government policy. Conversely, market forces, expressed through the decisions of purchasers, may threaten to close inefficient units that it is government policy to keep open. The turmoil of the internal market and the contradictions of the managed market increase as the government tries to implement two self-contradictory policies . . .' (p. 191–2).

Indeed, environmental issues are seen by many contemporary researchers as being responsible for the majority of variance in burnout studies (Kleiber *et al.*, 1995; Miller, 1995a; Bellani *et al.*, 1996; Visintini *et al.*, 1996). The relative absence of gender effects in HIV/AIDS burnout studies also supports this. Accordingly, as indicated in the foregoing discussion, attention in explaining burnout in HIV/ AIDS should be given more to issues of context in care-giving.

The context of caring

It has become clear that HIV/AIDS care does carry many significant burdens. Indeed, studies show that the work environment explains the majority of variance in HIV health worker burnout (Kleiber, Enzmann and Gusy, 1993). As we have seen, increasing numbers of reports describe the psychological toll of working in a context of multiple loss of patients and bereavement within peer groups, of being unable to 'escape' from work, feeling a lack of trust in colleagues, and of finding problems in moving from the supportive role to being supported. Psychological distress may also arise from working within a relatively young staff population, and experiencing a proportionally increasing lack of resources and lack of ability to participate in decision-making about management of individuals or the wider social aspects of epidemic administration. Health workers on lower scales of the career ladder may find themselves trapped in positions with high expectations placed upon them, feeling the weight of *responsibility without sufficient authority* to perform the way they would wish. And always, the pressure to fight against time, political inertia or lassitude, social stigma, media fashion, and sometimes bewildering role expansion follows the daily routine of many HIV/AIDS workers, exerting further expectations on and by HIV/AIDS health workers.

It is also important to recognise that the potential for burnout or occupational stress and morbidity may be an *institutional* experience, as well as an individual one. Barbour (1995) describes difficulties in undertaking general changes on an organisational level from specific to holistic nursing care in managing people with HIV. A review of the stages of response made by the drug abuse treatment system to HIV/AIDS in New York (des Jarlais, 1990) identifies institutional stages of denial, panic and coping as the realities of the HIV pandemic are avoided, recognised and accommodated. However, a potential fourth stage is described as burnout, where perhaps the combined and unremitting imperatives of HIV/AIDS responses, care and management overwhelm services and the personnel within them. The actual experience of the closure of a major peer-led community service for people with AIDS in London, 'Frontliners' (Moreland and Legg, 1991), highlighted the particular vulnerabilities of volunteer and peer-led bodies that struggle to accommodate the burgeoning imperatives and demands placed on them by a grateful public. In many instances it will be community-based, focal programmes that tackle the acute needs of people at risk, perhaps in a manner that is more accessible and even relevant to the needs of those for and by whom they have been developed. However, when the shape of the pandemic changes and responses need to change with them, problems may then arise that can eventually cripple the organisation. This was part of the reason for the closure of Frontliners – the three key factors identified were:

1   The lack of relevant management experience in those leading the organisation.
2   The very rapid expansion of the organisation in response to the demands of members and funders.
3   The transition from self-help (for people with AIDS by people with AIDS) to service provision, undertaken without sufficient research or planning (Moreland and Legg, 1991).

It certainly follows that systems or institutions may look after their own staff by ensuring that they are appropriately equipped with skills and clear roles with which to express them (Kleiber *et al.*, 1992), as well as with support on an emotional and professional level. Those that do so will, it is assumed, be able to provide a better quality of care for people affected by HIV/AIDS over the longer term. However, even that may not be sufficient, particularly where seroprevalence is still relatively **low** (Miller, 1992b; Miller and Gillies, 1993):

- Where there are fewer identified people with HIV stigma may correspondingly be higher.
- Prevention activity may be taking place in a context of indifference.
- There may be a greater tendency to externalise responsibility for HIV prevention and care, making HIV activities undervalued.
- Where responses to HIV identification are infrequent, there may be no clear occupational network or management structure, so professional expectations, roles and boundaries may be unclear.
- Lack of experience may be reflected in a lack of confidence, in a context of insufficient work.
- Where facilities are eager to learn and develop HIV/AIDS expertise, there may be competition for resources, skills and patients.
- Existing professional skills and established procedures are frequently being challenged.
- Every new case may be seen as a crisis.

As for the difficulties associated with role expansion and ambiguity, the discussion of the development of counselling (below) is a case in point. It may also be the case that the increasingly reported issue of difficulties with colleagues reflects the tensions of role overlap, as has been noted in qualitative studies of multi-disciplinary HIV/AIDS care (e.g., Barbour, 1995) in which professional rivalries and boundary-testing emerge. Research reports from the MOMS study in England (Miller and Gillies, 1993; Miller, 1995a, 1996) have identified how professional rivalry and mistrust can lead to serious problems in burnout prevention, as colleagues fear disclosing personal vulnerability to each other.

Context matters – the pressures of HIV/AIDS counselling

The difficulties of innovation when responding to a major new health threat, particularly in contexts of political denial and imperfect technical and clinical understanding, have been well-rehearsed in HIV/AIDS. Furthermore, health care workers in the HIV/AIDS field, particularly in the first few years of the epidemic, have experienced often unavoidable role expansion as the novel pressures of their work have demanded unprecedented and sometimes acute advocacy, media participation, involvement in health policy formation and teaching of colleagues (Miller and Brown, 1988). Role expansion and the development of new professional responsibilities have been seen particularly in the case of HIV/AIDS counselling.

Counselling was almost unheard of as a cornerstone approach to public health management in *any* field prior to the emergence of HIV/AIDS. Yet, particularly in the earliest years of the unfolding pandemic in most countries, the absence or inaccessability of viable interventions for treatment, and for prevention – both often based on governmental denial – and the shock of diagnosis and recognition of the social impact of HIV diagnoses, had many groups of those most directly affected (patients and their loved-ones) clamouring for psychosocial support and developing support groups, models of which became refined into contemporary approaches to HIV/AIDS counselling (Carballo and Miller, 1990; Miller *et al.*, 1999).

As global responses to HIV coalesced through the World Health Organization's Global Programme on AIDS, counselling became established as an early part of the foundation response at country levels. Soon, training followed as National AIDS Programmes quickly responded to imperatives for action. However, difficulties in implementing such a novel response to HIV management and control soon emerged, with very serious consequences for those most directly involved – that is, for those trained to counsel and charged with implementing what they knew.

Difficulties in HIV/AIDS counselling implementation had previously been summarised by Carballo and Miller (1990):

- *Lack of prior definition* and characterisation of counselling, resulting in often *ad hoc* and non-integrated service provision.
- The absence of a clear *professional identity* and structure for counsellors, making training and organisation of counsellors problematic.
- Absence of clear *policies* on the content and provision of counselling.
- Dilemmas in meeting the needs for *confidentiality* in counselling.
- Few opportunities to assess systematically counselling *efficacy* in prevention and psychosocial impact reduction.
- Lack of awareness of resources required in counselling *development*.
- Lack of awareness of needs, personnel, and authority in counselling *staffing*.

Additionally, Miller (1989) identified additional constraints and challenges to counselling implementation in developing and developed countries, such as: mobility of target groups being counselled; ensuring adequate funding; developing services that appear attractive, relevant and accessible; overcoming staff fears and negative attitudes towards those they counsel; staff exhaustion and burnout. Additionally, inter-country and national HIV/AIDS counselling training activities did not give additional status to health workers doing it, did not lead to substantive posts or even job descriptions that included acknowledgement of the extra work – and stresses – involved, and counselling was usually under the control of the health worker in charge – not those actually counselling patients (Osborne, van Praag and Jackson, 1997). These all combined to create a vicious circle that in many countries actually maintained a lack of professional coherence and professional identity where counselling was being implemented (Figure 5.1). This circle had the capacity to waste significant amounts of national effort in settings where counselling training was required for health staff who would then emerge from training with commitment and enthusiasm, only to find they had insufficient authority to implement services they now felt responsible for – an ideal basis for generating frustration, hopelessness and burnout (Bennett, Miller, Ross, 1995; Kalibala, 1995).

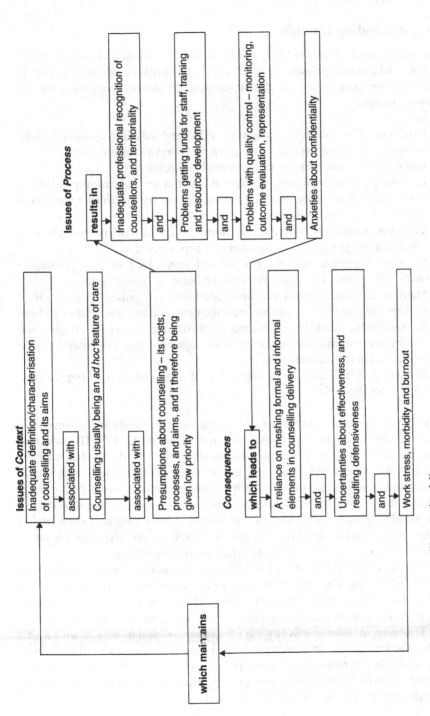

Figure 5.1 Problems in counselling service delivery.
Source: Miller, 1989.

Issues of *Process*

results in

Inadequate professional recognition of counsellors, and territoriality

and

Problems getting funds for staff, training and resource development

and

Problems with quality control – monitoring, outcome evaluation, representation

and

Anxieties about confidentiality

Issues of *Context*

Inadequate definition/characterisation of counselling and its aims

associated with

Counselling usually being an *ad hoc* feature of care

associated with

Presumptions about counselling – its costs, processes, and aims, and it therefore being given low priority

Consequences

which leads to

A reliance on meshing formal and informal elements in counselling delivery

and

Uncertainties about effectiveness, and resulting defensiveness

and

Work stress, morbidity and burnout

which maintains

Some concluding thoughts

As noted in recent reviews (Miller, 1992b; Mann, Tarantola and Netter, 1992), the potential for occupational stress in HIV care workers can be expected to *increase* in the near future, in developed and developing countries, for the following reasons:

- Numbers of people with recognised HIV and AIDS are rising rapidly, mortality in many areas is more frequent and overwork is increasing.
- Resources in many areas are proportionally decreasing.
- In many parts of the world, whole communities are increasingly becoming implicated – there is less possibility in such places for health care workers to find distance from the disease.
- Patient presenting characteristics are altering – the 'patient' increasingly is the whole family, groups and communities of orphans, etc.
- Many management uncertainties remain unresolved or are growing – treatment options, care capacity, resource-building capacity, etc.
- Many overt psychological pressures are being recognised increasingly as evident and important in care and management, and in communities without the specialised resources to manage such manifestations (although community mechanisms for psychosocial management and care may be well-established in related contexts).
- Many HIV/AIDS carers are complaining of stress and recognising the need for care for themselves.

It is clear that there are many reasons for predicting the possibility of burnout in populations of health care workers working in the context of HIV/AIDS, and that many of these relate to the psychosocial context in which the disease has emerged and taken hold since 1981. The pressures attendant on those designing, implementing and maintaining care seem likely to only become greater in future years. Thus, the need to be able to characterise work pressures and burnout responses in these populations *now* is considerable – quality of care for patients means having quality staff, and achieving this also requires a burden of care that administrators and organisations appear to have been reluctant to acknowledge.

Of course, HIV/AIDS is still a young field. But in many ways, this adds to the need to know what is happening in terms of impact of work on staff, and if this field can be a laboratory for characterisation and development of burnout and its prevention for areas of health care with similar characteristics – such as oncology care. However, in order to ensure we get the best possible data we can with which to plan the best prevention strategies, it is important to consider the methodological pitfalls that research to date has failed to avoid. Thus, the next chapter will describe methodological issues and give possible suggestions for improving research designs to boost their utility.

6 Methodological limitations and issues raised in burnout research to date

Burnout research – whether in the context of HIV/AIDS or in other fields of health care – has some notable limitations. While all research has limitations, not least when enquiry associated with relatively new concepts and constructs is ploughing the virgin fields of empiricism, it is useful to be aware of what can be done to improve the quality of data. This will hopefully lead to more relevant information for management and prevention of burnout in HIV/AIDS, and in other fields of health care. Accordingly, this brief review will highlight some of the suggestions that have emerged from research and commentaries to date.

Limitations of questionnaire-only studies

From the literature on occupational morbidity and burnout, and reviews made to date (e.g., Maslach and Jackson, 1982; Perlman and Hartman, 1982; Miller, 1991; Cordes and Dougherty, 1993), at least two *procedural* issues emerge consistently:

1 The overwhelming majority of surveys involve only the administration of self-report, self-administered (and often postal) questionnaires.
2 Reporting of burnout-associated or morbidity-associated stressors has been predetermined by the researchers requiring respondents to identify such stressors from a predetermined list or by using instruments that identify only those features that bolster the constructs upon which the instrument is based (Handy, 1988; Miller, 1993).

Both of these may work to limit observable detail that may shed light on under-lying issues possibly fuelling the development and eventual recognition of chronic occupational morbidity. In her qualitative survey of Scottish HIV/AIDS health workers, Barbour (1995) makes the ringing point that:

'Scant attention . . . has been paid to *contextualising* AIDS-related work. Much of the research to date . . . has assumed that the demands of AIDS-related work are self-evident and unique to this field of work. In order adequately to understand the experiences and responses of staff we need to know a great deal more about their expectations of AIDS work, their level of preparedness, and the ways in which the perceived demands of AIDS-related work interact with requirements of individuals in their parallel roles as citizens and family members. Workers' experiences must be studied with reference to:

- The work setting.
- The pattern of epidemic spread.
- Client group/s involved.
- Nature and content of services.
- Division of professional responsibilities.
- Professional background and training of staff.
- Previous work experience.
- Staff's career plans and interests.
- Routes into AIDS-related work.
- Social and family circumstances of staff.' (p. 522)

The point is well-made, particularly given the evidence so far for differential responses to stress according to HIV/AIDS service, profession, levels of training, family and marital status, and so on. Roth (1995) would extend the variables of interest further to include the social, structural characteristics central to the individual staff members's sense of self-identity, and their sense of place in their social, domestic and professional communities.

This point also has particular relevance for planning of burnout management and prevention – as Chapters 8 and 10 indicate, targeting staff support to the *specific* needs of particular staff groups is critical in ensuring their success. These needs cannot be specified without having a detailed apreciation of the work contexts in which they arise. Such appreciation is not something that emerges from examination of grouped scores from standardised psychometric scales. Standardised psychometric instruments need to be complemented with qualitative *observational and interview* data.

In reviewing the methodologies of life-event studies in persons with psychiatric illness, Paykel (1983) concluded:

'. . . when careful interviews are carried out, reliable and valid data are obtained. Methods which are intermediate between interview and self-report produce intermediate results. When self-report checklists are used, there are serious deficiencies in data collection. Future studies will need to concentrate on interview methods' (p. 347).

Interviews also offer the potential to describe more precisely or even *explain* the process of response to individually experienced occupational stressors. Questionnaires may not adequately identify the *meaning* attached to concepts identified by respondents (Gillies, 1991), in the way that an interview allows by following the path that the respondent selects in answering structured questions. For example,

Leiter (1990) has suggested that 'burnout' is a social phenomenon, with responses to occupational stressors probably being a function of particular relationship dynamics associated with specific institutions. Interviewing about such issues most likely enables more relevant data to be gleaned while also saving time, as Gillies (1991) has concluded:

'By interviewing, an awareness of the seemingly nebulous aspects of some behavioural problems can be gained. Inconsistencies in attitudes and opinions are more apparent, and the value of particular social relationships connected with the behaviour and how they operate are more easily identified'.

In an earlier review relating to HIV/AIDS carers, Miller (1991) argued that a sole reliance on standardised psychometric survey methodologies led the risk of missing the often meaningful, subclinical psychological morbidity that can come to define the perspective of the health worker, even if distress never rises to levels that might cause breakdown of functioning, or be revealed as extreme subscale scores on the MBI.

Limitations of cross-sectional studies

A related limitation is that of the cross-sectional study. Although much of the published research in this field reveals correlations between stress and specific characteristics of the health workers involved, there is much yet to learn about why these results emerge – something only longitudinal qualitative and quantitative studies could reveal (Schaufeli, Maslach and Marek, 1993). Indeed, Leiter (1993) has gone further:

'. . . the viability of burnout as a research area depends on a thorough understanding of the full range of experiences assessed in burnout studies. This goal will be facilitated by the development of models that articulate the relationships among components of burnout and their relationships with organisational and personal conditions'(p. 238).

There have been relatively few studies of this type in the HIV/AIDS literature, those of Bennett (1992b), Kleiber, Enzmann and Gusy (1995), and Miller, Gillies and Elliott (1996) being among the notable exceptions.[The study by Kleiber, Enzmann and Gusy (1995) was not qualitative in the sense that it was supplemented by interview methods.] Also, where such studies have been undertaken, they rarely last beyond six months (a point shared in research on the impact of educational interventions for HIV/AIDS workers) (Horsman and Sheeran, 1995). Studies in other fields of health care employing psychometric and interview data over periods of five to ten years have shown the value of longitudinal approaches by, for example, identifying periods in medical staffs' training that render them vulnerable to psychological vulnerability, despite the added expense of such methodologies (e.g., Baldwin, Dodd and Wrate, 1997).

Potential bias of burnout research volunteers

One issue that has been neglected in studies to date is the self-selection of staff for arduous occupations or specialisms, and the significance of this for proneness or vulnerability to burnout. As we have seen in studies of HIV/AIDS health workers, some health staff may identify closely with groups identified as being at greater risk for HIV/AIDS transmission. This identification and commitment may contribute significantly to structural and contextual stressors, including interpersonal relationships, processes of accountability, and numbers of staff involved and issues raised in care, which in turn lead to psychological and occupational morbidity in themselves, their colleagues and their non-work relationships.

It may certainly have an impact on the quality of information received from studies in which respondents are study volunteers, opting in to a discussion of why their work is stressful. The use of volunteers in surveys of stress is problematic for interpretation and generalisability of findings. Barbour (1994) noted that about one-quarter of studies on health workers impact of HIV/AIDS care showing their response rates achieved rates of 50 per cent or less, and just less than half had 60 per cent or less response rates. In an early report from the UK MOMS study, Miller (1995) noted

'Put most simply, we must ask if those who volunteer to participate in research on work stress do so because they are more stressed, and/or possess a desire to complain about their working circumstances, and therefore we must question if their responses are truly representative of the populations eligible for participation'(p. 219).

Miller (1995a) examined for possible biases by sending short, self-report postal questionnaires to non-volunteers in the fields of HIV/AIDS and oncology using questions with high face validity replicated from the structured interview schedule employed in interviews with volunteer participants. Overall, statistically significant differences were found between volunteers and non-volunteer populations. A greater proportion of volunteers found their work stressful, non-volunteers saying their work was only 'sometimes' stressful ($P = <0.001$). The same result was seen for current experiences of work-related stress – volunteers were currently stressed by work. Significant differences were found with regard to time available to do work properly – the majority of non-volunteers said they did have enough time, whereas volunteers said they did not ($P = 0.009$). HIV/AIDS non-volunteers identified fewer frustrations in their work activities related to clinical autonomy, clinical decision-making, and relationships with senior colleagues ($P = 0.001$), and both HIV/AIDS and oncology study non-volunteers were more likely to be physicians and not paramedical or nursing staff ($P = 0.03$ for HIV/AIDS; $P = 0.02$ for oncology). The conclusion is that in this case, study volunteers were different, and the generalisability of results must be more cautiously considered as a result.

Barbour (1994) also notes that many UK studies, particularly with regard to health workers attitudes and beliefs about HIV/AIDS care, had been undertaken *before* they were exposed to HIV-infected patients! Clearly, levels of actual experience need to be quantified and cut-offs need to be applied before staff can be admitted to studies that reflect their presumed responses to that work.

Problems with interpreting burnout measures

Self-report measures are the predominant forms in use in the literature, and they frequently have a negative loading in items, so only the negative or destructive aspects of work are assessed (Kahill, 1988). A wider range of items and a use of different measures may help to strengthen validity, and therefore the predictive value and generalisability of research in which such instruments are used. A good example of an instrument employing a broader scope for HIV/AIDS impact measurement is the AIDS Impact Scale (Bennett, Kelaher and Ross, 1994), which identifies both the burdens and rewards of HIV/AIDS care through its five scale factors (see Chapters 4 and 5).

This also highlights the value of corroborative approaches, such as structured interviewing, in research of this type, particularly where staff are being asked to define their own stressors. In particular, the possibility of social desirability influencing the answers to self-report instruments has been implicated in research by Ursprung (1986), leading to calls for the use of behavioural correlates in measuring workers' adaptation to work stress, such as third-party ratings by colleagues or supervisors. Jackson and Maslach's (1982) study of police officers and their spouses, and Cherniss's (1992) study involving interviews of confidantes of study subjects, are rare though important examples of verification applied beyond the immediate work environment.

As many burnout studies employ different measures, it is difficult to know if each study is measuring the same thing. As van Servellen and Leake (1993) noted, summarising results of earlier studies is difficult because the measures of job-related stress and burnout employed are often very different, and predictors of burnout, e.g., head nurse leadership style, longer hours/shorter work week, life events/unit stressors, social support, coping, noise, and hardiness, are often idiosyncratic to the studies reporting them. Also, many studies do not have comparison groups, and their results are often inconclusive, making meaningful generalizations difficult or impossible. A further problem with many of the studies cited – particularly in the HIV/AIDS stress and burnout literature – is that sample sizes are often too small to achieve powerful measures of significance. Instruments employed in the literature include self-report questionnaires, and 'open-ended' structured interviews, yet these are frequently not specified (e.g., as in Stewart *et al.*, 1982; Horstman and McKusick, 1986; Trieber *et al.*, 1987; Ross and Seeger, 1988). Similarly, where such measures are specified – whether for measuring stress or burnout – there is often no information on the validity or reliability of the instruments used, and frequently no discussion of sample selection or response rate. Comparisons between studies and meaningful conclusions are thus impossible.

Wallace and Brinkerhoff (1991) reccommend that we beware of interpreting the MBI too literally. They note the MBI subscale of depersonalisation may in fact reflect a coping technique, like 'detatched concern' (Pines and Maslach, 1978) for some, and be a symptom of burnout for others. It was found to be equally associated with both high and low levels of the same variable (work-related stress). Thus, a fundamental dimension of burnout may also be a technique used in attempting to combat it. It is also the case that workers may feel a low sense of personal accomplishment and not be suffering from burnout – work may simply fail to provide a sense of competence and accomplishment and yet not be especially stressful or related to the occurrence of burnout.

Aggregated norms on the MBI may obscure the real clinical and subjective experiences that coalesce to generate the burnout experience. For example, Rogers and Dodson (1987) found this with occupational therapists scoring significantly lower overall than the norms for health workers would lead one to otherwise expect. Additionally, Arthur (1990) argues that the arbitary use of cut-off points on the MBI subscales produces little insight into the factors that take a professional from a 'low-risk' to a 'high-risk' category for burnout. This point has been echoed by Leiter (1991), who questions the clinical basis for the use of present cut-off points in MBI scoring. Pines, Aronson and Kafry (1981) have suggested comparing individual scores with median scores by profession as an alternative – this may provide a more accurate picture of the degree of MBI burnout experienced by individuals.

Additionally, while many studies use the Maslach Burnout Inventory (MBI) (Maslach and Jackson, 1982) as a basis for identifying potential or actual burnout in health, educational and industrial workers, deriving a score relative to norms with such an instrument may *not* be the same as identifying real or potential burnout. Certainly, the process of identifying a clinical syndrome based on the application of questionnaire-based methodologies has been seriously questioned in this and other arenas (Miller, 1993), and it seems important to at least compare MBI subscale scores with scores on reliable and valid clinical mood scales, such as the General Health Questionnaire (Goldberg, 1981), if only in order to assess the degree to which the two compare.

A related point is the need for a clearer notion of criterion levels for burnout, not least because the jury seems still to be out on whether burnout really matters in the long term:

'In other words, it has not been shown conclusively that burnout is causally related to objective outcomes of consequence and importance. Thus, another task for researchers is to provide empirical evidence for the seriousness of burnout as a social problem.' (Schaufeli, Maslach and Marek, 1993, p. 258)

The necessity for clear characterisations and appropriate measures

One way to be clear about what is being measured – and to have confidence in the results – is to ensure there has been an adequate characterisation of the needs for support and/or prevention, and a clear idea of what the staff themselves want from an intervention. This emphasises the need for consultation with staffs of individual facilities to ensure that intervention packages reflect what is wanted and needed by the staffs and the organisations to whom they are directed. The UK burnout and prevention studies described in Chapters 7 and 8 show the feasibility of doing so. Specifically, before starting on any burnout prevention strategy, we need to have a focus on the information that can both: (a) inform the implementation of staff support (the organisational dynamics, contextual structural and procedural issues, foci of stress, etc.), and (b) enable evaluation of outcomes (both organisational and staff elements such as absenteeism, turnover, mood, quality of relationships and social support, etc.).

For coping with the development of HIV/AIDS care in the context of a San Francisco Drug Abuse Treatment Programme, Sorensen, Constantini and London (1989) first examined the problem areas for staff, and then intervened accordingly. For *fears of infection*, they suggested developing very clear infection control guidelines, universal precautions being adopted, and regular staff seminars reviewing and updating such issues. They described the use of 'process group support sessions' having 'mixed success' (no further details were given). In managing *confidentiality*, dilemmas over appropriate limits of information management and confidentiality (e.g., associated with partner notification) were addressed by regular staff seminars and updates on confidentiality laws and guidelines, frequently with visiting experts and close liaison with companion HIV/AIDS and legal services. Recognition of and adherence to *appropriate treatment goals* was facilitated by the development of a distinct clinic treatment philosophy featuring 'low threshold treatment' to ensure wider service coverage and use by its targetted consumers. The specific clinical needs of workers managing HIV patients were also addressed by service management, including a lowering of counsellor caseloads and provision of on-going education where required. Finally, *recognising the limits of treatment* was facilitated by staff training on recognising the signs of burnout and development of staff self-care plans, including aerobic exercise, a nutritional diet, opportunities for rest and recreation, sufficient periods of unstructured time, hobbies, time-management techniques, and nurturing friendships and family relationships.

Measuring levels of organisational and staff morbidity have been turned into substantial industries in non-health occupational settings. While it is easy in some contexts to become cynical about the reasons for this (see Briner, 1997, for a trenchant review), the appropriateness of baseline and replicable measurement is beyond doubt – as long as the appropriate things are being measured. In the UK Burnout Prevention study (Chapter 8), longitudinal measures were taken of mood (GHQ-28), and burnout (MBI). Additionally, staff were asked to identify their work stressors, and the answers were subjected to content analysis and clustering. The structured interview schedule provided quantifiable qualitative information on staff demographics, experiences of and approaches to stress management, perceptions of the nature, appropriateness of, and satisfaction with staff support activities, and preferences for change. Individual health indices, including stress-related behaviours common in studies of this type included, smoking, alcohol consumption, use of recreational and prescription drugs, and other 'leisure' pursuits (the MOMS study included the opportunity to reveal frequency of high-risk sex). The wider-ranging MOMS study also considered subjectively rated quality of work tasks, work environment, staff–staff and staff–patient relationships, motivations for HIV/AIDS (and oncology) work, the best and the most difficult parts of work, reasons for absence, and so on (see Chapter 7). As the methodological discussion in Chapter 7 shows, despite the interview schedule being non-standardised, it was possible to include measures of both reliability and validity into the interview process, both of which yielded meaningful results (Miller, 1995a).

Briner's (1997) analysis suggests dividing information-gathering into three distinct but related groups:

1   Well-being
2   Work conditions
3   Stress responses

Each of these will have both subjective and objective data – both of which are valuable and ascribable to organisations and individuals and teams within them. The useful thing about this tryptich is that each of the categories provides opportunities for measurement, they can change in positive and negative directions, and they all have usable indices that can be used before and after supportive interventions have been put in place.

Well-being

As the MOMS and UK Prevention studies show, subjective assessment of well-being (and responses to stressful work conditions) are easy to undertake with informed questions of high face validity. Objective ratings may be more difficult, although some of the earliest research by Jackson and Maslach (1982) used ratings by spouses of police officers alongside MBI measures of each to determine levels of work stress and adjustment. Cherniss (1992) also employed interviews of confidantes of staff to validate staffs' descriptions of their responses to work stress. Other indicators of routine functioning (e.g., self-care, satisfaction with life, and with work life) may also be employed, alongside ratings by colleagues. Cooper and Cartwright (1994) argue for the application of stress audits, sampling different jobs, departments, and sections of the workforce, using increasingly well-standardised psychometric instruments such as the Occupational Stress Indicator (OSI) (Cooper, Sloan and Williams, 1988). Such instruments enable repeated measures on key indices of occupational well-being and functioning. Other psychometric measures that are not frequently reported in this context, but which would be useful in particular circumstances, include alternative measures of mood, for example the Hospital Anxiety and Depression (HAD) scale, as well as scales measuring locus of control, quality of life, satisfaction with life, adjustment to HIV/AIDS work (i.e., the AIDS Impact Scale; Bennett, Kelaher and Ross, 1994) and level of social connectedness or interaction.

Work conditions

Again, while subjective assessments of work conditions are relatively straight-forward, they also have familiar limitations – they may be influenced by non-work issues or conditions (e.g., Spector, 1992), by mood states (e.g., Salovey *et al.*, 1991), and by individual differences (e.g., Burke, Brief and George, 1993). On the other hand, objective measures can be a vital supplement – for example, use of office space, use of facilities (e.g., pressure on key technology or supplies), frequency, duration and focus of staff disputes, frequency and nature of complaints by service users, ratios of permanent to agency staff, numbers of relapses – and of deaths – of service users, levels of measured productivity, ward atmosphere scales, etc.

Stress responses

As for the previous two areas of measurement, in charting stress responses, subjective indices may be gleaned relatively straightforwardly from staff interviews. These may include staff in post, as well as staff who are leaving ('exit interviews' – as has been used successfully in charting HIV risk behaviour in prisons), or who have left. Aside from subjective, self-report statements about stress and its causes, objective indices of response to chronic and acute work stresses may include levels of absence and certified sickness, staff turnover, numbers of disciplinary hearings, reductions in job performance, costs incurred for support, and for covering staff shortages due to absence. Further indicators of staff satisfaction – in repeated measure designs – could include use of compassionate leave, demand for use of staff support (where such support is already available), attendance, content, and staff satisfaction with it, and quality of care as measures by, for example, patient satisfaction and quality of life measures.

A problem in the majority of outcome studies is the difficulty with identifying causality, and the true nature of relationships between inferred stressors and inferred responses to them. For this reason, *longitudinal studies* are necessary if we are to have reliable data that will be useful and practically transferrable in staff support designs. Again, Briner (1997) and his colleagues have some useful ideas:

- Charting naturally occurring experiments, where assessments are made over the cycle of natural or imposed fluctuations in objective job characteristics, such as integration of new treatment approaches, staff reductions, changes of work premises, etc.
- Completing baseline assessments, then implementing tailored interventions, then repeating baseline measures to ascertain levels of change.
- Having staff complete qualitative daily diaries that include self-reports of well-being and work conditions and experiences, in addition to the objective

assessments of working conditions associated with 'natural' or tailored interventions. Frost *et al.* (1991) describe using diaries in the context of a staff support group, both for personal reflection and for evaluating the content of groups). An ethnographic approach was used successfully over time to assess qualitative features of response to burnout prevention by 'survival bonding' in HIV/AIDS health workers (Wade and Perlman Simon, 1993).

The important corollary to implementing any such form(s) of data-gathering is that they be applied *systematically*. The MOMS study revealed the surprising, though reportedly common (Briner, 1998), lack of systematic data-gathering on even basic staff-related indices by hospital personnel departments – such as recording routine sickness absence!.

Recognising that HIV/AIDS is new

Despite the growth of studies focusing on health worker impact of HIV/AIDS, this is still a relatively new area in which the need for clear characterisation of stresses faced by staff remains, particularly in under-researched HIV/AIDS care environments – for example, in developing country settings where specifics of care and intervention may be very different to those found in Western/Northern contexts (Kalibala, 1995; Osborne, Van Praag and Jackson, 1997). As such, it is not clear if findings from other areas of medicine can be generalised to HIV/AIDS work. Indeed, it seems more likely at present that HIV/AIDS will be the vehicle for developing awareness and insight about burnout management and prevention in health care generally (Mann, 1995). Be that as it may, reliance on findings from standardised instruments developed for use in Western/Northern general medical and other settings may not reveal the full spectrum of issues relevant to the development, maintenance and amelioration of morbidity in HIV/AIDS health staff in other cultures. Even if they do, this needs to be further verified. As noted above, the use of structured interview schedules to accompany administration of standardised instruments (and other means of establishing reliability and validity of responses, such as analysis of personnel and general practice records) therefore seems appropriate.

How has previous work informed interventions

Information on implementation of support programmes for health staff is relatively rare in comparison to the amount of literature to date characterising stresses faced by this workforce. In the context of HIV/AIDS, interventions are presented predominantly as forms of information provision designed to reduce staffs' anxieties about working in this setting (Brimlow, 1995). Despite this, as Horsman and Sheeran (1995) and Schaufeli, Maslach and Marek (1993) have noted, there are few if any studies which measure actual changes in behaviour arising from educational initiatives. Additionally, as the paradoxes outlined in

Chapter 10 suggest, the fit between previous research findings on staff stress and subsequent interventions usually has been suboptimal.

A further point is the rarity of studies published to date in which the people for whom staff support has been designed or implemented have actually been consulted about what forms of intervention they would prefer (e.g., Shinn *et al.*, 1984; Horstman and McKusick, 1986; Bennett, 1992a; Miller, 1995a). As conditions under which work stress and burnout occur may vary according to organisational and national culture (Roth, 1995), it is important to determine the conditions under which staff would most use the support on offer – to identify the characteristics that would lead to the greatest cost-benefit being achieved.

Letting staff define their stressors

Much more work is necessary to develop methods for defining and measuring subject-defined stressors and consequences in this field (Bennett and Kelaher, 1993), particularly as the true scale and severity of responses to occupational stresses needs clarification (Miller, 1991), perhaps because 'notions of stress in the workplace are still often conceptually confused, and do not readily read across to concepts of illness' (Jenkins, 1993, p. 66). Jenkins (1993) has highlighted the remarkable and evident lack of epidemiological evidence on the psychiatric status of health professions in the UK, and Schaufeli, Enzmann and Girault (1993) have similarly noted

> '. . . the great need for epidemiological knowledge of burnout in order to identify specific (sub)groups at risk. For instance, virtually no studies exist that provide the sort of information that would be necessary for planning appropriate interventions' (p. 214).

The true nature of identified occupational stress cannot therefore be placed in a clear context in health work, although estimates of costs for long-term (i.e., certified) sickness absence in the UK associated with anxiety and depression have been made in the region of two billion pounds annually! (Banham, 1992). The same review reported that 30 times as many working days are lost through stress and mental illness than through industrial disputes (Jenkins, 1993). Nevertheless, it may be the case that burnout syndromes defined earlier are extreme manifestations only, and therefore much less prevalent, for example, than chronic subclinical psychological morbidity occasioned by unremitting anxieties and frustrations associated with the changing structures and delivery of contemporary health care in the UK (Miller, 1993).

For these reasons, there should be a conscious attempt to allow subjects to explicate their own perceptions of the stressors they have identified within – and as a consequence of working in – their workplaces. Research to date has imposed stress lists on subjects, perhaps limiting choices and thus understanding of stressors experienced. Attention needs to be increased, if not initiated, on the experiences of those who have actually been through severe work stress and/or burnout. A sound clinical maxim is this: 'If you want to know what's wrong, ask the patient'. If the staff member (or ex-staff-member) has been 'the patient', we could be wasting valuable experiential information about symptoms, causes, and *processes* of burnout that clinical and academic researchers have hitherto reported on the basis of those with on-going experience (and hence those skilled at adaptation and surviving).

An important corollary to this is the need also to allow staff to state their vocational values, and expectations of their work and role, so that the levels of 'fit' with organisational imperatives can be assessed more precisely. This issue may explain the differences in response to organisational and role variables found in some surveys of nurses versus physicians, and paid staff versus volunteer staff, in HIV/AIDS burnout research (e.g., Miller, 1995a). Professional values may also have a direct bearing on the way we can appropriately interpret 'depersonalisation' in observed work stress responses.

In addition, it has become clear that we need to expand the range of staff groups consulted and recruited in the context of stress and burnout studies (Barbour, 1995; Horsman and Sheeran, 1995). Hitherto neglected staff groups, such as porters and housekeeping staff, and staff working in community settings perhaps single-handedly, will also have their own perceptions of risk, of need and of support. For example, Barbour (1995) found that ancillary staff were the staff group most likely to consider that AIDS work made unique demands on them, particularly as their jobs may carry very high but unrecognised levels of patient (and patient family) contact. By including such groups, organisational perspectives on the impact of HIV care will be more thorough and findings more relevant.

It is also evident that more attention needs to be given to staff responses to work with increasing varieties of communities directly affected by HIV/AIDS, such as IDUs, sex workers, women, children, and families, of all cultures and socioeconomic levels.

Relationships and communication

Given the acknowledged issues regarding interpersonal communication and relationships, and the development of work stress, this area of work needs far more precise explication than the glib generalising that has been a hallmark of reports to date. Communication includes the quality and content of communication with supervisors, bosses, managers, colleagues and junior colleagues. Communication links directly with notions of self-esteem and perceptions of value within an organisation, and the sense of initiative and creative flexibility available to the individual worker. Group processes also therefore become a critical aspect of future burnout research, rather than an inferential variable.

Linked to these crucial issues is the notion of how work is communicated externally, and the degree to which public or community perceptions of HIV/AIDS work are mediated by stigma. Greater stigma will presumably lead to greater discriminatory practice against people with HIV, and also against their carers. In this regard, if identified capacity for communication does not equal the demonstrated need for it, additional work pressures will emerge as a fruitful ground for additional research.

Demographic and other information

As the foregoing discussion has identified, while demograpic variables are routinely examined, they are given no emphasis in burnout studies. It is important that standardised and non-standardised measures are cross-tabulated against gender, age, professional group, length of time since qualifying, length of time in current position, and seniority (rank), to see if they influence the nature of peoples' experiences of work stress and burnout, and their preferences for prevention of burnout. Not doing so materially inhibits the generalisability of study findings, not least in the design of appropriate prevention activities.

A continuing grey area in burnout research is the issue of personality and its link to work stress responses. While personality research is seriously controversial in many ways, the ubiquity of occupational personality profiles and assessments suggests that substantial normative data could be used very constructively in predicting and preventing burnout in individual workers and groups.

Additionally, very little is known as yet about the impact of work on non-work lives and relationships, particularly in the context of HIV/AIDS. Until the scale of impact external to the workplace is appreciated, the appropriateness of the content of prevention strategies can never be certainly known. Research in the non-HIV/AIDS arena points to the potentially buffering effects on work stress of marriage and having children, and expanding enquiry to this arena would help to broaden notions of self-efficacy and social support, while clarifying their relevance for management.

Characterising staffs' perceptions of available support, both inside and outside the workplace, is a critical element in determining their actual quality of response to work stress and burnout, and this has not adequately been done to date. Identifying how they use what they have – both positively and negatively (e.g., drug and alcohol use) – will also help in the design and tailoring of prevention approaches.

And, of course, models of work stress and burnout management and prevention are urgently needed against which to assess outcomes. Miller's First Law states, 'The value of a good idea is in direct proportion to the ease with which it can be expressed'. If we do not express and test available (and successful) models of care for staff, based on what we increasingly know of work stress and its management in this large and tragically mushrooming arena, then our work ultimately has no value.

Conclusions

These issues really determine the 'next step' of development in quality research on HIV/AIDS burnout, and it was in the light of this analysis that two national, multi-centre studies were initiated in England in the mid-1990s. While neither satisfies all the suggestions made above, they were the first substantial studies of this type in this field in the UK, and attempted to provide a comprehensive start in doing so. The first study to be described (Chapter 7) is the 'UK Multi-centre Occupational Morbidity Study' (MOMS); the second (Chapter 8) is the study entitled 'Prevention of Occupational Morbidity and Burnout in Management of HIV Infection and Disease'.

7 The UK Multi-centre Occupational Morbidity Study (MOMS)

Experiences and independent predictors of workplace stress and burnout

Aims and objectives

As the previous chapters have shown, the issue of occupational morbidity and burnout is an important health care issue, and seems to be of considerable relevance to workers in the field of HIV/AIDS. Health care in HIV/AIDS embodies particular features of management and service provision which encourage expectations that burnout may be a significant problem. However, research and understanding of staff stress and burnout issues in the field of HIV/AIDS is at an early stage, and more opportunities are needed to explore staffs' own perceptions of how they may best be helped in avoiding or managing work stress and burnout. In addition, comparative studies of staff populations in HIV/AIDS and e.g., oncology, are important because we need to know if HIV/AIDS is 'special' or embodies particular and unique features – this is necessary to understand if specific aspects must be included in the design of interventions for burnout prevention or management.

Additionally, many limitations have been identified in methodologies employed to date (Chapter 6). Accordingly, a cross-sectional study of HIV/AIDS and oncology health staff – the MOMS study – was undertaken with the following specific objectives:

- Identify the general characteristics of the populations of HIV/AIDS and oncology health workers volunteering for a study of this type.
- Establish the characteristics of occupational morbidity in statutory health workers caring for people with HIV infection and disease, including AIDS and cancer, using systemmatically recorded subjective perceptions of current work stressors and the levels of stress experienced, and standardised instruments of measurement.
- Examine the interactions between characteristics of work stress and morbidity, and issues known or considered to have strong associations with MBI-reported burnout and/or findings in burnout-related research in HIV/AIDS and oncology staff.
- Identify the main predictors of self-reported stress in the workplace, and to identify those which were independently significant for both HIV/AIDS and for oncology staff.

- Assess the relationship between HIV/AIDS and oncology workers' work and self-reported domestic and social relationships outside the work setting, in order to identify the degree to which work appeared to affect non-work relationships.
- Identify and record preferences, and circumstances for use of, staff support programmes to reduce future work stress and morbidity, in order that relevant staff support regimes may be designed and implemented in future.

Characteristics of the populations were examined to assess for the degree of similarity and difference in the fields of HIV/AIDS and oncology. Then, self-reported experiences of work stress were examined, in relation to scores on the MBI subscales, and the GHQ, and the demographic variables described. Independently significant predictors of self-reported workplace stress were examined by cross-tabulating specified variables for each group with all questions asked at interview, and with psychometric scores. Family and social responses to working in HIV/AIDS and oncology were assessed, and preferences for staff support examined in relation to demographic characteristics.

As family and social responses and consequences of working in HIV/AIDS care have already been described briefly (Chapter 5) and published elsewhere in detail (Miller and Gillies, 1996), the results of this aspect of the MOMS project will not be repeated here. Also, the findings on preferences for staff support will be covered in detail in Chapter 8, as they fit closely with the results of the second UK study reported in this book.

Methods

This was a cross-sectional comparative study of health care workers managing HIV/AIDS patients, and those managing oncology patients. A total of 103 HIV/AIDS health workers employed in seven London hospitals and out-patient services providing specialist expertise in HIV/AIDS management were compared with 100 oncology health workers employed in two split sites of a national cancer research and treatment hospital. Health workers' responses to a structured interview schedule and a series of standardised questionnaires designed to assess psychological vulnerability and occupational 'burnout' were examined in order to determine their perceived stresses in the workplace, their self-reported responses to such stressors and the consequences they experienced in their workplace activity, and in their professional and personal relationships. Data were also sought from General Practice and Personnel Department records of a randomly selected 20 per cent of the study sample in order to enable verification of self-reported information on GP attendance, prescriptions given, and days off work for sickness and other reasons in the six months prior to being interviewed. The aim was to derive an indication of the validity of self-reported morbidity.

A further sub-study compared volunteers for the study with non-volunteers from the HIV and oncology study sites fitting eligibility criteria, in order to assess the representativeness of the volunteer populations, and therefore the generalisability of the study results (the results of this process were described in Chapter 6).

HIV and oncology staff were recruited from 'high-profile' specialist management centres in order to minimise the possibility of health staff having managed the care of both HIV and oncology patients at the same time. In this way it was hoped to achieve the clearest possible picture of the specific factors influencing occupational morbidity in each field. As the oncology sites also comprised a national treatment and research centre, the geographical location of the two oncology sites under observation was not an issue of concern because these sites accept patients from all over the UK. *All* care facilities surveyed were located within the Greater London area, and their catchment areas covered much common ground – all clinics of genitourinary medicine (GUM) in the UK are empowered to accept any self-referrals, so patients at any of the hospital-based study sites could have come from anywhere within the Greater London area, or from outside it as well. Departments of GUM also act as the major routes of referral to HIV in-patient treatment facilities in the major hospitals studied.

Criteria for inclusion of study participants

HIV and oncology health workers are appropriate populations for comparison because:

- Illnesses managed by both are often chronic and debilitating.
- Many interventions and treatments are experimental, with uncertain efficacy.
- Both fields of care are emotive, and stigma is reported anecdotally by health workers to be significant in each field.
- Each field has high reported mortality.
- Families and loved-ones are closely involved in care of patients in each field.
- Both fields encourage multi-disciplinary care and support.
- Health workers have repeated and long-term contact with patients (and their loved-ones).
- Much of the earlier literature on burnout in health workers has been based on studies of oncology staff, particularly nurses (see Chapter 3).

Participants seen in both fields manage a broad spectrum of clinical manifestations, and both patient populations may have extended asymptomatic states, depending on their diagnoses. Accordingly, study participants in both fields manage diverse clinical populations, some managing more asymptomatic patients than colleagues in related teams, and some managing more end-stage disease. Where clinical states are asymptomatic, however, patient recognition of long-term implications of HIV infection, for example, may occasion often intense psychosocial disturbance (Miller and Riccio, 1990), requiring often intensive clinical interventions for patients and their families (Miller and Green, 1986).

Health workers were eligible for the study if they satisfied the following criteria for inclusion and for having:

- Work experience continuously for six months or more in the field (HIV or oncology) *and* for six months or more at the site from which recruitment was undertaken.
- A qualification enabling full practice of their discipline (i.e., non-students/ trainees).
- A recognised role in facilitating clinical care (this allowed admission of two receptionist-administrators into the overall sample, as they were deemed by their clinical team directors to be vital parts of the clinical care process, and they had frequent, direct contact with patients and their relatives).

These criteria were imposed in order to ensure that data were derived from health care workers with sufficient levels of experience as a practitioner, and with a long-term understanding of their work environment. The criteria also helped to minimise other elements, such as level of training, that might otherwise have biased the nature of responses. Thus, the need to have worked for six months or longer at the site where interviewed eliminated junior medical staff on six-month rotations, whose elevated rates of stress and occupational morbidity are already characterised, and whose responses might have skewed the overall results (Firth-Cozens, 1987; Firth-Cozens and Morrison, 1989). Relative inexperience has also been identified as a possible cause of 'burnout' in earlier, questionnaire-based studies in HIV health staff (see Chapter 5). Having a clear role in facilitating clinical care is important to minimise possible role confusion that might additionally and adversely affect inter-disciplinary relationships (Kleiber *et al.*, 1992). Study populations comprised physicians, nurses and paramedical staff (clinical psychologists, social workers, health advisers, radiographers, counsellors, receptionists) primarily because they are the professions most closely involved in HIV/AIDS and oncology clinical care. Their clinical roles also differentiate them *en masse* from the roles of non-clinical and trainee staff, for whom lower reported stress has been found in relation to role conflict, ambiguity and work overload (Bates and Moore, 1975). These professional groups also form the dominant medically affiliated populations studied in earlier burnout and occupational stress research (Miller, 1996). The group of paramedical staff in the HIV/AIDS sample was grouped together because they all had roles that overlap significantly in function (e.g., provision of information and counselling) and separately they were numerically insufficient in this study to enable meaningful interpretation of data.

Data collection instruments

The study samples from each site were asked to complete an identical series of short self-report questionnaires, standardised and validated in previous studies of psychological and other stresses (Maslach and Jackson, 1986; Goldberg and Williams, 1988). The questionnaires included:

- *The Maslach Burnout Inventory* (MBI)(Maslach and Jackson, 1982). This 22-item questionnaire consists of three subscales measuring the constructs of emotional exhaustion, depersonalisation, and personal accomplishment. As shown in Chapters 3 and 4, the MBI is the most widely used instrument in research of this type.

- *The General Health Questionnaire-28* (GHQ-28) (Goldberg, 1981). This 28-item self-report questionnaire is an adaptation of the original 60-item General Health Questionnaire published in 1978 (Goldberg, 1978). It is an instrument that enables screening for 'state' (not 'trait') psychological and psychiatric vulnerability, by focusing on 'inability to continue to carry out one's normal "healthy" functions, and the appearance of new phenomena of a distressing nature' (Goldberg and Williams, 1988). Although the GHQ is not designed to make diagnoses of clinical severity, it is designed to differentiate psychiatric patients as a class from non-cases as a class.

Administration of the self-completed standardised questionnaires described above was preceded by a face-to-face structured interview using a purpose-designed structured interview schedule. This structured interview schedule examined the following issues:

- Personal demographics (age, sex, work status, etc.).
- Family experiences of health work.
- Family history of chronic or life-threatening illness.
- Personal history of potential exposure to HIV.
- HIV antibody test history.
- Professional demographics (occupation, length of experience, hours worked, etc.).
- Motivations for working in their field.
- History of voluntary (non-paid) work.
- Type and level of patient contacts.
- Work environment issues affecting work satisfaction.
- Levels and adequacy of training in their present specialism.
- Experiences of breaking bad news.
- Perceived workplace stressors.
- Nature and frequency of available staff emotional support.
- Preferences for staff emotional support.
- Job security and recognition experienced.
- The best and the most difficult parts of work.
- Symptoms and experiences of stress and coping strategies at work.
- Time taken off work and why.
- General health indices (drinking, smoking, medication, GP visits).
- Professional relations with colleagues, and with patients
- Experiences of burnout since qualifying.
- Impact of work on relationships outside the workplace.

The content of the interview schedule was determined by consulting:

- Literature to date on burnout, occupational stress and occupational psychological morbidity.

- Specialists in staff counselling, particularly those working with HIV workers and oncology workers.
- Staff working in these fields (discussions held on an individual, confidential basis).

Internal reliability was assessed by comparing responses to key questions replicated (with modifications) in the interview schedule. In addition, a retrospective study of personnel and GP records of a randomly selected 20 per cent of each of the study samples was made in order to verify the self-reported information on GP attendance, prescriptions given, days off work for sickness and other reasons in the six months prior to interview. The data obtained provided an indication of the validity of self-reported morbidity.

Overall, the structured interview schedule, together with the purpose-designed short questionnaires, and the standardised quantitative instruments, took approximately 75–90 minutes to complete in each case.

Administration of data collection instruments

All data were collected by one researcher. This avoided any concerns about the consistency of approach across sites and subjects, and inter-interviewer variance (Moser and Kalton, 1979). Additionally, the researcher was a qualified clinical psychologist, trained and certified in clinical history-taking and administration of standardised psychometric instruments, and bound by a professional code of conduct regarding the management of confidential information. Additionally, the researcher was able to apply clinical judgement to interpretations of psychometric scale and interview results while the interview was taking place – in this way, those emerging as having serious psychological vulnerability could be referred immediately to a clinical colleague, without the requirement for third parties intervening (a requirement of ethical committees at all sites).

All interviews were conducted in quiet, comfortable, sound-proofed rooms in which confidentiality was assured.

Results

Response rates

Overall, 64 per cent (n = 103/161) of the eligible HIV/AIDS staff, and 22 per cent (n = 100/450) of those approached for the oncology sample, volunteered to participate in the study.

Sample characteristics

The range of professional groups participating was significantly different between HIV and oncology, with the HIV group having significantly more physicians and fewer nurses participating than the oncology group (χ^2 = 14.71, 2 d.f., P = 0.0006) (see Table 7.1).

Table 7.1 Health worker samples by gender, age, seniority, profession and experience

Characteristics	HIV/AIDS staff sample (+% of study sample) n = 103	Oncology staff sample (+% of study sample) n = 100
Gender: Male	34 (33%)	8 (8%)
Female	69 (67%)	92 (92%)
Age: Mean	33.10	34.40
Standard deviation	7.52	8.47
Range	22–57	22–58
Median	31.00	32.00
Seniority:		
Consultant + Equivalent	10 (10%)	7 (7%)
Senior/Principal	28 (27%)	48 (38%)
Junior/Clinician	59 (57%)	55 (55%)
Other	6 (6%)	0 (0%)
Months since qualification:		
Range	6–420	24–408
Median	84	120
Profession:		
Physician	20	7
Nurse	51	75
Paramedic	32	18
Months *in situ*:		
Range	6–312	6–240
Median	24	36

HIV/AIDS and oncology staff were largely comparable in relation to age (t = –1.16, d.f. = 201, P = 0.25). However, there were significantly more male staff in the HIV group than in the oncology group (χ^2 = 19.34, 1 d.f., P = <0.001). There was a significant difference between HIV and oncology samples both in months since qualifying, and in months in situ. Regarding months since qualifying, the HIV/AIDS median was 84 months (range 6 to 420); the oncology median was 120 months (range 24 to 408) (Mann–Whitney test, P = <0.001).

The HIV/AIDS and oncology samples were also significantly different regarding median months in their present setting. The HIV sample had spent significantly less time (median = 24 months, range = 6 to 312 months) than the oncology sample (median = 36 months, range = 6 to 240 months) (Mann–Whitney test, P = <0.001).

Psychometric category scores

Total individual scores on the GHQ-28 were divided according to the modal division employed in previous published research cited by the authors, i.e., 0–4 = 'non-case', 5–24 = 'case'. A 'case' is considered to be a person showing sufficient

Table 7.2 Psychometric category scores on GHQ-28 and MBI

Variable	Category	HIV/AIDS (n = 103)	Oncology (n=100)	χ^2	d.f.	P
GHQ total scores*	Non-case (0–4)	61 (60%)	58 (58%)	0.04	1	0.84
	Case (5–24)	40 (40%)	42 (42%)			
MBI Emotional exhaustion subscale*	Low (0–16)	28 (28%)	34 (34%)	2.76	2	0.25
	Moderate (17–26)	37 (37%)	41 (41%)			
	High (27 or over)	36 (35%)	25 (25%)			
MBI Depersonalisation subscale*	Low (0–6)	60 (59%)	67 (67%)	1.27	2	0.53
	Moderate (7–12)	28 (28%)	22 (22%)			
	High (13 or over)	13 (13%)	11 (11%)			
MBI Personal accomplishment subscale *	Low (39 or over)	47 (47%)	37 (37%)	2.21	2	0.33
	Moderate (32–38)	35 (35%)	44 (44%)			
	High (0–31)	19 (18%)	19 (19%)			

* Two missing values in HIV/AIDS sample.

psychological vulnerability to merit possible referral to mental health specialist staff. When overall scores were thus grouped, 59 per cent (n = 119) scored as 'non-cases', and 41 per cent (n = 82) scored as 'cases on the GHQ-28.

On the MBI subscale categories, there were no differences found on any of the subscales between HIV/AIDS and oncology groups. Combined HIV and oncology participant category scores for Emotional Exhaustion were as follows: High = 30 per cent (n = 61); Moderate = 39 per cent (n = 78); Low = 31 per cent (n = 62). In subsequent 2 × 2 tests of association, 'high' and 'moderate' scores were grouped – hence, 69 per cent (n = 139) overall scored in the 'high/moderate' range of the MBI EE subscale.

Category scores grouped for Depersonalisation were as follows: High = 12 per cent (n = 24); Moderate = 25 per cent (n = 50); and Low = 63 per cent (n = 127). A total of 37 per cent (n = 74) therefore scored in the 'high/moderate' range of the MBI DP subscale. Finally, category scores for Personal Accomplishment were as follows: High = 19 per cent (n = 38); Moderate = 39 per cent (n = 79); and Low = 42 per cent (n = 84). A total of 58 per cent (n = 117) therefore scored in the 'high/moderate' range of the MBI PA subscale.

Associations with self-reported and psychometric measures of work-related stress

In order to assess current level of reported work stress and its impact, all participants were asked to indicate self-reported stress symptoms, to report on experiences of self-defined burnout, to identify how work-related stresses had risen or fallen in the six months prior to interview, and to complete the MBI and the GHQ-28. Frequency data obtained on these issues follow.

Univariate analyses were subsequently performed to test the null hypotheses that for the interview and psychometric variables indicating work-related stress, there would be no differences in outcome according to those issues previously identified in the literature as possible sources of difference:

- Field of work (HIV/AIDS or oncology).
- Gender.
- Age.
- Professional group.
- Professional seniority.
- Length of professional experience.

Continuity corrections were used for 2×2 tables, and a test for trend was used where appropriate. Where differences were found to be significant at the 1 per cent level, a multivariate analysis was done to adjust for potential confounding variables. Results from univariate and multivariate analyses are tabulated in the Appendix at the end of the book[1].

Present and previous work stress reported by HIV/AIDS and oncology groups combined

Overall, 91 per cent (n = 185) reported that at the time of their interview they were finding work continuously stressful. For 63 per cent (n = 118), work stress had increased in the six months prior to being interviewed, while for 22 per cent (n = 42) it had decreased, and for 14 per cent (n = 27) work stress had remained at the same level. Where reported changes in levels of work stress in the prior six months had occurred, they were described as being due to either: (a) clinical and managerial problems with patients and patients' families, loss of experienced colleagues or relationship difficulties with those remaining, or work having been re-organised (55 per cent, n = 87); or (b) to personal (non-work) issues, the impact of new National Health Service re-structuring, or (more positively) having finally mastered new aspects of their work (45 per cent, n = 72).

While all staff reported that there were work stresses they endured and responded to, work stresses ranked as being 'most important' to participants could be encompassed within four categories:

1   Issues concerning inadequacies and tensions of providing clinical management, e.g., 'Overwork', 'Uncertainty about clinical management', 'Having nothing new to offer' (48 per cent, n = 95).
2   Relationships with patients and with staff, and issues of identifying with patients, e.g., 'Relationships with staff', 'Identification with patients from own age/peer groups' (19 per cent, n = 38).
3   Issues concerning patients' deaths and decline, e.g., 'Deaths of patients', 'Psychological difficulties in patients' (17 per cent, n = 34).
4   Other issues concerning service executive management, and staff, e.g., 'Attitudes of some staff' (15 per cent, n = 30).

When asked to rank which issues were the most problemmatic in relationships with patients, staff responses included:

- The deaths and decline of patients, e.g., 'To have to watch the physical and psychological decline of my patients' (45 per cent, n = 90).
- Self-reported inadequacies associated with giving clinical care and support, e.g., 'That I cannot sufficiently diminish the distress of patients' loved-ones', and 'To have to break bad news to patients or relatives/loved-ones' (38 per cent, n = 76).
- Identifying with and maintaining relationships with patients, e.g., 'That I form close relationships with some of my patients' (17 per cent, n = 35).

In considering possible environmental influences on experienced work stress, 66 per cent overall (n = 134) reported they did not have enough *time* to do the work they were required to do, and 60 per cent (n = 122) reported that their work *premises were inadequate* for the work they had to do. Only 34 per cent (n = 70) of staff questioned said they had access to a quiet rest room away from patients, while 55 per cent (n = 111) reported they had no privacy for doing their clinical work and 53 per cent (n = 106) said they had insufficient privacy for doing their necessary administrative work. Overall, the work atmosphere, however, was described as 'good' by 78 per cent (n = 159), while 22 per cent (n = 44) said it was 'poor'.

The other main aspect of work that could affect work stress levels was relations with colleagues. Some 32 per cent (n = 64) reported having serious disagreements with colleagues in the workplace. Where reported, these disagreements concerned mainly issues relating to patient and staff management (60 per cent, n = 38), and service executive management (40 per cent, n = 25). Additionally, 76 per cent (n = 154) reported having felt professionally obstructed by colleagues at some time, and 82 per cent (n = 163) reported feeling difficulties in showing distress about work issues to colleagues. The quality of cooperation across professions was described as 'poor' by 81 per cent (n = 163) overall, and as 'good' by 19 per cent (n = 38). On the other hand, 89 per cent (n = 177) said they could participate in decision-making regarding clinical management.

Self-reported physical, behavioural and cognitive/affective stress symptoms

Participants had been asked to complete a handout listing symptoms of stress, and requiring them to indicate whether they experienced any of these symptoms in their current work. Overall, more than 50 per cent of the study participants said 'yes' to the majority of items, indicating that they experienced the symptoms listed between 'sometimes' to 'all the time' in relation to their work.

For *physical* stress symptoms, 98 per cent (n = 200) reported tiredness; sleeplessness was reported by 69 per cent (n = 139); muscle pains were reported by 62 per cent (n = 126); lingering minor illnesses were reported by 55 per cent (n = 111); and malaise was self-reported by 54 per cent (n = 109). Some

46 per cent (n = 94) self-reported experiencing gastrointestinal disturbances as symptoms of work stress, 42 per cent (n = 86) reported skin complaints, 29 per cent (n = 59) reported palpitations, and 21 per cent (n = 43) reported 'other' physical symptoms of work-related stress.

The most-cited self-reported *behavioural* stress symptom experienced in relation to work was 'readiness to be irritated/frustrated' (97 per cent, n = 198). Then came problems in communication with colleagues (79 per cent, n = 161), and agitation/nervousness, reported by 75 per cent (n = 152). Some 64 per cent (n = 130) overall reported problems in communication with patients, and 62 per cent (n = 126) reported proneness to anger/prejudice as behavioural stress symptoms. Overall, 58 per cent (n = 117) reported rigidity or inflexibility in problem-solving, 51 per cent (n = 104) cited withdrawal from non-involved colleagues and friends, and 50 per cent (n = 101) reported anxiety/anxiety attacks as behavioural symptoms of their work-related stress.

Just under half the overall study sample self-reported self-righteousness ('heroism') as a behavioural symptom of their work-related stress (49 per cent, n = 99), 44 per cent (n = 89) said 'yes' to impulsive acts, and 21 per cent (n = 42) reported victimisation or blaming of patients.

Self-reported *cognitive/affective* stress symptoms experienced in relation to work added up as follows: 96 per cent (n = 194) reported sadness, 95 per cent (n = 192) reported frustration, 82 per cent (n = 166) reported experiencing grief, 79 per cent (n = 160) reported concentration problems, 78 per cent (n = 158) reported experiencing hypersensitivity, and 76 per cent (n = 155) reported experiencing indecision as a work-related stress symptom. Some 71 per cent (n = 145) reported 'a sense of failure' as a cognitive/affective stress symptom, and 70 per cent (n = 141) reported inattention and distractability. Overall, 67 per cent (n = 135) reported experiencing pessimism and hopelessness, 64 per cent (n = 127) reported over-identification with patients' needs, 63 per cent (n = 128) reported emotional numbness/indifference, and 61 per cent (n = 124) reported cynicism as a work-related stress symptom. In total, 59 per cent (n = 120) reported experiencing depression as a symptom of their work stress, and 56 per cent (n = 114) reported fatalism as a symptom.

Self-reported responses to work stress

Overall, when asked 'If you could describe how you generally feel in a word or a phrase, what would it be?', grouped answers showed that 38 per cent (n = 77) said they felt 'vulnerable/exhausted/miserable', and 62 per cent (n = 126) said they felt 'fine/okay'. Some 70 per cent (n = 141) described their ability to distance themselves from their patients' difficulties as either 'fairly good' or 'very good', while for the remaining 30 per cent (n = 61), their abilities to do so were self-reported as 'poor' or 'uncertain'. Similarly, 52 per cent (n = 106) reported they usually found it 'easy' to shut off from work, while 48 per cent (n = 97) found it 'difficult'.

When asked about alcohol and tobacco consumption, 6 per cent (n = 13) overall said they were non-drinkers. Of the remainder, 17 per cent (n = 33) said they had been drinking more alcohol since working in their present field. Actual reported consumption was as follows: 75 per cent (n = 152) reported consuming 1–14 units weekly, and 19 per cent (n = 38) reported consuming 15 or more units weekly. Overall, 71 per cent (n = 143) described themselves as 'non-smokers'. However, of those 29 per cent (n = 60) who reported smoking, 32 per cent (n = 19) reported smoking more since coming to their present job, 9 per cent overall (n = 18) reported smoking 1–9 cigarettes daily, and 20 per cent (n = 42) reported smoking 10 or more cigarettes daily.

Overall, 60 per cent of the study population (n = 121) reported having seen their GP or a physician at some time during the six months before being interviewed. Of these, 9 per cent (n = 11) reported having been prescribed medication for the treatment of anxiety or depression, 22 per cent (n = 27) reported having no prescriptions made, and 69 per cent (n = 83) reported receiving prescriptions for other medication (e.g., pain killers, contraceptives, antibiotics).

Concerning self-reported experiences of burnout at work, 21 per cent (n = 43) of staff said they had known no colleagues to burn out since they were qualified, 49 per cent (n = 99) said 1–5 colleagues had burned out since they had qualified, and 30 per cent (n = 61) reported that six or more had done so. When asked how many colleagues had burned out since they had worked in their present field, 39 per cent (n = 79) reported none having done so, 32 per cent (n = 65) said 1–2, and 29 per cent (n = 59) reported three or more. When asked if they had ever suffered burnout, 65 per cent (n = 132) said either 'no' or 'uncertain', and 35 per cent (n = 71) said 'yes'.

In terms of responses to possible dangers of HIV infection associated with contemporary health care and other sources, frequency analyses showed that 62 per cent (n = 64) of the HIV/AIDS study population self-identified a history of possible exposure to HIV since 1980. Of these, 81 per cent (n = 52) reported that their possible exposure was sexual, 2 per cent (n = 2) felt it was through blood transfusion, and 22 per cent (n = 23) felt their possible exposure was occupational. In contrast, only 27 per cent of the oncology sample felt they had possible exposure to HIV in the same period, mainly occupationally (17 per cent), and sexually (16 per cent). While 40 per cent of the HIV/AIDS sample had undergone an HIV antibody test (83 per cent of these did so on their own initiative), 23 per cent of the oncology sample had been tested, and it was on the initiative of only 22 per cent of those who had done so (others were tested because of blood donation, etc.).

Differences between HIV/AIDS and oncology staff regarding self-reported and psychometric measures of work-related stress
(Table 1 in the Appendix)

Results from univariate analyses found to be significant at the 0.01 level or less are shown in the Appendix (Table 1). As it shows, people working in HIV/AIDS were significantly *more* likely than those working in oncology to:

- Smoke 10 or more cigarettes daily (29 per cent of HIV/AIDS staff, versus 12 per cent of oncology staff).
- Report skin complaints as stress symptoms (52 per cent versus 32 per cent).
- Be stressed by the appearance of patients' repeated or new infections (53 per cent versus 31 per cent).
- Feel concerned that their work overlaps with that of other professions (58 per cent versus 35 per cent), and that concerns raised by this are resolved less than half the time (39 per cent versus 11 per cent).
- Feel they participate in decision-making over changes in their professional activities and conditions (90 per cent versus 78 per cent).

These findings all remained significant at the 5 per cent level after adjusting for age, sex and professional group.

On the other hand, people working in HIV/AIDS were significantly *less* likely than those working in oncology to:

- Report having adequate work premises (30 per cent versus 50 per cent).
- Have adequate material resources at work (82 per cent versus 93 per cent).
- Participate in sport to shut off after work (12 per cent versus 31 per cent).

These all remained significant at the 5 per cent level after adjusting for age, sex and professional group.

In all other respects of occupational stress and morbidity, there were no other significant differences found between HIV/AIDS and oncology groups.

Differences between sexes regarding self-reported and psychometric measures of work stress (Table 2 in the Appendix)

Women were significantly ($P < 0.01$) *more* likely than men to find it difficult to show distress about work-related issues (84 per cent versus 66 per cent of men). Conversely, women were significantly (<1 per cent) *less* likely than men to consume 15 or more units of alcohol weekly (33 per cent of men versus 15 per cent of women), or be concerned about their work overlapping with that of other professions (41 per cent of women versus 69 per cent of men). After adjustment by HIV/oncology group, age and professional group, these all remained significant at the 5 per cent level. There were no significant interactions (effect modifications). In other words, associations were the same in the HIV and oncology groups. There were no differences significant at the 1 per cent level or less between men and women on psychometric measures of burnout or psychological vulnerability (GHQ-28 and MBI category scores).

Differences between age groups (<30 and 30+ years) regarding self-reported and psychometric measures of work stress (Table 3 in the Appendix)

People aged 30 years and over were significantly (<1 per cent) *more* likely than those aged 29 or less to:

- Be prone to anger and prejudice (72 per cent versus 44 per cent of younger staff).
- Over-identify with patients' needs.
- Know six or more people who have experienced burnout since qualifying (35 per cent versus 18 per cent).
- Know three or more people who have experienced burnout since working in their present field (37 per cent versus 14 per cent).

These findings all remained significant at the 1 per cent level after stratifying by HIV/oncology group, sex and professional group. The associations were not significantly different across HIV and oncology groups.

Differences between physicians and nurses regarding self-reported and psychometric measures of work stress (Table 4 in the Appendix).

At the 1 per cent level of significance, nurses were more likely than physicians to have consulted a physician in the six months prior to interview, and thought that their stress would be reduced by having more staff. Physicians, on the other hand, were more likely than nurses to think better service management and fewer patients would reduce work stress. No other differences were found. All remained significant at the 5 per cent level after adjusting for work in HIV/oncology, age, sex, professional experience and seniority, except 'Having seen a GP in the last six months'. There were no significant differences between the HIV and Oncology groups.

Differences between nurses and paramedics regarding self-reported and psychometric measures of work stress (Table 5 in the Appendix)

Nurses were significantly *more* likely than paramedical staff to find breaking bad news contributes to stress (74 per cent versus 36 per cent); and to find breaking bad news to patients' loved-ones/families is a problemmatic element in relationships with patients; and to think more resources/staff will reduce work stress. Paramedics were significantly *more* likely than nursing staff to feel personally obstructed by colleagues, and to feel that better service management will reduce work stress. No other differences between nurses and paramedics were found at the 1 per cent level or less, and all findings remained significant at the 1 per cent level after adjusting by HIV/oncology, age, sex, months of professional experience and seniority.

Differences between senior and junior staff concerning self-reported and psychometric measures of work stress (Table 6 in the Appendix)

Senior staff included those at the consultant or equivalent, senior/principal medical, nursing and paramedical levels. Junior staff were those at the registrar/clinician, junior nursing and other levels. Senior staff were significantly *more* likely than junior staff to:

- Do 11 or more hours overtime (22 per cent versus 4 per cent).
- Rate their work atmosphere highly.
- Have a 'low' MBI PA category score (i.e., they feel a higher sense of personal accomplishment on the MBI).

Senior staff were significantly *less* likely than junior staff to:

- Experience emotional numbness/indifference as a stress symptom (51 per cent versus 72 per cent).
- Find the involvement of patients' loved-ones/families stressful (48 per cent versus 67 per cent).
- Find it problematic that they form close relationships with patients.
- Find breaking bad news to patients problematic in relationships with them.
- Find lack of training in death and dying a work stress (36 per cent versus 57 per cent).
- Have difficulty in showing distress about work-related issues.
- Score in the 'high/moderate' categories of the MBI PA subscale (46 per cent versus 71 per cent).

All remained significant at the 1 per cent level after adjusting by age, HIV/ Oncology, sex and professional group, except 'Breaking bad news to relatives of patients is a problem' ($P = 0.079$). After further adjustments by months of professional experience, 'Difficulties in showing distress to colleagues' ($P = 0.059$) was no longer significant at the 5 per cent level. There were no interactions with HIV/oncology, except 'Emotional numbness/indifference'. Junior HIV/ AIDS staff were significantly more likely to experience 'emotional numbness/ indifference' than senior staff ($\chi^2 = 11.16$, 1 d.f., $P = <0.001$), whereas there was no significant difference between senior and junior staffs' experiences of 'emotional numbness/indifference' in the oncology sample ($\chi^2 = 0.336$, 1 d.f., $P = 0.562$).

Differences between those with less than 96 months versus those with 96 or more months of professional experience regarding self-reported and psychometric measures of work stress (Table 7 in the Appendix)

Those staff with more professional experience were *more* likely to score in the 'low' category of the MBI Depersonalisation subscale (76 per cent versus 51 per cent). However, those with less than eight years experience were significantly *more* likely to:

- Report emotional numbness/indifference as a stress symptom (52 per cent versus 75 per cent).
- Have enough time to do their required work (25 per cent versus 44 per cent).
- Experience lack of training in death and dying as a work stress (37 per cent versus 61 per cent).

- Find it difficult to show distress about work-related issues.
- Score as 'High/moderate' on the Depersonalisation scale of the MBI (24 per cent versus 49 per cent).
- Shut off from work by socialising (36 per cent versus 57 per cent).

After adjusting by HIV/Oncology, age, sex and professional group, all remained statistically significant at the 5 per cent level. After further adjustment by seniority, 'Shutting off from work by socialising' lost significance ($P = 0.16$), while for 'Emotional numbness/indifference' ($P = 0.059$) and 'Lack of training in death and dying' ($P = 0.062$), significance was borderline.

There were no significant differences (interactions) between these associations in the HIV/AIDS and oncology groups, except for 'Difficulties in showing work-related distress to colleagues' ($P = 0.006$). HIV/AIDS staff with less than eight years' experience had much more difficulty showing distress about work-related issues (93 per cent versus 57 per cent, $\chi^2 = 16.47$, 1 d.f., $P = <0.001$). Oncology staff, however, revealed no differences between more and less-experienced staff in reporting difficulties associated with showing distress about work-related issues (85 per cent versus 83 per cent, $\chi^2 = 0.00$, 1 d.f., $P = 1.000$).

Overall summary of self-reported occupational morbidity

Overall, no differences could be detected at the 1 per cent level regarding GHQ-28 scores, or in MBI 'Emotional exhaustion' subscale scores. Those working in HIV/AIDS, junior and less-experienced staff reported more stresses in their work, and more physical, cognitive/affective and behavioural responses to those stresses. Those over 30 years report knowing more people who have experienced burnout, although no differences were seen on experience of burnout between any groups. Reports of how work stress could be reduced differed according to professional group – physicians suggested having fewer patients, nurses suggested having more staff, and paramedical staff suggested having better service management.

Independently significant predictors of self-reported workplace stress

For each of the variables concerning self-reported work stress and psychometric category scores, cross-tabulated with the whole variable set, the following procedures were undertaken:

1 Chi-square tests of association were performed.
2 All variables significant at the 1 per cent level were tabulated in order to avoid possible common errors arising from misapplication of significance tests to survey analysis (Moser and Kalton, 1979), and Type I errors.
3 Odds ratios (ORs) and their associated 95 per cent confidence intervals were calculated for each of these variables.
4 Variables which were significant at the 0.1 per cent level were entered into a multi-variate logistic model to determine independent significant variables.

This significance level was chosen for the models because it would offer a greater likelihood of identifying truly independent variables more efficiently.

These outcome variables were of interest because they enabled a systematic study of the symptoms and consequences of occupational morbidity in these populations of health workers, based upon their self-reports of work stresses. Additionally, the significance of MBI subscale scores in relation to subject self-defined stresses and to a standardised clinical measure was possible by this approach. As described earlier, such an approach has not been taken in the majority of studies in this field, yet the information from an analysis of independently significant predictors of self-reported stress at work is particularly necessary if appropriate weight is to be given to subscale scores on the MBI, and relevant interventions are to be designed.

For each of the analyses, summaries will be given, and the tabulated data shown in the Appendix.

Identifying variables independently associated with experiencing work stress

HIV/AIDS STAFF SUMMARY
(Tables 8a and 8b, 10a and 10b in the Appendix)

Scoring in the high/moderate range of the MBI EE subscale, having more than one colleague experiencing burnout, and finding deaths of patients a work stress, were all independently significant predictors of *finding work stressful for HIV/AIDS staff*. Unadjusted ORs revealed that people in each of these categories are over five times more likely to find work stressful than those who are not. Adjusted ORs revealed that staff finding deaths of patients a work stress, and having colleagues who have burned out, are more than eight times more likely to find work stressful than those who do not. Those scoring as an MBI EE 'case' are almost four times more likely to report finding work stressful than 'non-cases'.

For HIV/AIDS staff, the only independently significant predictor of *currently experiencing stress at work* was having had a history of potential exposure to HIV since 1980. ORs adjusted for proneness to anger and prejudice, and inattention and distractibility, showed that HIV workers with a history of potential exposure to HIV since 1980 were over 12 times more likely than those who did not to currently experience stress associated with work.

ONCOLOGY STAFF SUMMARY
(Tables 9a and 9b, 11a and 11b in the Appendix)

For *oncology staff*, feeling 'vulnerable/exhausted/miserable', scoring in the range for 'caseness' on the GHQ-28, and finding the work *environment* stressful, were all independently significant predictors of *finding work stressful*. ORs adjusted for these variables show that staff reporting they generally feel 'vulnerable/exhausted/miserable' are six times more likely than those who feel 'fine/okay' to report finding work stressful. Those scoring as GHQ-28 'cases' are over three times more likely, and those finding the work environment stressful are over four times more likely, to report finding work stressful.

Independently significant predictors of *currently experiencing stress associated with work* for oncology staff included having problems in communicating with colleagues, and reporting depression as a stress symptom. After adjusting for each other, ORs showed that people in each of these categories were more than four times more likely than those who were not to currently experience stress associated with their work in oncology.

Identifying variables independently associated with self-reported health state

HIV/AIDS STAFF
(Tables 12a and 12b in the Appendix)

Those HIV/AIDS staff who reported that their primary emotional relationship had suffered as a result of their work in the field were over seven times more likely to self-report their present state as 'vulnerable/exhausted/miserable' than those who had not had such relationship problems. People scoring as 'cases' on the GHQ-28 were just over five times more likely to describe their present state as 'vulnerable/exhausted/miserable' than those who were 'non-cases'. People describing themselves as being 'vulnerable/exhausted/miserable' were between four and five times more likely to experience malaise lingering minor illnesses, skin complaints, and palpitations as stress symptoms than those who said they were generally feeling 'fine/okay'. Those experiencing anxiety and anxiety attacks, and withdrawal from non-involved colleagues and/or friends were over three times more likely to describe their general state as 'vulnerable/exhausted/miserable', than those who reported they were 'fine/okay'.

For HIV/AIDS staff, after logistic regressions were performed, independently significant predictors of generally feeling 'vulnerable/exhausted/miserable' were scoring as a 'case' on the GHQ-28, and reporting malaise as a stress symptom. ORs adjusted for each variable showed that staff in each of these categories were over three times more likely, than those not in these categories, to report generally feeling 'vulnerable/miserable/exhausted'.

ONCOLOGY STAFF
(Tables 13a, 13b, and 13c in the Appendix)

Oncology staff were over ten times more likely to report feeling 'vulnerable/ exhausted/miserable' if they experienced agitation/nervousness as a behavioural stress symptom. Similarly, staff were over seven times more likely to feel 'vulnerable/exhausted/miserable' if they also reported lingering minor illnesses and sleeplessness as stress symptoms. Oncology staff were over six times more likely to feel 'vulnerable/exhausted/miserable' if they experienced pessimism and hopelessness, muscle pains, and gastrointestinal disturbances, than if they did not do so. Similarly, they were over six times more likely to report feeling 'vulnerable/ exhausted/miserable' if they scored as 'cases' on the GHQ-28, than if they were 'non-cases'. Oncology staff reporting inattention and distractibility, and malaise, were over five times more likely than those not reporting these symptoms to say they were feeling 'vulnerable/exhausted/miserable'. Those for whom maintaining confidence in their clinical skills was a work stress were over four times more likely than those for whom it was not to report feeling 'vulnerable/exhausted/miserable', as were those reporting depression as a stress symptom. Staff reporting anxiety attacks were over three times more likely than those not doing so to report feeling vulnerable, and those reporting being unable to make decisions about changes in professional activities and conditions were much less likely than those who could to report feeling 'fine/okay' when asked to report their general health state.

An independently significant predictor of generally feeling 'vulnerable/ exhausted/miserable' was having reported lingering minor illnesses as stress symptoms (adjusted ORs showed those who did were more than seven times more likely to feel 'vulnerable/exhausted/miserable'). A second independently significant predictor on this variable was being unable to make decisions about future changes in one's professional activities and conditions. For these staff, adjusted ORs showed they were over five times more likely to generally feel 'vulnerable/exhausted/miserable', than those who could make such decisions.

Indentifying variables independently associated with GHQ-28 total scores

HIV/AIDS STAFF
(Tables 14a and 14b in the Appendix)

Table 14a in the Appendix identifies those variables which were significantly associated with scoring as a 'case' on the GHQ-28 at the 1 per cent level or less. Those staff reporting depression as a stress symptom were over six times more likely than those not reporting this symptom to score as a 'case' on this measure. HIV/AIDS staff were also over five times more likely to score as a case on the GHQ-28 if they reported feeling professionally obstructed by colleagues, felt a sense of failure when stressed, experienced pessimism and hopelessness, and reported generally feeling 'vulnerable/exhausted/miserable'. HIV/AIDS staff were over three times more likely to score as a case on the GHQ-28 if they reported a poor ability to distance themselves from patients' difficulties, reported muscle pains, and anxiety/anxiety attacks, as stress symptoms, found the work environment stressful, and reported lingering minor illnesses, and self-righteousness ('heroism') as stress symptoms.

Independently significant predictors of scoring as a 'case' on the GHQ-28 for HIV/AIDS staff (Table 14b in the Appendix) were having reported generally feeling 'vulnerable/exhausted/miserable', and reporting depression as a stress symptom. ORs adjusted for each show that those reporting depression were over six times more likely to score as a GHQ-28 'case', and those reporting feeling 'vulnerable/exhausted/miserable' were over four times more likely to do so.

ONCOLOGY STAFF
(Tables 15a and 15b in the Appendix)

Oncology staff were 17 times more likely to score as a 'case' on the GHQ-28 if they reported hypersensitivity as a stress symptom, than if they did not. Those reporting sleeplessness were over 16 times more likely to be a GHQ-28 'case' than those presumably sleeping well. Oncology staff were more than six times more likely to appear as a GHQ-28 'case' if they reported maintaining confidence in clinical skills a work stress, reported malaise as a stress symptom, or feeling generally 'vulnerable/exhausted/miserable', than if they did not report these things. Staff reporting not having control over future professional circumstances were over five times more likely to appear as a GHQ-28 'case' than those who did have such control. Staff were more than four times more likely to score as a GHQ-28 'case' if they reported experiencing palpitations, anxiety/anxiety attacks, muscle pains, withdrawal, and depression, than those who did not report these things. Where staff reported patient relations becoming problematic when patients challenged their work, or when knowing patients would die, they were more than four times more likely to score as a 'case' on the GHQ-28, than if patient relations were unaffected by these things. Lastly, staff who had broken bad news more than 11 times in the past six months, and who reported feeling professionally inadequate, were more than three times more likely to score as a 'case' on the GHQ-28 than those who had broken bad news 10 times or less, and who did not feel professionally inadequate.

For oncology staff, *independently significant predictors* of scoring as a 'case' on the GHQ-28 were having reported withdrawal from non-involved colleagues and friends, and sleeplessness, as self-reported stress symptoms, and having reported that maintaining confidence in clinical skills was a work stress. Adjusted ORs showed that those reporting sleeplessness were nine times more likely to score as a 'case', whereas those who reported withdrawal and stress with maintaining confidence in clinical skills were each over four times more likely to score as a GHQ-28 'case'.

Identifying variables independently associated with MBI emotional exhaustion (EE) subscale category scores

HIV/AIDS STAFF
(Tables 16a and 16b in the Appendix)

For HIV/AIDS staff, the ORs reveal that the highest increased odds of scoring in the high–moderate range of the MBI EE subscale occurs in those experiencing self-righteousness ('heroism') as a self-reported stress symptom – they are over six times more likely to score in this range than those not reporting this symptom. Similarly, those reporting they found work stressful were also six times more likely to score in the high–moderate MBI EE range. HIV/AIDS staff reporting grief were over five times more likely than those not doing so to score in this range.

Staff were more than four times more likely to score in the high/moderate categories of the MBI EE subscale if they reported a sense of failure or pessimism and hopelessness as stress symptoms, if they reported communication problems with colleagues, or with patients, reported feeling professionally obstructed or found the work environment stressful, compared with those who did not make such reports. Staff who reported stress symptoms of withdrawal, anxiety attacks, or depression, and over-identifying with patients' needs, were all more than three times more likely than non-reporters to score high–moderate on the MBI EE subscale.

For HIV/AIDS staff, *independently significant predictors* of scoring in the 'high–moderate' range of the MBI EE subscale were reporting finding work stressful, and reporting self-righteousness ('heroism'), and pessimism and hopelessness, as stress symptoms. ORs adjusted for each of the modelled variables revealed that those who found work stressful were almost seven times more likely than those who did not to score as an MBI EE 'case'. Those reporting self-righteousness were five times more likely, and those who reported pessimism and hopelessness were over three times more likely to score as an MBI EE 'case' than those not reporting these stress symptoms.

ONCOLOGY STAFF
(Tables 17a and 17b in the Appendix)

For oncology staff, Table 17a in the Appendix shows that oncology staff reporting palpitations as stress symptoms are over 10 times more likely to score in the high–moderate categories (i.e., as 'cases' in this analysis) of the MBI EE than non-reporters of these symptoms. Those reporting more than 50 per cent of their colleagues being stressed are seven times more likely to score as cases on the MBI EE subscale. Those for whom coping with work technology is a stress are six-and-a-half times more likely to score as cases, and those for whom a lack of training in death and dying, and overwork, are work stresses, are more than five times more likely to score as MBI EE cases. Oncology staff reporting anxiety attacks, and scoring as 'cases' on the GHQ-28, are more than four times more likely to score as MBI EE cases than those who do not. Staff were more than three times more likely to score as cases on the MBI EE subscale if they reported feeling professionally inadequate, reported seeing dying patients – and/or knowing patients will die – was problematic in relations with patients, reported finding maintaining clinical confidence stressful, and reported depression as a stress symptom, than those who did not report these issues.

For oncology staff, independently significant predictors of scoring as a 'case' – in the 'high–moderate' range of the MBI EE subscale (Table 17b in the Appendix) – were having reported experiencing palpitations as a stress symptom, having more than half ones' work colleagues stressed, and having reported lack of training in death and dying, and overwork, as work stresses. For the latter, adjusted ORs show that those reporting such stresses were seven and six times respectively more likely to score as an MBI EE 'case'. Reporting over half of your work colleagues as stressed, and having palpitations, are each associated with being nine times more likely to be an MBI EE 'case'.

Identifying variables independently associated with MBI depersonalisation (DP) subscale category scores

HIV/AIDS STAFF
(Tables 18a and 18b in the Appendix)

Table 18a in the Appendix shows those variables significantly associated with scoring in the 'high–moderate' range (i.e., as 'cases' in this analysis) of the MBI DP (depersonalisation) subscale at the 1 per cent level or less. HIV/AIDS staff reporting emotional numbness and indifference as a stress symptom were over 16 times more likely than those not doing so to score as MBI DP cases. Staff reporting cynicism as a symptom of stress were over seven-and-a-half times more likely to score as MBI DP cases, while staff reporting that relations separately with staff and with patients were work stresses were five times more likely than those not doing so to score as MBI DP cases. Staff reporting lingering minor illnesses, withdrawal, and gastrointestinal disturbances, and those reporting difficulties in emotional support-seeking, were all more than four times more likely than those who did not to score as cases on the MBI DP subscale. Those reporting palpitations were three times more likely to score as an MBI DP 'case', and senior staff were significantly less likely to score as an MBI DP 'case' than junior staff.

For HIV/AIDS staff, the only *independently significant* variable predicting a 'high–moderate' score on the MBI DP subscale was having reported emotional numbness/indifference as a stress symptom (Table 18b in the Appendix). Those doing so were, after ORs had been adjusted for all the modelled variables, over nine times more likely to score as a 'case' on this variable.

ONCOLOGY STAFF
(Tables 19a and 19b in the Appendix)

As Table 19a in the Appendix shows, those reporting cynicism as a stress symptom were 24 times more likely than those not doing so to score in the 'high/moderate' categories (i.e., as 'cases' in this analysis) of the MBI DP subscale. Those reporting emotional numbness/indifference were over nine times more likely than those who did not to score as an MBI DP 'case', while those reporting anxiety attacks as stress symptoms were over five times more likely to be so. Oncology staff were more than four times more likely to score as an MBI DP 'case' if they reported experiencing pessimism and hopelessness, and gastrointestinal disturbances as stress symptoms, and if they had found maintaining clinical confidence a work stress. Oncology staff were more than three times more likely to score as an MBI DP 'case' if they experienced problems in relations with patients associated with seeing them die, and with knowing they will die, and if they reported palpitations as stress symptoms.

For oncology staff, *independently significant predictors* of scoring as a 'case' (i.e., in the 'high–moderate' range) on the MBI DP subscale were having reported cynicism, emotional numbness/indifference, and anxiety attacks, as stress symptoms. ORs adjusted for all the modelled variables showed those self-reporting cynicism were over 21 times more likely to score as an MBI DP 'case' than those who did not. Those reporting emotional numbness were nine times more likely, and those reporting anxiety attacks were over four times more likely, to appear as an MBI DP 'case' than those not reporting these stress symptoms.

Identifying variables independently associated with MBI personal accomplishment (PA) subscale category scores

HIV/AIDS STAFF
(Tables 20a and 20b in the Appendix)

As summarised in Table 20a of the Appendix, HIV/AIDS staff taking six or more days off work for reasons other than holidays in the six months prior to interview were over 12 times more likely than those who had not done so to score as a 'case' on the MBI PA subscale – that is, to report a 'reduced sense of personal accomplishment'. Those staff having personal reasons for seeking work elsewhere than their current position were significantly less likely than those with work-related reasons to score as a 'case' on the MBI PA subscale.

For HIV/AIDS staff, neither of the variables modelled in Table 20b of the Appendix could reliably be described as independently significant predictors (at the 0.1 level) of scoring as a 'case' on the MBI PA subscale.

ONCOLOGY STAFF
(Tables 21a and 21b in the Appendix)

As shown in Table 21a of the Appendix, oncology staff were over four times more likely to score within the 'high-moderate' range of MBI PA subscale categories if they agreed that watching the physical decline of their patients was problematic in their relations with patients, than if they disagreed that this was so. Senior staff were significantly less likely to score as an MBI PA 'case' – i.e., within the 'high–moderate' range – than junior staff. When the cell was re-ordered, junior staff were found to be over four times more likely to score as having 'high–moderate' levels of reduced personal accomplishment on the MBI PA subscale (OR = 4.10, CI = 1.58 to 10.76; χ^2 = 9.36, 1 d.f., P = 0.002 not tabulated).

For oncology staff, both 'Problems with watching the physical decline of patients' and 'Professional seniority' were independently significant predictors of scoring as a 'case' on the MBI PA subscale (Table 21b in the Appendix). ORs adjusted for each show that those agreeing with the former were four times more likely to score as an MBI PA 'case', while senior staff were 0.26 times less likely to score thus than junior staff.

*Overall summary of results of assessment of independently significant
predictors of workplace stress*

The independently significant predictors of 'caseness' on both the self-report and
psychometric variables, based on logistic regressions, are summarised in Table 7.3.

Multi-variate analyses using the logistic regression method were subsequently
performed to see if each of these variables remained independently significant
after adjusting for sex, age, professional group, months of professional experience, and seniority. In all cases, they did so.

Overall, each of the seven variables assessed had independently significant
predictors, with the exception of MBI PA 'caseness' for the HIV/AIDS sample –
no independently significant predictors were found.

The HIV/AIDS sample revealed ten separate independently significant predictors on measures of work-related stress. MBI EE subscale category scores
predicted finding work stressful overall, while a history of potential exposure to

Table 7.3 Independently significant predictors of 'caseness' on selected variables

Variable + Question no.	HIV/AIDS	Oncology
Q.25. Work is stressful	MBI EE category score	103. How you generally feel; GHQ-28 total score; 37. Work environment is stressful
Q.87. Currently experiencing stress associated with work	9. Potential exposure to HIV since 1980	144.6. Problems communicating with colleagues; 145.9. Depression
Q.103. Generally feeling vulnerable/exhausted/ miserable	GHQ-28 total score; 143.8. Malaise	143.2. Lingering minor illnesses; 154. Making decisions about professional circumstances
GHQ-28 'Caseness'	103. Generally feeling vulnerable/exhaused/ miserable/; 145.9. Depression	144.10. Withdrawal; 143.6. Sleeplessness; 141.16. Maintaining clinical confidence is a work stress
MBI EE 'Caseness'	144.9. Self-righteousness ('heroism') 25. Finding work stressful 145.6. Pessimism and hopelessness	143.5. Palpitations; 93. More than 50% of colleagues are stressed; 141.20. Lack of training in death and dying; 141.18. Overwork
MBI DP 'Caseness'	145.1. Emotional numbness/ indifference	145.8. Cynicism; 145.1. Emotional numbness/ indifference
MBI PA 'Caseness'		155.6. Problems from watching the physical decline of patients

HIV since 1980 predicted currently experiencing work-related stress in HIV/ AIDS staff. Independently significant predictors of generally feeling 'vulnerable/ exhausted/miserable' were GHQ-28 'caseness', and malaise as a self-reported stress symptom. Predictors of GHQ-28 'caseness', on the other hand, were self-reported feeling 'vulnerable/exhausted/miserable', and depression as a self-reported stress symptom. Independently significant predictors of MBI EE subscale 'caseness' were finding work stressful, and self-righteousness ('heroism') and pessimism and hopelessness as self-reported stress symptoms. Finally, MBI DP 'caseness' for HIV/AIDS staff was independently predicted by self-reported emotional numbness/indifference as a stress symptom.

For oncology staff, there was only one independently significant predictor shared in common with HIV/AIDS staff – emotional numbness/indifference as a predictor of MBI DP 'caseness'.

Predictors of oncology staff reporting they found work stressful were feeling 'vulnerable/exhausted/miserable', scoring as a 'case' on the GHQ-28, and reporting that the work environment is stressful. Independently significant predictors of currently experiencing work-related stress included having problems communicating with colleagues, and the self-reported stress symptom of depression. Independently significant predictors of oncology staff feeling 'vulnerable/ exhausted/miserable' included the self-reported stress symptom of lingering minor illnesses, and reported difficulties in being able to make decisions about future professional circumstances. GHQ-28 'caseness' for oncology staff was independently significantly predicted by self-reported stress symptoms of withdrawal from non-involved colleagues and friends, and sleeplessness, and finding that maintaining clinical confidence was a work stress. MBI EE subscale 'caseness' was independently predicted by reporting palpitations, overwork, having more than 50 per cent of one's colleagues stressed, and reporting that a lack of training in death and dying is a work stress. MBI DP subscale 'caseness' in oncology workers was independently significantly predicted by self-reported stress symptoms of cynicism, and emotional numbness/indifference (the only predictor shared with HIV/AIDS staff). Finally, reporting staff–patient relationship problems associated with watching the physical decline of patients was the only independently significant predictor of MBI PA 'caseness' for oncology staff.

Discussion

Overall findings

All staff surveyed in this study reported physical work-related stress symptoms such as fatigue, behavioural problems such as irritation and agitation, and cognitive/affective work-related stress symptoms, including sadness and having problems concentrating. More than one-third overall reported feeling generally vulnerable, exhausted or miserable, and just under one-half overall scored as being vulnerable to psychological or psychiatric disturbance. A minority reported drinking and smoking to excess, but just over one-third reported they had experienced self-defined burnout in their jobs. Therefore, stress at work appeared to be a problem for those populations surveyed.

In considering characteristics associated with self-reported occupational morbidity, in staff working either in HIV/AIDS or oncology, only three areas of difference between the two groups were found. HIV/AIDS staff were significantly more likely to be stressed by the appearance of repeated or new infections in their patients, and by the way their work overlapped across professions, such as between physicians and paramedical staff. HIV/AIDS staff were significantly more likely than oncology staff to show stress as skin complaints, and by higher levels of cigarette smoking. On the other hand, HIV/AIDS staff also reported having more of a say in decision-making over their work than oncology staff.

There were few significant gender differences in self-reported work stress, although female staff reported more problems than males in revealing distress to work colleagues, they reportedly drank less alcohol, as do women in the general population (Smyth and Browne, 1992), and were less worried than males about how their work roles overlapped across professions. There were no significant differences between the sexes on psychometric indices of psychological vulnerability or work burnout. People 30 years of age and over were more likely than those younger to have known someone with burnout, and to see anger and prejudice within themselves as work stress symptoms. Also, they were more likely to over-identify with patients' needs.

Professional group differences primarily concerned the main professional groups' suggestions for reducing staff stress, whether by having fewer patients, more staff, or better National Health Service (NHS) service management. These are discussed in terms of social support and boosting the sense of professional efficacy.

More senior staff reported lower levels of work stress than juniors, and also reported lower levels of MBI-measured reduced personal accomplishment than junior staff – seniors felt higher levels of personal accomplishment. Junior staff reported more stress in work tasks with an emotional component, and were more likely to show emotional numbness or indifference as a stress symptom. More experienced staff (who were also more senior) were, however, more in touch with patients' needs, and were able to use a wider range of options for shutting off from work. Those with less experience reported more emotionally laden issues causing work stress.

In considering independently significant predictors of work-related stress, the HIV/AIDS population had 10 separate predictors emerging, and the oncology group had 17 – the only one shared between the two groups was emotional numbness/indifference being associated with scoring as a case on the MBI DP subscale. For both groups, MBI emotional exhaustion revealed the greatest number of independently significant associations. For oncology, there were more such associations in work-related issues than was the case for HIV/AIDS, where individual symptomatology predominated. These findings endorse the centrality of emotional exhaustion in the expression of reported workplace stress, and may indicate the relative individual isolation perceived by individual health care workers in oncology when compared with the binding focus and ethos shared by HIV/AIDS workers (formed as a consequence of the social and political dimensions associated with working in this field).

Signs and symptoms of workplace stress

Self-reported workplace stress was experienced by the majority of staff surveyed. Some 91 per cent overall reported they currently experience work-related stress, and two-thirds of these said their work stress had increased in the six months prior to being interviewed. Of those who said workplace stress had recently increased, almost one-half blamed structural changes in the NHS. This issue is discussed further below.

For most, stress was experienced as a fundamentally physical process involving symptoms associated with physical tension, fatigue or depletion. This is in keeping with the findings of Ullrich and FitzGerald (1990) in their study of Bavarian oncology physicians and nurses, although they were looking mainly for physical symptoms of stress and their correlates in these groups. In the MOMS study the most commonly reported physical symptoms of workplace stress included tiredness, sleeplessness, muscle pains, lingering minor illnesses and malaise.

In considering the range of self-reported stress symptoms, there is much consistency with earlier findings in the literature regarding symtoms of burnout, as summarised in Chapter 4. Indeed, although Maslach and Schaufeli (1993) emphasise 'mental and behavioural symptoms rather than physical symptoms' as typical of burnout presentations, the findings from this study were more in accord with the subjective diagnostic criteria for burnout proposed by Bibeau et al. (1989).

Overall, while two-thirds of those participating in this study said they generally felt 'fine or okay' when asked to describe their general (not just work-related) health state, it is a matter of concern that just over one-third of the frontline clinical staff participating said they generally felt 'vulnerable or exhausted or miserable'. These findings show that stress in the workplace does exist to a clinically measurable degree for a large minority of staff. Of interest is the degree to which these self-reported stress features associated with health worker characteristics match those found in assessing independently significant associations with burnout measures, as reported below. Also, these levels of self-reported stress imply that it is necessary to do something to reduce workplace stress if quality of care for patients is to be maintained or improved. Just what needs to be done depends on how stress does impact on staff.

For example, earlier research (Chapter 4) suggests that work stress is associated with behaviours that may potentially lead to ill health, such as drinking and smoking. In the present study, however, 19 per cent of alcohol drinkers said they were consuming 15 or more units of alcohol weekly – a smaller percentage than the 29 per cent and 30 per cent found on the General Household Survey (Smyth and Browne, 1992) and 1991 Health Survey respectively for the general population. Additionally, 20 per cent overall said they smoked 10 or more cigarettes daily, a proportion comparable with that found for the same occupational classes in each of the above-mentioned surveys of the general population. When looking at the associations between smoking and drinking levels, and scores on the GHQ-28 and MBI indicating the experience of work-related stress, no independent associations were found. Similarly, of those who had seen a physician in the six months prior to interview, 9 per cent had received prescriptions for the treatment of anxiety and/or depression (5 per cent overall) – a figure within global epidemiological trends suggesting no differences with normal population samples (Carnwath and Miller, 1986). Therefore, the findings from this study are not in agreement with those of Plant, Plant and Foster (1992), as smoking and drinking do not appear to be associated with workplace stress. One possible major contextual influence on workplace stress has been the recent NHS structural 'reforms'. Half those with recently increased workplace stress attributed the increase to NHS structural changes. At the time of the study, much concern was being expressed about how these changes were generating uncertainty over the merging of hospitals and departments, the pressure for staff to perform in a bewildering new 'market' culture with new jargon and the new rules, and fears for down-grading of professional status and of redundancies (Sheldon and Borowitz, 1993; Dickinson, 1995; Halton, 1995). For many staff, these structural changes in the NHS were occurring after their careers were established. Thus, the culture of their organisation was changing around them.

Such potential mismatching of organisational culture and personal aspirations was held by Cherniss (1980) to be at the heart of the development of burnout. Given the proportions of staff suggesting that such issues are generating an increase in work stress, it seems likely that organisational conditions that reflect wider structural changes would contribute independently to burnout in these populations. This matter is considered in view of the independently significant associations with burnout measures, below.

Differences in stress issues and levels between HIV/AIDS and oncology

Perhaps the most interesting feature of comparisons between the HIV/AIDS and oncology staff groups was how rarely significant differences were identified between the two. HIV/AIDS staff were significantly more stressed than oncology staff by the appearance of new or repeated infections in particular, and by the way their work overlapped across professions. HIV/AIDS staff did, however, report having more of a say in decision-making about their work circumstances. Stress appeared significantly more for HIV/AIDS staff as skin complaints, and they reported smoking more cigarettes each day than oncology staff, after sex, age and professional group were adjusted for. In all other respects, there were no significant differences found between HIV/AIDS and oncology groups. In considering why, attention will first be given to possible differences between the fields of HIV/AIDS and oncology, and then to possible similarities, that may have led to the results achieved.

As a clinical issue, the appearance of repeated or new infections in HIV/AIDS care would be an expected finding in each of the groups of HIV/AIDS and oncology, given the chronic, episodic nature of disease expression in each field (Gray-Toft and Anderson, 1980; Miller and Green, 1986). However, uncertainty about the appearance of serious, challenging infections and diseases, many of which have no adequately characterised management regimes, has been identified in this study as a source of significant stress in HIV/AIDS care. Perhaps this is significantly more so in HIV/AIDS because the appearance of HIV diseases can be so multifarious and unpredictable, implicating so many different body systems (Miller, Weber and Green, 1986).

Additionally, given the high level of identification of staff with patients reported in earlier studies of HIV/AIDS staff (e.g., Horstman and McKusick, 1986; Bennett, Michie and Kippax, 1991), the sense of being de-skilled and of having to witness seemingly inevitable physical decline with people who are seen regularly over periods of years, *and* of having additionally to up-date bad news, can be seen to compound the burden of both HIV/AIDS and oncology care. Findings in this study of independently significant associations with caseness on the GHQ-28, and the MBI emotional exhaustion and personal accomplishment subscales for oncology staff in particular, suggest that facing these issues could usefully be a component of a generic programme for staff stress management for those managing chronic, life-threatening disease.

As with the present study, Kleiber, Enzmann and Gusy (1995) found greater latitude and autonomy in decision-making in HIV/AIDS staff than in oncology staff. They also concluded that AIDS care management and its problems promotes a sense of professional identity, what anthropologists call *communitas*. Of course, it is important to be clear about those issues one's views can realistically influence. Being able to determine the colour of the staff room walls is possibly less gratifying potentially than being able to participate meaningfully in decisions about the conduct of clinical management on a daily basis. In this study, HIV/AIDS staff had more participation than oncology staff in decision-making over professional conditions and their professional future, but not over clinical decision-making. Further, so much of the ethos of HIV/AIDS care is multi-disciplinary, and this inevitably will involve role overlap and perhaps a blurring of management responsibility in some professions. Thus, increased self-reported stress associated with the way work overlaps across professions in this group is not surprising.

Although these findings are important for characterising stressors in care, the differences found between HIV/AIDS and oncology are relatively few in number. The findings of independently significant associations between MBI subscale scores and stress symptoms and issues in either field would suggest that the experience of stress is differently attributed by each, and that the experience of MBI-defined burnout may be more related to the institutional context of care than to specific topics of clinical management, or characteristics of the health worker. Independently significant associations of self-reported work stress and psycho-metrically measured burnout with field of care are discussed further in detail below.

Finally, if it is the case that reported stresses experienced in the two fields are largely comparable, this has important implications for management of occupational stress in these fields. For example, it means that options for management of occupational stress are very similar in each – while acknowledging issues of special significance to each.

Before such conclusions can be drawn, however, it is necessary to consider the roles that previously identified areas of importance for stress characterisation may play in shaping the design of occupational staff support programmes. These areas include gender, age, seniority, and professional experience.

Gender and workplace stress

It is likely that women actually predominate numerically in studies of health workplace stress and burnout, because a majority of nurses are female, and most such studies have involved nursing populations (Miller, 1991). Despite the gender imbalance in favour of women in research of this type, as in this study, the role of gender in the development of work stress and burnout is not yet well understood or well characterised. Recent work (Cordes and Dougherty, 1993; Roth, 1995) has begun to address this issue by emphasising the importance of sex-role socialisation and similar societal imperatives in gender-based reponses to workplace stress. For example, Roth (1995) suggests that societal imperatives, including sex-role socialisation, would influence the personal aims and expectations of work, and therefore vulnerability to burnout, if these embedded values are brought into confrontation with occupational values that do not acknowledge sex-role socialisation.

In the present study, gender differences in self-reported workplace stress included women finding it significantly more difficult than men to show distress about work-related issues, being significantly less likely than men to consume more than 15 units of alcohol weekly, and less likely to be concerned about how their work overlapped with that of other professions. No other gender differences significant at the 1 per cent level or less were found. Thus, only one of the significant differences, that concerning women reporting more difficulty in showing and communicating work-based distress, does not appear to conform to what might be expected from conventional sex-role stereotypes. Such stereotypes would predict that women are more likely to open up about problems, and are therefore more likely to report problems of an emotional nature in conversation.

If women are expected to disclose personal issues more openly, they may also disclose difficulties concerning their expected disclosure more as well. It may therefore be that women *reported* such difficulties in showing work-related distress proportionally more than men in the structured interview in this study, as a constrained expression of sex stereotyping.

Additionally, the lower concern among women about their work overlapping with work of other professions may also be a reflection of the preponderance of female nursing staff in this study. As suggested in Chapter 5, nurses have less agency over their role as health staff than other professions do – they have less authority to change their roles or work content, or how their work intersects with that of allied professions. It is conceivable therefore that, in knowing this, nurses have a lower investment in professional territorial overlap, because they know there is little they can do about it – hence the apparent lack of concern revealed in this study.

There was a noteworthy absence of any gender effects on MBI subscale scores. While other studies in health workers, such as those by Lemkau *et al.* (1987), and Bennett, Michie and Kippax (1991), also found no such gender effects, the fact that some studies have suggests that further evidence is required. Well-controlled studies in health workers by Maslach and Jackson (1985), and van Servellen and Leake (1993), suggest that men are more likely to have higher levels of depersonalisation, and Maslach and Jackson (1985) reported that female health workers are more likely to report higher levels of emotional exhaustion (although subsequent findings by Maslach and Jackson did not replicate this latter result). Thus, these present findings do not clarify this issue. Further explication of any gender effects on MBI subscale scores may require higher numbers of subjects so multivariate analyses have a better chance of demonstrating specific gender differences.

Age, seniority, professional experience and workplace stress

There were many similarities across these three variables, as might be expected given that seniority tends to increase with increasing age and experience. Indeed, it may be unnecessary to separate these factors in future studies. In examining the results of multivariate analyses involving these variables, there were few surprises.

As might be anticipated given their probable longer exposure to colleagues in related health services, at the 1 per cent level, people aged 30 years and over were significantly more likely than those aged less than 30 years to know colleagues who had experience of burnout.

Increasing professional experience was found by Bennett, Michie and Kippax (1991) to be a buffer for work stress – more experienced health staff were found to be less stressed by work – a result this study has confirmed. Senior staff were found to report lower stress levels at work, and to have an increased sense of personal accomplishment, compared with junior staff. Those with more experience were found to have lower levels of MBI-rated depersonalisation than less experienced staff, which corresponds with the finding that those 30 years of age and over were significantly more likely to over-identify with patients' needs.

The lower levels of stress among senior staff equates with the finding that those with eight years' experience or more reported significantly more options for shutting off from work – they appeared to have more ways of ensuring stress amelioration or avoidance. Perhaps they could afford their recreation more than those who were less experienced, less senior, and therefore earning lower salaries. Both Leiter (1991) and Cordes and Dougherty (1993) place considerable emphasis on those with more experience having more coping resources, and the results of this study tend to endorse this.

The increased depersonalisation and reduced personal accomplishment of the less experienced and junior staff fits Handy's (1987) observations of junior nurses being troubled by the apparent discrepancies between their therapeutic ideals and the conduct of daily ward routines. Increased levels of depersonalisation in junior staff also accords with Maslach and Jackson's (1981) MBI validation results. On the other hand, findings of significantly lower likelihood of having *reduced* personal accomplishment with more experience (i.e., being less alienated from, and more in touch with, patients' issues and needs, and feeling appropriately aware of achievements and successes in the work arena) run counter to the results of van Servellen and Leake (1993) – they found that older, more experienced nurses had significantly lower MBI emotional exhaustion scores, and those with more experience were significantly more likely to have lower personal accomplishment scores. While van Servellen and Leake (1993) suggested that increasing age and experience blunts a sense of professional accomplishment, the findings of the present study tend to suggest that experience brings heightened satisfaction and lower stress.

This finding appears ever more curious in view of increased age being significantly associated with anger and prejudice as a self-reported stress symptom in this study. While it is easy to suggest that this may be a consequence of the more experienced being less flexible, it is worth noting that the stress symptom was not directly attributed. That is, the anger and prejudice reported by staff may be directed at patients, or at colleagues, or perhaps more likely at NHS management changes. The latter is most likely, given that just under half those who reported an increase in stress in the six months prior to being interviewed said their stress was related to structural and management changes in the NHS. Those over 30 years of age were significantly more likely to over-identify with patients' needs – a finding which corroborates with the decreased depersonalisation in those with eight or more years experience: if they knew that structural changes placed the meeting of patients' needs in jeopardy, the potential for identification is obvious. It is also worth remembering that epidemiological data for the UK demonstrate that the majority of patients with HIV disease fall in the age range of 30 to 39 years.

Age alone did not appear to influence likelihood of appearing as a 'case' on the GHQ-28 or MBI subscales.

Junior and less experienced staff were united in being significantly more likely to report work stress associated with a lack of training in death and dying, having difficulties in showing work-related distress to colleagues, and reporting emotional numbness/indifference as a stress symptom. Junior staff were also significantly more likely to report work stress associated with a sense of danger in work tasks, involvements of patients' loved-ones, forming close relationships with patients, and breaking bad news to patients. Each of these issues can be viewed as indicative of the perils of inexperience, of being required to do greater proportions of 'hands-on' clinical work without a break, or without sufficient authority to manipulate personal work schedules, and with not having fully learned coping skills to assist in maintaining personal distance and a sense of informed, sympathetic professional confidence that only good experience can bring. Not surprisingly, therefore, junior staff were significantly more likely to score as having a reduced sense of personal accomplishment on the MBI PA subscale.

The pressure on junior staff to 'sink or swim' was also reflected in the finding that those with less than eight years' professional experience reported having less time to do their work, which generated work stress for them. They were more likely to score as a 'case' on the MBI depersonalisation subscale. This is also to be expected, given that the force of such stresses and work pressures conspires to alienate the health worker from those on whose behalf they work – patients are a main source of overwork, after all.

Finally, it is noteworthy that the sources of work stress in those with less clinical experience are largely features attributable to organisational circumstances, as Cordes and Dougherty (1993) predict. These include relevant training opportunities, danger-minimisation and clinical task demands. The lack of association of emotional exhaustion with either age, seniority or months of professional experience is, however, perhaps surprising, given that the trend in the results of this study is to equate higher levels and broader ranges of work stress with being junior, or having less health care workplace experience. Similar trends have been revealed in other studies reviewed in this book.

Professional group differences and workplace stress

The general lack of significant differences between professional groups at the 1 per cent level found in this study is not as may have been expected, given the different clinical responsibilities, levels of professional autonomy, roles, job security and organisational structures associated with health care work as physicians, nurses and paramedical staff (Cooper and Davidson, 1987). Some significant differences were found, however. Nurses were significantly more likely than physicians to have consulted a physician about their personal health in the six months prior to interview. Nurses were significantly more likely than paramedical staff to report work stress associated with breaking bad news, to both patients and their families.

Although few in number, these results indicate – contrary to those of Kleiber, Enzmann and Gusy (1995) in their study of health workers across the fields of HIV/AIDS, oncology and geriatrics – that there are professional differences in reported susceptibility to stress effects. Such differences had been found in a 1990 study by Ullrich and FitzGerald. They reported that nurses had more physical complaints than physicians because of the levels of physical exertion in their work. They also noted that proximity to dying patients was not related to reported stress symptomatology, however. For physicians, Ullrich and FitzGerald noted that identification with patients resulted in stress effects normally associated with patient rejection (what Maslach and Jackson [1981] would refer to as symptoms of depersonalisation). For nurses, however, over-identification with patients was associated with over-tiredness.

Important professional group differences emerging in this present study concerned ideas endorsed for reducing stress in the workplace: nurses thought that their work stress would be reduced by having more staff to work with. Physicians and paramedics, on the other hand, were more likely than nurses to think better service management and fewer patients would reduce work stress. It is interesting that in all three groups, options for work stress management are externalised – they are placed within the aegis of the organisation, not individual staff members. This runs contrary to conventional organisational approaches to staff stress management, which tend to posit responsibility for change within the stressed individual. Such staff suggestions fit those of Leiter (1991), who reccommends basing staff appraisals on group performance, or the performance of the staff unit (e.g., ward), reducing the harsh and inappropriate focus on individuals facing organisational stress.

In the current study, it seems that nursing staff were in fact asking for a bigger group to work with. Such an approach would offer greater opportunities for collegiality, and thus more scope for personal staff support. With physicians, on the other hand, having fewer patients would result in increased attention to those patients seen, with correspondingly increased opportunities for focusing on options for care and management, and closer therapeutic relationships. In addition, having more time for individual patients would also mean, for those physicians in out-patient services, being under less pressure to deal with people waiting in clinic waiting rooms immediately. Having fewer patients to see may accordingly increase the sense of professional and personal efficacy necessary for personal work stress reduction or management.

To summarise thus far, while the issues of field of health work, gender, age and professional group are all associated with self-reported stressors in the workplace, only seniority and professional experience appear to be significantly associated with burnout as measured on subscales of the MBI. This is surprising, given the findings from previously reviewed studies suggesting that all such issues may play a part in the development of burnout, and the parallels between stress symptoms identified in this study and burnout symptoms previously reviewed. Does this then mean that work stress is really different from burnout and, if so, how? In order to identify how these issues could be reconciled, characteristics of workplace stress (as opposed to health worker characteristics) were associated with self-reports of responses to current work stress and psychometric subscale scores on the GHQ-28, and the MBI, in order to identify those associations that were independently significant.

Factors independently associated with workplace stress and burnout

The main themes to emerge from the analyses of independently significant predictors of workplace stress and MBI-measured burnout in this study concerned the centrality of MBI emotional exhaustion as a core focus of identifiable self-reported burnout, and the significance of the GHQ-28 scores as a correlate of self-reported workplace stress. Additional themes included the significance of exposure to HIV as a stress predictor, and the relationship of stress symptoms based in the individual to those based in the organisational or institutional environment.

The centrality of emotional exhaustion

When asked 'is work stressful?', for HIV/AIDS staff, the only independently significant association was achieving a 'high/moderate' category score on the MBI emotional exhaustion (EE) subscale. This is perhaps surprising, given the variety of suggested stressors that HIV/AIDS staff encounter, and results found in earlier research (see Chapters 4 and 5). Kleiber, Enzmann and Gusy (1995), for example, found that emotional exhaustion was associated in HIV/AIDS staff with time pressure, lack of autonomy over decision-making, problems interacting with clients, and confrontation with death and dying. On the other hand, analyses of associations made between field of health care and MBI subscale scores revealed no significant associations with HIV/AIDS work. Maslach and Ozer (1995), in reviewing the potential significance of MBI-based research for HIV/AIDS workers, suggest that emotional exhaustion could be the *end-stage* experience of health staff having to face emotionally stressful activities, including working with difficult or unpleasant patients (and unpleasant disease states), breaking bad news, dealing with patients' deaths, and conflicts with co-workers and/or supervisors. HIV/AIDS staffs' responses to 'is your work stressful?' revealed significant associations that confirm the suggestion of Maslach and Ozer (1995) about links between occupational experience, in this instance deaths of patients, and MBI-measured emotional exhaustion.

When looking directly at independently significant associations with MBI EE subscale scores, for HIV/AIDS staff, self-reported stress symptoms of self-righteousness ('heroism'), and pessimism and hopelessness, were both independently significant. These variables are expected corollaries of emotional exhaustion – being stressed generally but affectively in particular, having communication difficulties with patients and with colleagues, needing to withdraw, while still over-identifying with the needs of the clinical situation, and feeling a sense of failure, depressed and pessimistic as a consequence (Cherniss, 1980; Maslach and Jackson, 1982; Cox, Kuk and Leiter, 1993). In this study, each of these issues are significant associations with MBI EE subscale scores for HIV/AIDS staff. As Cordes and Dougherty (1993) have characterised the burnout process, these features found in this study are what might be expected in the light of unrealistic personal demands in the face of mounting work pressure. The combination of these significant associations suggests strongly that this central aspect of the burnout experience is, for HIV/AIDS staff, focused around individually experienced consequences of stress and this, in turn, suggests that burnout and stress prevention must take account of the depth of emotional intensity and individual emotional isolation that can accompany the burnout process. The independently significant associations with MBI EE 'caseness' also reflect the psychological vulnerabilities that lead to scoring as a case on the GHQ-28 – a significant association with feeling generally exhausted, vulnerable and/or miserable. This is discussed further below.

It is noteworthy that the issues found to be independently associated with emotional exhaustion in HIV/AIDS staff by Kleiber, Enzmann and Gusy (1995) reflect quite closely those stressors associated both with MBI emotional exhaustion subscale scores, and generally feeling vulnerable, exhausted and/or miserable, in oncology staff. For oncology staff, independently significant associations with MBI EE subscale 'caseness' reflect expected symptom states and, more interestingly, contextual deficits not otherwise represented. Independently significant predictors of MBI EE subscale 'caseness' in oncology staff include 'Palpitations' and 'Overwork', both of which are unsurprising correlates of the states described earlier. The less expected predictors were 'Having more than 50 per cent of colleagues stressed', and 'Lack of training in death and dying'. Reporting more than half of one's colleagues as being stressed may be explicable insofar as working within a stressed milieu reduces opportunities for support from colleagues. Indeed, many staff reported that with their colleagues being stressed, they themselves felt it was inappropriate to take time away to receive support as this would simply increase the stresses on their already overstressed colleagues. As Leiter (1990) has noted, burnout appears to be a social pheno-menon – a shared experience reflecting the specific organisational dynamics. As a major element of the triumvirate of emotional exhaustion, depersonalisation, and reduced sense of personal accomplishment, the appearance of these independent predictors of emotional exhaustion fulfils in part expectations from earlier research findings.

In oncology staff, independently significant associations with MBI EE 'caseness' are predominantly environmentally based. That is, they concern circumstances of work rather than symptoms consequential to work, as many of the HIV/AIDS staffs' associations do. This highlights the importance of *context* in generating MBI-measured burnout (Cherniss, 1980; Leiter, 1991).

One of the consequences of having a broader range of environmental stressors associated independently with stress and burnout in oncology, as Kleiber, Enzmann and Gusy (1995) have noted, is that options for intervention are also correspondingly broader. Before arguing for the need to incorporate organisa-tional environmental awareness into the design of staff support, however, it is necessary to see the extent to which this is consistent, and how much this environmental focus may contrast with burnout associations in the HIV/AIDS sample.

Independently significant associations with other MBI subscale scores

The only independently significant association with 'caseness' on the MBI de-personalisation subscale, among HIV/AIDS staff, was the one most expected – 'Emotional numbness/indifference'. Depersonalisation is a process of detatch-ment, of avoiding over-involvement, of distancing oneself psychologically from patients, seeing them as symptom clusters whose views may be derogated. Significant associations with this variable in the present study reflected many of these issues and their corollaries – seniority (which frequently equates with increasing distance from closer and detailed relations with patients), relations becoming stressful with staff and with patients, difficulties in emotional support-seeking, and more familiar stress symptoms of lingering minor illnesses, gastro-intestinal disturbances and palpitations. Handy (1988) suggested that psychiatric nurses may employ avoidance and distancing from patients as a coping mechanism to help manage stresses including boredom and fatigue assciated with alternating periods of slackness and acute overwork. Cordes and Dougherty (1993) have also suggested that depersonalisation is also a socialised response in health professionals – it is something that enables vital distance from the intensity of patient distress, while also working to preserve appropriate professional detatchment.

The same findings apply for oncology staff, the only additional independently significant association with depersonalisation being the stress symptom, 'Cynicism'. A cynic is defined in *The Oxford English Dictionary* as 'one who shows a disposition to disbelieve in the sincerity or goodness of human motives and actions, and is wont to express this by sneers and sarcasms; a sneering fault-finder'. As such, cynicism appears an expected and appropriate association with deperson-alisation as defined under the auspices of the MBI! Given such entymological precedents, it is perhaps hardly surprising that Kleiber, Enzmann and Gusy (1995) reported depersonalisation in HIV/AIDS workers being significantly associated with problems in interacting with clients, much as one might expect with the emotional numbness/indifference reported in the present study.

For oncology staff, findings on the MBI reduced personal accomplishment variable apply as they do for HIV/AIDS staff. The expectations placed upon health workers, especially those working in specialist centres of publicly acknowledged prominence, to cure and to save and to fulfill instantly the promises of 'high-tech' medicine must be considerable. When they cannot be met, when patients continue to deteriorate and die, and when those patients are often known to staff for long periods of time so that their losses are felt not only professionally, one would expect problems to arise, not least a reduced sense of personal accomplishment. In view of this, finding that having problems from watching the physical decline of patients was an independently significant predictor for this variable was not unexpected. What *was* unexpected is that it was the only such predictor identified. A strong but not independently significant association was also found with professional seniority, with junior staff being 0.24 times as likely to score as a case on reduced personal accomplishment than senior staff. This is consistent with findings by seniority generally in this study – as opposed to findings only with oncology staff. Senior staff overall were found to have higher levels of personal accomplishment (that is, lower MBI reduced personal accomplishment scores) than junior staff, who were more likely than senior staff to have high–moderate scores on this variable indicating lower levels of personal accomplishment.

A further point relates to Leiter's (1991) suggestion that reduced sense of personal accomplishment develops in parallel with emotional exhaustion, as both are mediated in their development largely by the availability of social support. The opposite of emotional support in the workplace might be identified as having difficulties or problems communicating with colleagues, and the finding that this was an independently significant feature associated with oncology staff currently feeling work stress suggests that the development of reduced personal accomplishment was to be expected in this group. HIV/AIDS staff had no independently significant features associated with MBI reduced sense of personal accomplishment, but they also reported no problems communicating with colleagues. Given that Leiter's (1991) social support buffering hypothesis appears to have some confirmation with these results, it seems possible that provision of mechanisms for increasing social support in the oncology workplace (and in any other field of care) may help to immunise work settings against burnout among colleagues. As if to provide further support for this, an independently significant association with MBI emotional exhaustion in oncology staff was reporting that more than 50 per cent of colleagues are stressed at the time of the structured interview.

GHQ-28 scores and other correlates of workplace stress

The cluster of issues independently significantly associated with scoring as psychologically vulnerable on the GHQ-28, and with generally feeling vulnerable/exhausted/miserable, are internally consistent clinically. Together they reflect a sense of largely physical depletion that the GHQ-28 has a tendency to pick up. People with many physical symptoms associated with, for example, sleeplessness, agitation and distress, will usually be high scorers on the GHQ-28 as it is sensitive to responses reflecting these.

For the HIV/AIDS sample, independently significant associations with caseness on GHQ-28 total scores included generally feeling vulnerable/exhausted/miserable, and depression. In view of the relatively high numbers of associations with physical and cognitive/affective symptoms of anxiety at the 1 per cent level on this variable (see Table 14a in the Appendix), these findings are not surprising as the GHQ-28 contains a high loading of somatic indices that would normally be expected to identify such an associated symptom cluster (Goldberg and Williams, 1988).

The same conclusions may be drawn for the oncology staffs' as for those working in HIV/AIDS. The independently significant predictors 'Withdrawal', and 'Sleeplessness' are both to be expected as elements of the profile of psychological vulnerability that the GHQ-28 would identify. Further, associations at the 1 per cent level with issues concerning problematic relations with patients, sense of control over professional circumstances, confidence in clinical skills, and physical, behavioural and cogitive/affective stress symptoms reflect many of the major themes associated with anecdotal and empirical reports of health worker psychosocial vulnerability (see Chapters 4 and 5).

The independently significant associations with generally feeling vulnerable/exhausted/miserable for HIV/AIDS staff are those that would be expected for people suffering physical depletion and emotional stress, scoring as psychologically vulnerable on the GHQ-28, and malaise. It is noteworthy that these factors emerge from a group of variables (in Table 12a in the Appendix) describing many of the characteristics mentioned in the GHQ-28, and that are also correlates of social distress, such as a suffering primary emotional relationship, and withdrawal from others not involved in work in HIV/AIDS. Depression is clinically associated with social withdrawal, so its independently significant association in this context is to be expected. For oncology staff, the significant independent predictors on this variable – 'Lingering minor illnesses', and 'Being unable to make decisions about changes in professional activities and conditions' – emerge from a long list of physical, cognitive/affective, and behavioural stress symptoms (see Table 13b in the Appendix). What is surprising, therefore, is the lack of correlation with GHQ-28 total scores, or at least subscale category scores on the MBI.

While HIV/AIDS staff responses to work being stressful were independently associated only with MBI EE subscale category scores, oncology staffs' responses to agreeing that work is stressful were significantly independently associated with describing their general feeling at work as 'Vulnerable/exhausted/miserable'; also, by scoring as being psychologically vulnerable on the GHQ-28; and by reporting that the work environment is stressful. However, in looking again at the findings in Table 9a of the Appendix, many of the factors hypothesised as contributing to work stress by Cooper (1983), and by Warr (1990), and as confirmed in research involving oncology staffs discussed in Chapter 3, were indeed also identified as significant before these logistic regressions were performed. In addition to the variables identified above, currently experiencing stress at work, having more than 50 per cent of colleagues stressed at work, having insufficient time to work, feeling depressed, overworked, finding shutting off from work difficult and experiencing sleeplessness are all cited at the 1 per cent level.

As such, those variables that are independently significant predictors may be seen to represent 'clusters' of the issues that are not independently significant: The GHQ-28 is sensitive to physical symptoms and sequelae of stress, and has subscales for depressive phenomena. This shares many features that might encourage a respondent to report feeling vulnerable, exhausted, and/or miserable. The stress of a work environment may be compounded by time pressure, the stress of colleagues, and feeling overworked, as Kleiber, Enzmann and Gusy (1995), Leiter (1991) and Bennett, Michie and Kippax (1991) reported.

The importance of prior potential exposure to HIV as a stress predictor

The only independent significant predictor for HIV/AIDS staff currently experiencing stress at work was having 'a history of potential exposure to HIV since 1980'. This predictor was identified from a context including two stress symptom variables: inattention and distractability, and anger.

Even where there has been no prior self-identified risk of HIV exposure, studies have regularly shown that fear of HIV infection from patient (body fluid) contact is sufficient to generate and maintain prejudice against patients with HIV/AIDS (see Chapters 5 and 6). Teaching regimes to reduce stigma, prejudice and fear of patients with HIV/AIDS – and of managing them – are constantly, necessarily being reviewed and re-developed in order to reduce such concern for self-risk at work (e.g., Brimlow, 1995; Gallop and Taerk, 1995).

These results in the HIV/AIDS sample may therefore be explained by the closer proximity to HIV disease, and to the physical, psychological and psychosocial effects that people affected by HIV endure. Once again, where a population of staff has identified its potential for risk, and the consequences of that potential are drammatically and unavoidably expressed before (and by) them on a daily basis, perhaps their self-identified possibility of one day being on the receiving end of the care such as they provide is a more understandable cause of stress than otherwise might appear.

Stress in the individual and in the environment

The most commonly reported work stresses overall included overwork and having little new to offer, relationships with patients and with staff, deaths and decline in patients, and attitudes of some colleagues – one-third of those surveyed reported serious disagreements with colleagues. The most important issues giving rise to problems in relations with patients included having to watch patients decline and die, feeling professionally inadequate, and forming close relations with patients. Each of these reflect the expected litany of reasons for work stress consistently identified in studies reviewed earlier (Chapters 3–5).

Environmental variables reported overall to be contributing to work stress included having insufficient time to complete required work, and having inadequate working premises. Being able to relate openly to colleagues was problematic for many – three-quarters of respondents reported having felt professionally obstructed by colleagues at some time, and eight in ten overall reported feeling difficulties in showing work-related distress to colleagues. Quality of co-operation across professions was described as 'poor' by a similar number, although only one in ten said they could not participate to some degree in decision-making over clinical management.

As has been described frequently above, occupational stresses, and personally driven stresses such as professional expectations and demands on self-competence, are the issues that fuel the development of emotional exhaustion, either in parallel with, or soon followed by, depersonalisation and reduced sense of personal accomplishment (Leiter, 1991; Cordes and Dougherty, 1993). Yet in examining the independently significant associations found above, those associated with the HIV/AIDS staff group were based almost entirely in stress symptoms, and those found for oncology comprised a combination of physical, behavioural and affective stress symptoms, *and* environmental or contextual variables such as stressful conditions of work, lack of training, and difficulties with colleagues.

Possible reasons why this might be so have already emerged from a number of arenas. For example, the study by Kleiber, Enzmann and Gusy (1995), contrasting HIV/AIDS workers and oncology workers' responses to their jobs, found that HIV/AIDS staff had greater latitude and autonomy in decision-making than did oncology staff. These authors made the conclusion that HIV/AIDS care staffs' responses revealed a greater sense of professional identity. Similar suggestions have come from the work of Bennett and colleagues, using the AIDS Impact Scale to emphasise the notion that in addition to being stressful, HIV/AIDS work can also be very rewarding: peer identification and involvement is one of the structures upon which both reward and stress can be built.

Whether stress or reward comes from interaction with colleagues has been shown in this and other studies to be related to the degree of social support perceived in collegiate interactions. Having problems communicating with colleagues was independently significantly associated in this study with oncology staff currently finding work stressful. In addition, the unreported part of this study also revealed that friends of HIV/AIDS staff were significantly more supportive of their involvement in this work, than were oncology staffs' friends of their work arena (Miller and Gillies, 1996).

A further force in creating a sense of professional identity is shared adversity (Shilts, 1987; Sontag, 1990; Grimshaw, 1995). The newness of HIV has generated an ethos the world over of a continuum of care from hospital clinic to community (WHO, 1992, 1995), an ethos that has been welded in the socially cauterising fires of astonishing media attention and political and social marginalisation (Green and Miller, 1987; Shilts, 1987). It seems possible that while sympathetic others in oncology care may include extended families and loved-ones, in HIV/AIDS for so many the extended family by the bedside is the wider, equally marginalised community of peers, pressure groups, advocates and support groups. In other words, for those working and living with HIV, from marginalisation has grown a sense of social and professional cohesion. Where there is such social identity and movement, reflected in global awareness and political resource provision, work is a more dynamic environment where individual influence can perhaps be more likely. It seems not unlikely that where such conditions do exist, criticism is probably going to be directed at personal incapacity to sustain personal and social agendas, rather than towards the circumstances in which personal commitments are daily re-enacted. And where work attracts sympathy and social sanction, as in oncology, it seems probable that obstructive working circumstances are more likely to be isolated as stressors than personal consequences of them.

Of course, a feature of organisational development previously alluded to is the NHS structural changes that have occurred and been threatened in the services surveyed (Tomlinson, 1993). As suggested earlier, given the proportions of staff overall reporting that organisational changes have increased work stress, it would seem likely that organisational conditions reflecting wider structural change would contribute independently to burnout in the groups surveyed. However, while the oncology sites were certainly facing the reportedly unpalatable prospect of amalgamation and significant service retrenchment, HIV/AIDS had been a growth area in health in the UK during the period of the study, with ring-fenced monies for research and service development being curtailed only in 1995. Thus, it could be argued that to a significant degree, HIV/AIDS services had prospered while those for oncology had faced the threat of decline.

Additionally, the design of HIV/AIDS services has been shaped to a large degree by active collaboration between service-providers of all categories, and patients and patient advocate groups (Kaleeba, Ray, and Willmore, 1991). Oncology services may have much less flexibility – they are more established, and therefore probably less able to respond to suggestions for structural adjustment, wherever such suggestions may come from. In burnout terms, Leiter (1991) has described how increased capacity for participation in decision-making over work conditions in health care is equated with lower MBI scores. A reduced capacity would therefore be expected to appear as increased MBI subscale scores. This reflects the structural distinctions that can be drawn between HIV/AIDS and oncology. Once again, the contextual imperatives for attribution of workplace stress are unequal.

In terms of what this means for the distinction between burnout and work stress, these analyses support the notion of burnout being (a) a sub-category of stress, with (b) physical, cognitive/affective and behavioural sequelae (c) experienced differently in different settings. Only by applying associations with burnout subscales of the MBI have the social imperatives driving the expression of burnout been clarified. In this study it has been found, as suggested by Leiter (1991), that the experience of MBI-defined burnout appears to be more related to the institutional context of care than to specific topics of clinical management, or characteristics of the health worker. The burnout tryptich of emotional exhaustion, depersonalisation and reduced personal accomplishment therefore seems to be a very useful structure with which to tease apart social and organisational imperatives operating on the expression of individually felt, and organisationally experienced, workplace stressors and their consequences.

The question of how these findings may usefully influence the design of stress and burnout prevention strategies is addressed in detail in Chapter 10.

Note

1 In each of the data tables from the MOMS study in Chapters 7 and 8, and in the Appendix, the numbers before variables indicate the listing of the questions or variable in the Structured Interview Schedule and associated questionnaires.

8 The UK studies on staff preferences for support, and burnout management and prevention

A key element of the Multi-Centre Occupational Morbidity Study (MOMS) investigation concerned identifying staffs' current strategies for managing the stresses they experienced (Chapter 7), and their preferences for future staff support. In this aspect, the MOMS study was a forerunner to the later, qualitative UK Burnout Prevention Study, reported later below.

The methodology of the MOMS study has been described in detail in Chapter 7. The findings and discussion relevant to staff support will be presented below, and the second part of this chapter will consider the qualitative project of English HIV/AIDS staff support programmes known as the UK Burnout Prevention study.

MOMS: stress management and support preferences

Results

Present strategies for managing work-related stress

All staff were asked in their structured interview how they presently dealt with work-related stress. When asked if they had coping strategies which they used for managing moments of stress, 88 per cent overall (n = 179) said 'yes', and 12 per cent (n = 24) said 'no' or 'uncertain'. Overall,

- 48 per cent (n = 97) managed work-related stress by 'active management' – distracting activities (e.g., exercise, socialising, holidays), stress-prevention and management (including sleeping, relaxation, withdrawal), drinking and sex.
- 33 per cent (n = 68) dealt with work-related stress by talking about it with selected colleagues and/or friends.
- 19 per cent (n = 38) reported that their main strategies for managing work-related stress included attempting to focus more on work, working harder, re-organising, confronting stressful issues, or they don't have a strategy – they just 'keep going'.

Chi square tests of association were performed to determine the influence of age, sex, months of professional experience, professional group, seniority, HIV/AIDS or oncology work, GHQ-28 'caseness', and MBI subscale category scores on strategies chosen. Results are presented in Table 8.1.

As Table 8.1 shows, choice of main work stress-management strategy was not associated with differences according to 'caseness' on the GHQ-28, MBI EE or MBI DP subscale categories (despite high–moderate scorers on the MBI EE being much more likely to use stress prevention and relaxation strategies than low scorers), with seniority, months of professional experience, sex or age group. What this analysis does show can be summarised as follows:

- Males were significantly more likely than females (38 per cent versus 10 per cent) to use stress prevention and relaxation strategies, while females were more likely than males to use communication (37 per cent versus 21 per cent) and active distraction (35 per cent versus 20 per cent).
- Physicians were more likely to use work-focused strategies to manage work stress than nurses or paramedical staff (37 per cent versus 14 per cent and 22 per cent).
- Paramedical staff were more likely to use preventive and relaxation strategies than physicians or nurses (28 per cent versus 15 per cent and 12 per cent).
- Nurses were more likely to manage stress by methods of active distraction (37 per cent versus 18 per cent and 24 per cent).
- HIV/AIDS staff were more likely than oncology staff to rely on being more work-focused (29 per cent versus 8 per cent), and to employ stress-prevention and relaxation strategies (21 per cent versus 11 per cent).
- Oncology staff were more likely than HIV/AIDS staff to use communication (41 per cent versus 26 per cent) and active distraction (40 per cent versus 23 per cent) to manage work-related stress.
- Those scoring as 'high–moderate' on the MBI PA subscale were more likely to use communication (41 per cent versus 23 per cent), and less likely to use stress-prevention and relaxation strategies than people scoring 'low' (10 per cent versus 26 per cent).

When considering how strategies for managing work stress move from the workplace to the home environment, in order to see if they are different for the same people in different settings, those working harder in response to stress, and those with no work-stress management strategy, were not selected for the analyses. In taking the remainder of the two populations of HIV/AIDS and oncology workers together, 52 per cent (n = 59) cited 'communication with selected colleagues or friends' as their primary strategy overall, 32 per cent (n = 36) cited 'active distraction', and 16 per cent (n = 19) cited 'stress-prevention/ relaxation' as their main strategy. There was no significant difference between home and work-based strategies for managing work-related stress, where strategies were employed (χ^2 = 1.50, 4 d.f., P = 0.826).

Table 8.1 Main strategies for managing work-related stress

Variable	Category	Work stress management strategies:				χ^2	d.f.	P
		Work-focused	Communication	Active distraction	Relaxation/prevention			
Sex	Male	9 (21%)	9 (21%)	8 (20%)	16 (38%)	20.66	3	<0.001
	Female	29 (18%)	59 (37%)	56 (35%)	17 (10%)			
Age	0 – 30	14 (15%)	36 (39%)	32 (35%)	10 (11%)	6.26	3	0.099
	30 +	24 (22%)	32 (29%)	32 (29%)	23 (20%)			
Work field	HIV	30 (29%)	27 (26%)	24 (23%)	22 (21%)	23.25	3	<0.001
	Oncology	8 (8%)	41 (41%)	40 (40%)	11 (11%)			
Professional group	Physician	10 (37%)	8 (30%)	5 (18%)	4 (15%)	17.89	6	0.006
	Nurses	17 (14%)	47 (37%)	47 (37%)	15 (12%)			
	Paramedic	11 (22%)	13 (26%)	12 (24%)	14 (28%)			
Months of professional experience	0 – 48	10 (22%)	13 (28%)	14 (30%)	9 (20%)	3.82	6	0.701
	49–96	10 (16%)	26 (43%)	17 (28%)	8 (13%)			
	97 +	18 (19%)	29 (30%)	33 (34%)	16 (17%)			
Seniority	Senior	16 (19%)	24 (29%)	25 (30%)	18 (22%)	3.54	3	0.315
	Junior	22 (18%)	44 (37%)	39 (33%)	15 (12%)			
GHQ total scores*	0–4	21 (18%)	41 (34%)	37 (31%)	20 (17%)	0.12	3	0.988
	5–24	15 (18%)	27 (33%)	27 (33%)	13 (16%)			
MBI EE category scores*	High/Moderate	25 (18%)	44 (31%)	42 (30%)	29 (21%)	6.46	3	0.091
	Low	11 (18%)	24 (39%)	22 (36%)	4 (7%)			
MBI DP category scores*	High/Moderate	18 (25%)	22 (31%)	18 (25%)	14 (19%)	5.77	3	0.123
	Low	18 (14%)	46 (36%)	46 (36%)	19 (14%)			
MBI PA category scores*	High/Moderate	25 (20%)	50 (41%)	35 (29%)	12 (10%)	15.01	3	0.001
	Low	11 (14%)	18 (23%)	29 (37%)	21 (26%)			

*Two missing values

HIV/AIDS and oncology staff preferences for emotional staff support

OVERALL FINDINGS ON STAFF SUPPORT PREFERENCES

Overall, there were substantial levels of agreement on many of the variables presented in this section of the structured interview schedule. For example, 75 per cent of the total sample (n = 152) said there were *factors making emotional support-seeking difficult for them at work*. When asked what these factors were, results for combined categories (combined to enable sufficient numbers for univariate analyses) were as follows:

- 69 per cent (n = 105) said lack of trust in how colleagues would handle information about their vulnerability, together with the sense that expressions of emotion would be interpreted as a lack of professionalism or a sign of being unfit to do their job.
- 31 per cent (n = 47) cited a lack of resources, including no personnel cover, absence of a facilitator, and the sense of adding to the burden of stressed colleagues by taking time away to deal with their own stress.

Staff were also asked to 'construct' their preferred staff support programme. When asked 'where they would prefer their staff support to be provided from', 66 per cent (n = 134) said from *outside* their organisation or institution, 15 per cent (n = 30) said from *inside* their organisation or institution, 18 per cent (n = 36) said from both outside and inside, and the remaining 1 per cent (n = 3) said 'neither'. When asked why they had answered this way, 53 per cent (n = 106) cited *facilitator issues*, including the greater understanding and accessibility of insiders, and the greater neutrality, confidentiality and clarity of perspective of outside facilitators as their main reason; 36 per cent (n = 72) cited issues of lack of trust in colleagues' reactions, insider impartiality, and not wanting to burden colleagues as their main reason; and 11 per cent (n = 23) cited other reasons, including satisfaction with the present arrangements, and caution about the efficacy of some methods – e.g., group support – as their main reasons.

When asked their preferred *form* of staff support, 54 per cent (n = 109) stated 'Individual' support, 12 per cent (n = 25) replied 'Group' support, 10 per cent (n = 20) said 'Either', and 24 per cent (n = 48) said 'Both' (as long as individual support was combined with group support).

Those with no present access to a support programme were asked if they would like such a service to be made available to them. Of 173 replies, 96 per cent (n = 166) said 'Yes'. When asked 'what they personally would like to talk about' in the context of staff support, 56 per cent (n = 111) said 'Professional issues and coping' – reviewing coping strategies for problems at work; 27 per cent (n = 54) said 'Personal feelings and issues' – about patients, bereavements and relationships outside the workplace; and 17 per cent (n = 33) said 'Whatever arises', or 'NHS structural, management and ethos changes' as their preferred topics of discussion.

Staff cited the following *requirements they would have* of a staff support programme if they were to feel *confident* about using it:

- 57 per cent (n = 115) said 'Confidentiality' – no sharing of information arising in staff support sessions with anyone.
- 29 per cent (n = 59) said 'Structural and process issues' – having support completely unlinked to service management (i.e., no feedback to bosses), being accessible, with clear boundaries and carefully selected groups, clear expectations of what is happening and a constructive atmosphere.
- 14 per cent (n = 26) said 'Facilitator issues' – facilitators would need to be trustworthy, experienced, neutral, qualified, and understand hospital procedures and pressures.

In this vein, staff were asked if they felt able to turn to selected colleagues for emotional support at work: While 16 per cent (n = 32) said 'No' or were 'Uncertain', 84 per cent (n = 171) said 'Yes' or 'Sometimes'.

COMPARING HIV/AIDS AND ONCOLOGY STAFF GROUPS

First, both HIV/AIDS and oncology samples were compared on their grouped answers to questions in the structured interview schedule regarding their preferences for formal emotional staff support. Findings are presented in Table 8.2, and reveal statisticaly significant differences between the HIV/AIDS and oncology samples on a number of variables:

- HIV/AIDS staff reported formal programmes for providing emotional support to staff as being more available.
- More oncology staff reported factors making emotional support-seeking difficult at work (82 per cent versus 68 per cent of HIV staff).
- Issues of trust, professionalism and position were reported more often as factors making emotional support-seeking difficult by oncology staff (78 per cent versus 59 per cent).
- Oncology staff wanted more individual staff support than HIV/AIDS staff (64 per cent versus 44 per cent).
- HIV/AIDS staff wanted to discuss personal feelings and issues significantly more often than oncology staff (35 per cent versus 19 per cent), and significantly more oncology staff than HIV/AIDS staff had no fixed agenda, citing 'whatever arises/ethos issues' (23 per cent versus 10 per cent).

Multivariate analyses adjusting for age, sex, professional group, months of professional experience, seniority and 'caseness' on the GHQ-28 and MBI subscales were attempted with each of the variables whose associations with HIV/oncology were significant at the 5 per cent level or less. For question 62, 'Are there factors making emotional support-seeking difficult for you at work?', after adjusting for age, sex, professional group, months of professional experience, seniority and 'caseness' on the GHQ-28 and MBI subscales, scoring as a 'case' on the GHQ-28 remained significant (OR = 2.28, 95 per cent, CI = 1.05 to 4.95, P = 0.038, LRS on 2 d.f. = 61.29).

Table 8.2 Preferences for staff support by HIV/AIDS and oncology

Variable	HIV/AIDS	Oncology	χ^2	d.f.	P
Q.58. Do you have a formal programme for providing emotional support to staff in your workplace?					
No	69 (67%)	99 (99%)	34.22	1	<0.001
Yes	34 (33%)	1 (1%)			
Q.62. Are there factors making emotional support-seeking difficult for you at work?					
Yes	70 (68%)	82 (82%)	4.59	1	0.032
No	33 (32%)	18 (18%)			
Q.63. If yes, what are they?					
Trust/professionalism and position	41 (59%)	64 (78%)	5.82	1	0.015
Lack of resources	29 (41%)	18 (22%)			
Q.64. If you had the choice, would you rather have access to staff support:					
From outside	67 (66%)	67 (67%)	0.56	2	0.756
From inside	14 (14%)	16 (16%)			
From both	20 (20%)	16 (16%)			
Q.65. For what reasons?					
Lack of trust in colleagues	37 (37%)	35 (35%)			
Facilitator issues	50 (49%)	56 (56%)	1.48	2	0.477
Other issues	14 (14%)	9 (9%)			
Q.66. Would you prefer support in:					
A group	15 (15%)	10 (10%)			
Individually	45 (44%)	64 (64%)	8.09	3	0.044
Either	12 (12%)	8 (8%)			
Both	30 (29%)	18 (18%)			
Q.68. What issues would you personally like to talk about in the context of staff emotional support?					
Professional issues and coping	54 (55%)	57 (57%)	9.94	2	0.006
Personal feelings and issues	35 (35%)	19 (19%)			
Whatever arises/ethos issues	10 (10%)	23 (23%)			
Q.69. What requirements would you have to feel confident about using a staff support programme?					
Confidentiality	51 (50%)	64 (64%)	4.21	2	0.122
Structural and process issues	34 (34%)	25 (25%)			
Facilitator issues	16 (16%)	10 (10%)			
Q.70. Do you feel able to turn to some colleagues for emotional support at work?					
No	15 (15%)	17 (17%)	0.08	1	0.776
Yes	88 (85%)	83 (83%)			

Months of professional experience   As Table 8.3 shows, those HIV/AIDS staff with *less* professional experience (measured in months) found lack of resources to be the most important factor making emotional support-seeking difficult at work. Those with intermediate experience appeared less likely to report lack of trust in colleagues as a reason for wanting staff support from wherever they had chosen. Chi square tests of association were performed to test the hypothesis that this result might reflect a sense of greater job security with increased job experience. However, no significant results were found to confirm this hypothesis, either for the combined sample ($\chi^2 = 3.03$, 2 d.f., $P = 0.219$), or for HIV/AIDS ($\chi^2 = 0.36$, 2 d.f., $P = 0.832$) and oncology staff ($\chi^2 = 2.39$, 2 d.f., $P = 0.302$) separately. Finally, proportionally more staff with most professional experience wanted to talk about professional issues and professional coping than about other subjects. We should therefore expect MBI DP subscale category scores to be greater in those with more professional experience. This was not borne out in the multivariate analyses looking at months of professional experience (Chapter 7 and Tables 7, 18a and 18b in the Appendix). Furthermore, these analyses showed that people with more professional experience are actually less likely to show distress about work-related issues.

More of the *least experienced* in terms of time since qualification wanted to talk about personal feelings and issues, perhaps reflecting their relative lack of experience in learning to cope with emotionally challenging aspects of their work. While months of professional experience *per se* did not have an association with MBI EE subscale category scores at the 1 per cent level, many of the features associated with emotional exhaustion, including symptoms of stress, lowered clinical confidence, and difficulties in relations with patients, *and* scores indicating vulnerability and 'caseness' on the GHQ, did (Table 8.4).

Table 8.3 HIV/AIDS staff – months of professional experience

Variable	Professional experience (months)					
	0–48	49–96	>97	χ^2	d.f.	P
Q.63. Factors making emotional support-seeking difficult at work						
Trust/professionalism and position	9 (22%)	16 (39%)	16 (39%)	11.590	2	0.003
Lack of resources	18 (62%)	5 (17%)	6 (21%)			
Q.65. Why would you prefer staff support from outside, inside or both?						
Lack of trust in colleagues	15 (40%)	5 (14%)	17 (46%)	13.410	4	0.009
Facilitator issues	16 (32%)	19 (38%)	15 (30%)			
Other issues	2 (14%)	9 (64%)	3 (22%)			
Q.68. What issues would you personally like to talk about in the context of staff emotional support?						
Professional issues and coping	15 (28%)	17 (31%)	22 (41%)	8.941	4	0.062
Personal feelings and issues	16 (46%)	13 (37%)	6 (17%)			
Whatever arises/ethos issues	2 (20%)	2 (20%)	6 (60%)			

Table 8.4 Preferences for staff support – associations with GHQ-28 total scores

Variable	Cases >5	Control <4	χ^2	d.f.	P
Q.62. Are there factors making emotional support-seeking difficult for you at work?					
Yes	70 (46%)	81 (54%)	6.87	1	0.008
No	12 (24%)	38 (76%)			
Q.63. If yes, what are they?					
Trust/professionalism and position	45 (43%)	59 (57%)	0.91	1	0.339
Lack of resources	29 (41%)	18 (22%)			
Q.64. If you had the choice, would you rather have access to staff support:					
From outside	57 (43%)	75 (57%)	1.95	2	0.377
From inside	13 (43%)	17 (57%)			
From both	11 (31%)	25 (69%)			
Q.65. For what reasons?					
Lack of trust in colleagues	34 (47%)	38 (53%)	3.31	2	0.191
Facilitator issues	42 (40%)	63 (60%)			
Other issues	6 (26%)	17 (74%)			
Q.66. Would you prefer support in:					
A group	9 (36%)	16 (64%)	0.71	3	0.869
Individually	43 (40%)	65 (60%)			
Either	9 (45%)	11 (55%)			
Both	21 (45%)	26 (55%)			
Q.68. What issues would you personally like to talk about in the context of staff emotional support?					
Professional issues and coping	48 (44%)	61 (56%)	0.65	2	0.722
Personal feelings and issues	22 (41%)	32 (59%)			
Whatever arises/ethos issues	12 (36%)	21 (64%)			
Q.69. What requirements would you have to feel confident about using a staff support programme?					
Confidentiality	45 (40%)1	68 (60%)	0.67	2	0.715
Structural and process issues	27 (46%)	32 (54%)			
Facilitator issues	10 (38%)	16 (62%)			
Q.70. Do you feel able to turn to some colleagues for emotional support at work?					
No	16 (50%)	16 (50%)	0.92	1	0.337
Yes	66 (39%)	103 (61%)			

In a similar vein, less experienced HIV/AIDS staff were more likely to find factors making emotional support-seeking more difficult at work, although this was just outside the level of significance ($\chi^2 = 3.58$, 1 d.f., $P = 0.058$).

Level of professional experience (in months) had no statistically significant association with finding difficulties in emotional support-seeking, with decisions about where staff support should come from (i.e., from outside, inside or both), with preferences for modes of staff support, or with requirements for confident use of staff support. No multivariate analyses were therefore performed.

Professional group, gender, seniority and age   Overall, in considering preferences for staff support, no significant associations were found with professional group, gender, age or seniority for the HIV/AIDS group. Similarly, there were no significant associations with staff support variables for professional group, gender, age or seniority for the oncology group. Additionally, the oncology group showed no significant association between staff support variables and length of professional experience.

GHQ-28 total scores   Univariate analyses of responses to structured interview questions based on 'caseness' (i.e., scoring 5 or more) on the GHQ-28 were performed (see Table 8.4), and the only significant finding concerned question 62 ('Factors making emotional support-seeking difficult at work'). 'Cases' on the GHQ-28 (those scoring 5 or more) reported significantly more factors than 'non-cases' making emotional support-seeking difficult at work. This association no longer remained significant after subsequent multi-variate analyses adjusting for HIV/AIDS or oncology, age, gender, professional group, months of professional experience, and seniority.

MBI subscale category scores   In univariate analyses, only one significant association was found between MBI subscale category scores and preferences for staff support: People scoring in the low category of 'Personal accomplishment' subscale were significantly more likely to want to discuss personal feelings and issues in their staff support sessions ($\chi^2 = 10.28$, 2 d.f., $P = 0.005$).

This general absence of associations with MBI subscale category scores, apart from the MBIPA subscale, is perhaps surprising, given that total scores on the GHQ-28 were significantly associated with many of the symptoms associated with MBI EE 'caseness' (see Chapter 7).

Summary of findings on preferences for staff support

When examining strategies typically employed to reduce stress associated with work, significant differences in approach were found according to gender, professional group, HIV/Oncology, and MBI PA subscale category scores. There was no significant difference found between home-based and work-based strategies employed to manage work-related stress.

Overall, 75 per cent (n = 152) identified factors making emotional support-seeking difficult for them at work, the most commonly cited being a lack of trust in colleagues' use of information to be divulged, and anxiety that expressions of vulnerability would be seen as unprofessional, or indicating unsuitability for their work.

The majority of staff surveyed would prefer staff support to come from outside their organisation, and most wanted individual rather than group support. For content, just over one-half of those questioned wanted to use support sessions as an opportunity for learning how to cope better with work stress; personal feelings and issues were cited by one-quarter of those surveyed as preferred topics for staff support, indicating that non-work issues are also on the support agenda for a significant minority of staff. In order to feel comfortable about using staff support, confidentiality and well-designed and agreed procedures were required to be in place by potential users.

In examining the hypothesis that there were no differences between HIV/AIDS and oncology in preferences for staff support, significant differences between the two groups were found for factors making emotional support-seeking difficult at work – trust, professionalism and position were more obstructive for oncology staff. More oncology staff wanted individual support, and more HIV/AIDS than oncology staff wanted to discuss personal feelings and issues.

Preferences for staff support and experiences of its accessibility were also mediated by length of professional experience in the HIV/AIDS group. Scoring as a 'case' on the GHQ-28, and scoring as a 'non-case' on the MBI PA subscale was significantly associated with wanting to discuss personal feelings and issues (as these staff were presumably accomplishing work tasks more).

These findings will be discussed in the context of the models of staff support identified in the second study to be discussed – the UK Burnout Prevention study, and the relevance of earlier approaches will be questioned in view of them in Chapter 10.

The UK Burnout Prevention Study

Subsequent to the MOMS study, a second national multi-centre was undertaken (Miller, Gillies and Elliott, 1996), with the following aims:

- To identify and describe stresses arising from HIV/AIDS care, and the effects of these on the occupational setting.
- To characterise models of staff support for HIV/AIDS health workers currently operating.
- To examine the organisational features that affected the impact of these models over time.
- To assess the overall impact of structured models of staff support.
- To make recommendations for future staff support interventions.

Methods

This was a two-phase study. Phase I involved a detailed literature review, in-depth interviews of key staff from six national HIV/AIDS care sites, and a postal survey of key features of staff support activities in five more. The aim of Phase I was to identify and characterise the models of staff support available, and to select sites for Phase II.

The six sites selected for *Phase I* had the following organisational characteristics:

1   *Site 1* – A major hospital facility with a variety of linked but discrete services for specific patient groups, including a haemophilia unit, a ward for in-patients, an AIDS counselling unit (in- and out-patient counselling, and same-day HIV test counselling), and telephone counselling in a context of out-patient clinical management and monitoring.

2   *Site 2* – A Christian in-patient hospice providing palliative care for people with AIDS and their loved-ones. A total of 28 in-patient beds on three wards, and day care were provided. The ward teams had a ratio of 19 staff for eight beds, and there were 71 volunteer staff.

3   *Site 3* – A community-based peer-led HIV/AIDS support organisation comprising 25 paid staff and 115 volunteers. Direct services were provided in a day centre with administrative services based in a separate site. Volunteers worked either in the day centre, as transport volunteers, or by providing practical and emotional support in service users' homes.

4   *Site 4* – A major voluntary organisation (outside Greater London) providing practical HIV/AIDS services for people affected by HIV, including emotional support and counselling, practical home and community support, financial support, complementary therapies, advocacy, health education, campaign work and training. There were six full-time paid staff, and 116 volunteers.

5   *Site 5* – A charity providing an extensive range of in- and out-patient medical, respite and psychosocial services for people affected by HIV. Direct and indirect support is provided through a drop-in centre and cafe, counselling and support groups, creative and complementary therapies, day care, community services, education, training and residential activities. The total staff complement included 150 paid and 350 unpaid employees.

6   *Site 6* – A palliative care team providing an outreach service to people within central London – i.e., working with people with AIDS and their loved-ones in their own homes, responding to a wide network of liaison from the central London statutory health care establishment. Shortly after the study started, the team amalgamated with neighbouring palliative care services for oncology.

Phase II involved a longitudinal, prospective interview survey of HIV/AIDS staff at four selected sites (the first four sites described in Phase I), the eligible staff being interviewed at six-month intervals. By employing piloted structured interview schedules, the aim was to examine the 'life' of staff support activities over a six-month period, to determine outcomes relative to the models used, and to identify transferrable lessons for the design of prospective staff support activities. The structured interview schedule included questions on the following issues:

• Staff occupational demographic data and health indices.
• Experiences of workplace stress, and individual approaches to management.
• The nature of staff support currently provided.
• Satisfaction with staff support.
• Content of staff support.

- Difficulties and obstacles with staff support.
- Impact of staff support on workplace issues.
- Impact of workplace issues on the conduct and outcome of staff support.
- Suggestions and preferences for constructive change of staff support activities.

Phase II also involved repeated measures of staff morbidity using the GHQ-28, and the MBI, and the prospective examination of staff absence records. Interviews lasted about 50 minutes.

Staff were selected for Phase II according to the same applicable criteria as staff in the MOMS study.

Results

Phase I

Defining characteristics of staff support sites

Most of the organisations surveyed were relatively small (i.e., less than 20 full-time paid staff). Similarly, most had – whether statutory or non-statutory – highly respected and charismatic leadership which had taken a pro-active stance towards staff welfare. In the non-statutory services, *heirarchy* appeared to be less pronounced, and access to upper staff levels seemed easier and more immediate than in the statutory and hospital facilities.

In non-statutory services, professionalism appeared to embody a requirement that *personal vulnerability be acknowledged*, whereas in statutory services the opposite appeared to be the case. Also, what emerged clearly was the critical importance of management endorsing staff support procedures (even if very senior staff did not use them).

Professional mix did not appear to be considered controversial or an obstacle within service support activities, and many services' support activities were facilitated by 'other' professions on an external basis.

The content of support was not usually not pre-determined, and some services actively allowed discussion of external personal issues of relevance to the work-place. Only two services identified any theoretical underpinning to their staff support programme.

Models and content of staff support activities

The models and content of staff support employed in the six main sites (not in the postal survey) are shown in Table 8.5. In addition, the specific features potentially affecting the outcome of staff support at these sites were noted.

Costs and benefits of providing staff support

Most services maintained no records of the impact or outcomes of staff support activities. Few of the organisations contacted could identify specific costs associated with staff support. However, costs in terms of time appeared to be minimal, with monthly meetings for professional supervision being the norm. Having instant access in times of crisis was a feature of most organisations. Three of the sites suggested that the virtual absence of days taken off sick and staff turnover was attributable to provision of on-going and sympathetic staff support.

Much more work is clearly needed on quantification of costs associated with provision and non-provision of staff support.

Transferrable concepts and ensuring viability of staff support

A critical element in ensuring the success of staff support was maintaining *confidentiality* – with no direct feedback to management when emotional support is being given by external consultants. Similarly, maintaining confidentiality within support groups was seen as a vital ground-rule.

Support services were seen by most as requiring *multi-layering* – that is, more than one function was seen to be served by support programmes in the workplace. One leading staff support protagonist asserted that '. . . support for stress management actually needs to be placed in a context of broad staff management, including welfare and legal support, occupational development *and* supportive counselling.'

Support was seen by all those interviewed as something that belonged in the working week *as a part of the paid working week* – not an additional 'extra'. Support programmes were also considered to be most successful where they were designed into services from the start of those services.

Overall lessons and key criteria by which future staff support programmes may be characterised and assessed are summarised in Table 8.6.

Phase II

This section will confine itself to a discussion of respondents' characteristics, and consideration of some qualitative features regarding staff support. Quantitative data relate to two separate interviews of each respondent, separated by six months. Sites 1–4 in Phase I were used as the study sites in Phase II.

Response rates and demographic details

At the four sites, a total of 85 staff were recruited into the study. At the two non-statutory agencies all staff volunteered. At site B, where a recent staff re-organisation resulted in redundancies and generally perceived staff uncertainties and reluctance, only 25 per cent volunteered.

Participants came from a wide variety of professional groups, although this was not uniform across sites – non-statutory services, for example, had no medical or formal health personnel. Therefore, staff in these sites are included in the category of 'other', comprising administrative and clerical staff, outreach workers, managers, etc.

Table 8.5 Models and content of staff support at six UK sites

Staff support characteristics	Site 1	Site 2	Site 3
Staff support aims	To increase professional skills in managing crises and develop case management skills	• To enhance mutual appreciation in staff; • To deal with ward emergencies	• To provide regular support for staff; • To empower staff; • To resolve staff-related difficulties
Theoretical basis	Systemic Family Therapy Model	None defined	None defined
Nature of staff support	Varied according to service: • Weekly–monthly professional supervision; • Groups, and individual support if requested; • 4 × yearly individual performance review; • Case conferences as necessary	• Staff groups externally counselled 3-weekly; • Individual on-site counselling if required with counsellor or chaplain; • Staff masseur(euse) on request	• Fortnightly groups facilitated externally every third meeting; • Some complementary therapies available; • Management supervision every 2–3 weeks; • Up to six counselling individual sessions on request; • Volunteers' fortnightly group; • Volunteers' consultative group
Content of staff support	Biased towards development of professional capacities for conflict resolution	• Opportunities for discussion; • Affirmation exercises	• Open agenda – work and non-work issues; • Supervision work issues, personal development and emotional support; • Information for volunteers, also covering practical and policy issues
Recorded impact on staff illness, turnover and attendance	• No records available; • Impact informally measured by the number and quality of ideas gleaned from staff and groups per supervision session	• No records available during Phase I; • Variable attendance for support due to shiftwork	• 87% of staff attend support regularly; • No paid staff turnover in two years; • Sickness rates 'not high'
Specific features affecting outcome	• Absence of HIV/AIDS stigma in hospital; • Regular opportunity to off-load work issues; • Staff are trained in appropriate use of supervision time	• Staff closely bonded and mutually supportive (shared Christian ethos); • Professional hierarchy downplayed; • Small organisation with focused aims; • Managers look out for stress signs; • Ward staff breakfast together every day; • Adequate staff:patient ratios	• Small organisation + easy communication; • Much gay/lesbian mutual support; • Close identification + concern with clients; • Clear ground rules and boundaries re: confidentiality; • Complete management acceptance of support + stable frequency of meetings

Table 8.5 (continued)

Staff support characteristics	Site 4	Site 5	Site 6
Staff support aims	• Case-work monitoring; • Emotional support + affirmation (external)	• Supporting staff in their work; • To provide focus away from work, to relax	• Professional support; • Personal supervision
Theoretical basis	None defined	Co-counselling	None defined
Nature of staff support	• Monthly internal supervision by service Director; • External support on request; • Monthly volunteer support groups	Varies according to staff role: • Weekly entitlement of 1.5 hours group support, internally facilitated; • Supervision by group heads for counselling staff + paid external counselling as needed	• Weekly team meetings; • Weekly personal supervision by team Director; • 4 × yearly external group support; • Acute individual support as required
Content of staff support	• Review previous meeting notes and assess progress; • Staff inter-relationships; • Professional development; • Any personal issues raised by staff	Not available	• Difficult clinical situations; • Patients' family and relationship dynamics; • Responses to novel challenges
Recorded impact on staff absence and turnover	• 100% of paid staff in supervision; • Illness/absence/turnover 'rare'	• 80% of staff in support; • No data on staff absence or turnover	• No records available; • Attendance 'mandatory'
Specific features affecting outcome	• Recognised importance of staff support and making time for it; • Having staff support not seen as a sign of weakness; • Asking for help seen as a sign of strength	• Jobs not critically dependent on individuals; • Clear management structure and individual responsibilities; • 6 weeks paid holiday per year; • No overt 'tyranny of professionalism'; • Favourable sick-pay arrangements; • Good team spirit	• Trusting relationships among colleagues; • Regularity of sessions; • Committed attendance; • Adherence to confidentiality; • Relatively small unit size

Table 8.6 Key features contributing to the success of staff support

Management
- Management must lead by giving overt and consistent endorsement to staff support;
- Management must have a clear structure and be easily accessible by staff;
- Management should be honest with staff about the successes and difficulties being faced

Access
- Staff must be aware of how to access appropriate support;
- Differing types of support should be available and quickly accessible;
- Support should be available to all staff;
- Support should be part of work and take place within paid work time;
- Support should take place on a regular basis (fortnightly/monthly)

Confidentiality
- Support must be confidential and unlinked to management;
- Ground rules need to be established as regards confidentiality and reviewed regularly

Other features
- The aims and procedures for staff support must be clarified for those giving it and those receiving it in advance of it being started;
- Support is enhanced where there is a distinct organisation identity and ethos;
- Smaller-sized units appear to have better morale;
- Professional supervision must be distinguished from emotional support;
- Support by professional supervision should follow a clear format;
- Volunteers require different approaches in staff support;
- Content of support provisions should be flexible;
- Staff heirarchies should be de-emphasised;
- Staff should be trained in appropriate use of staff support

Groups
- Group confidentiality is paramount;
- Groups require experienced facilitation;
- Rules and processes for groups should be reviewed regularly;
- Membership should be constant with no 'dropping in or out';
- Groups should meet on a regular basis;
- Issues raised should be resolved – or a plan agreed – before the end of each group meeting.

Source: Miller, Gillies and Elliott, 1994.

Overall, 40 staff (47 per cent) were aged 29 years or less, and 45 (53 per cent) were aged 30 years or over. Twenty six (31 per cent) were male, and 59 (69 per cent) were female. There were eight physicians (9 per cent), 25 nurses (30 per cent), seven paramedics (8 per cent), and 45 'other' staff (53 per cent). Overall, 32 (38 per cent) were senior staff (using the MOMS criteria), and 53 (62 per cent) were junior staff.

Psychometric scores

Overall, 59 per cent (n = 50) scored above the cut-off level for psychological vulnerability on the GHQ-28. Additionally, using the scoring method indicating

Table 8.7 Study response rates, Phase II

Site	Eligible population	Response at first interview		Response at second interview	
	n	*n*	%	*n*	%
1	45	28	62	20	44
2	88	22	25	16	18
3	27	27	100	24	89
4	8	8	100	8	100
Totals	168	85	51	68	41

chronicity of vulnerability on this measure (Goldberg and Williams, 1988), 41 per cent overall scored at a level indicating chronic vulnerability. Across sites, percentages of vulnerable staff ranged from 52 per cent to 87 per cent. These figures are higher than in the MOMS study, although consistent with other surveys of statutory health service staff in the UK in the mid-1990s (e.g., Caplan, 1994).

Concerning the MBI scores, 31 per cent overall (n = 26) scored as suffering high levels of emotional exhaustion, 58 per cent (n = 47) scored with high levels of depersonalisation, and 34 per cent (n = 29) revealed low levels of personal accomplishment. Low sample sizes precluded any tests of association on this variable.

Perceptions of and preferences for staff support activities

ACCESSIBILITY

When staff were asked about any difficulties accessing their staff support, 49 per cent overall (n = 42) said there were problems with this. The main difficulties identified by 59 per cent (n = 25) concerned *resources* – lack of available time because of pressure of work, lack of dedicated staff support time, insufficient funding for support, lack of staff cover, and appropriate support being unavailable (e.g., for crisis intervention). Some 27 per cent (n = 11) suggested lack of confidentiality, and lack of management acknowledgement, made accessing staff support difficult.

AIMS

When asked what they felt their staff support programmes were trying to achieve, the following responses were given:

- A forum for dealing with work issues and problems – an opportunity for reflection and sharing views.
- Improving relationships between staff.
- Alleviating and controlling stress levels.

- Allowing time out from job stresses.
- Information gathering – management 'watching over' staff (25 per cent).
- 'No idea' (15 per cent).

Information gathering was seen as negative by those staff suggesting this – they were worried information might be used against them in the future.

IMPACT OF STAFF SUPPORT

Overall, 48 per cent (n = 41) felt that staff support was successful, 42 per cent (n = 36) said it was not, and 10 per cent (n = 8) were undecided. The staff at Sites 3 and 4 – the non-statutory organisations – were very positive in their views, while staff at Sites 1 and 2 – the hospital-based services – were not, indicating the variability across sites, and the idiocyncracy (and greater complexity with greater size) of organisational atmospheres.

Main beneficial effects were seen in staff support helping with problem-solving, with providing a 'safe place' away from the job, and with encouraging a sense and ethos of teamwork. Those viewing the impact as negative felt that regular discussions actually magnified or encouraged stresses in the workplace.

STRENGTHS AND WEAKNESSES OF STAFF SUPPORT

Identified strengths of the staff support programmes overall included:

- Priority/committment – accorded by management towards the welfare of staff, and of staff to the welfare of the organisation.
- Regularity – dedicated regular time for support sessions.
- Good facilitation (where it was judged an issue).
- Confidentiality.
- Flexibility – having choices about support modalities.

Overall, 62 per cent of staff (n = 53) felt that support sessions helped in relation-ships with colleagues by enabling better understanding of others' stresses and work problems, by fostering team building, and allowing mutual discussion.

Staff acknowledged that support helped them in their relationships with *patients*, by clarifying effective clinical management responses, by standardising elements of patient care, and that by managing staffs' personal stresses, quality of patient care would improve.

Reported weaknesses mirrored the strengths cited – i.e., it was the absence of qualities of strength (above) that was construed as the evidence of weakness.

PREFERENCES FOR STAFF SUPPORT

Almost half of the sample overall (47 per cent, n = 40) wanted the choice of either group or individual support as their primary preferred option. Group support was seen to offer opportunities to share ideas, experiences and opinions, and for team building. Individual support was considered better for professional supervision, for addressing specific work problems and for easier discussion of emotional problems. Some 28 per cent (n = 24) identified a first preference for group support, and 15 per cent (n = 13) wanted individual support.

These findings are contrary to the earlier MOMS survey, in which over one-half wanted individual support alone, 12 per cent wanted group support alone, and 24 per cent wanted both. This present result probably reflects the close binding ethos in two of the sites, and support-seeking being seen as a sign of strength in a third – groups were therefore less threatening overall than in statutory services with a more individually competitive atmosphere.

In terms of preferred frequency of staff support activities, the greatest overall preference was for monthly sessions (35 per cent, n = 25), closely followed by fortnightly (32 per cent, n = 23). This was a reflection of known difficulties in accessing adequate cover and work time in which to make use of staff support. However, for those wanting individual rather than group support as their first option, 42 per cent overall (n = 25) wanted it on demand at times of crisis.

Overall, 38 per cent (n = 32) opted for *external* facilitation, for the same reasons as given in the MOMS study – perceived impartiality and increased confidentiality. However, 27 per cent opted for *internal* facilitation because of the presumed greater familiarity of an internal facilitator with the true working conditions of staff.

The content of staff support

Issues discussed in staff support were categorised as follows:

- Patient/service user problems and individual/organisational responses.
- Staff relationships.
- General work issues.
- Staffs' personal issues.
- Service management issues.

Content varied considerably according to site, and appeared to reflect the type of support used and staffs' perceptions of what was allowable in discussion.

At *Site 1*, where confidence in the confidentiality of support procedures – and commitment to attendance – was low, issues predominantly included patient issues, general work issues, and staff relationships. Only two staff reported having discussed personal issues, and no-one discussed service management issues – not because there were none, but because they reportedly did not feel it safe to do so.

At *Site 2*, one-third of the participants reported discussing personal issues, in addition to the issues addressed in Site 1. Much of the general work discussion was undoubtedly associated with the recent staff restructuring and redundancies, which also forced a consideration of staff relationships. Personal issues were not easy for most people to raise, but an external counsellor was employed for this purpose to make it easier for them.

At *Site 3*, where the emphasis was on group support, most frequent subjects discussed were staff relationships and general work issues, followed by service user issues, and 50 per cent reported also discussing personal issues. The confidence of the staff in the confidentiality of support activities, and their trust in the internal supervisor, at this site led to greater willingness and readiness to address a wider variety of topics.

At Site 4, the main issues discussed concerned general work concerns. Support here was viewed by all as professional rather than emotional, so discussion of personal issues was rare (external counselling was made available for this when needed).

Support activities across time

Overall, there were no statistically significant changes in self-reported work stress, psychometric measures, or days of sickness/stress absence in the staff surveyed. Additionally, there were no significant changes in reported preferences for staff support, aside from a greater proportion overall wanting both individual and group support than at first interview (from 7 per cent to 65 per cent – $\chi^2 = 4.1$, 1 d.f., $P = 0.044$). There were no significant changes in levels of satisfaction with available staff support, nor in the support modalities actually available to staff at each site. The structure of support did change over the six-month observation period of the study, however.

ALTERATIONS IN STRUCTURE OF STAFF SUPPORT

These were as follows:

- Site 1: The HIV/AIDS facilities at this site were spread over three distinct units (with some staff overlap). In the day centre, there were changes in group support facilitation over time, with a facilitator unlinked to senior management being appointed (to staff acclaim). Unfortunately, this facilitator left after two months, and all staff support ceased. On the ward, fewer staff participated as groups appeared to lose aim and meaning. Nursing shifts also made attendance difficult. There were no changes in the out-patient clinic.
- Site 2: Over time, there was an increase in availability of externally facilitated counselling on the wards, and this counsellor was accessed more frequently as confidence of staff grew. Group support with the same facilitator was also being set up on each of the wards. Externally facilitated group support was put in place for paramedical staff (an innovation) and, aside from teething problems, the will to make it succeed in the long term was there.
- Site 3: The number of support groups for discrete staff clusters was reduced over time from three to two, as the facilitator was unable to maintain the same level of involvement. There was disagreement in the group affected about whether to integrate with the remaining two groups, or to stay without a facilitator and maintain the present trusting atmosphere.

- Site 4: The same support programme was maintained over the period of the study, with more staff accessing external individual support (paid for by the organisation).

The lesson from these observations is that support programmes are themselves dynamic institutions, subject to change and alterations in favour over short time periods. This may have significant consequences for the staff using them. Also, changes being planned or put in place by management have a considerable influence on the outlook of the staff, and prospective management changes may be complemented by appropriate, matched changes in staff support availability.

Summary of key findings relating to experiences of staff support

Based on the findings of this study (not all of which are reported here, and some of which overlap with the MOMS study), the following points may be summarised:

- Good models of staff support are hard to find.
- Because work stress and burnout are chronic clinical processes, management of burnout should be based in a long-term perspective.
- Organisational structures need to be considered in identifying what perpetuates stress in workers.
- Staff appear to have some clear ideas about their preferred approaches to staff support, and their requirements of them if they are to be used confidently.
- In keeping with related surveys, a significant proportion of the study population scored as being vulnerable to psychological morbidity on standardised psychometric measures validated in similar populations.
- One-half of the sample overall found emotional support-seeking difficult in the workplace.
- Staff are often confused about the type of support on offer, what it aims to achieve, and this confusion may impact on staff compliance.
- The majority of staff think provision of staff support is important for their work population.
- Workforces divided by geographical site, by profession and by pay status (paid versus volunteers) require particular attention to sharing of information across such divides.
- Access to and use of staff support is made difficult by resource difficulties – especially lack of time, and staff cover, and by fears of inappropriate disclosure.
- Staff support considered to convey strengths embodies the following:
  - (a) Showing that staff are cared for;
  - (b) Provision of competent facilitation;
  - (c) Allowing flexibility in meeting staffs' needs.
- Support appears to help staff in their relations with patients, and with colleagues.
- Confidentiality and lack of trust in colleagues are interlinked and both impact directly on the desire to engage in staff support.

- Content of staff support covers issues relating to patient management, relations between staff, general work issues, service management issues, and personal matters.
- Half the staff surveyed wanted a mixture of formats, ideally combining group and individual support – each is seen to have a different and related purpose.
- One in four wanted outside facilitation, and the same proportion wanted external and internal facilitation, as each is seen to embidy specific and necessary virtues.
- Groups are wanted monthly or fortnightly, and individual emotional support was seen to be desirable on demand – when crises hit.
- Staff support was not a constant process in the sites studied, and underwent considerable changes in a short period of time.

Discussion

Staff preferences for support for workplace stress

It is still unusual in the literature to find studies explicitly asking subjects about their coping strategies in the workplace, although those by Shinn *et al.* (1984), Bennett (1992a; 1995) and Horstman and McKusick (1986) are among notable exceptions. The MOMS study revealed that nearly 90 per cent of staff overall could identify coping strategies they consciously employed for managing workplace stress. Broadly speaking, just under half the participants in that study employed active management strategies, such as exercise, socialising, holidays, and stress prevention and management activities, including relaxation. A further one-third dealt with work stress by talking about it with selected colleagues or friends outside the workplace, and just under one-fifth managed work stress by re-focusing on work, re-organising, and/or doing more work. In contrast, communicating with colleagues and friends as a means of managing work stress was the most popular method identified among the physicians surveyed by Horstman and McKusick (1986). The 141 human service workers surveyed by Shinn *et al.* (1984) put focusing on family and friends as their most popular strategy, although when strategies were grouped together in the Shinn *et al.* study, those approaches directly focusing on improving work skills, changing work circumstances, and reviewing work priorities appeared equally often used.

Overall, the findings from asking participants about staff support in their workplace will be distilled into two areas: considerations regarding the targeting of staff support; and implications arising from staffs' stated preferences for the design of future staff support programmes.

The evidence in favour of targeted staff support

The results of the UK studies described here raise the issue of whether staff support programmes can be *generalisable* – that is, can one design meet the staff support needs of diverse populations from differing fields of health care? Or is it the case that staff support must be precisely targeted to meet the needs of *individual* staff populations, or even of individuals within staff populations? On the face of results obtained, the case for *targeting* staff support seems very strong, given that differences over staff support obstacles, preferences and outcomes were found 'between fields of care, levels of professional experience and seniority, professions, gender and organisations.

Differences were found, for example, in comparing HIV/AIDS and oncology staffs' preferences for staff support, and why they had such preferences. Oncology staff were significantly more likely than HIV/AIDS staff to cite issues of trust, professionalism and position (seniority) as providing obstacles to their seeking emotional support in the workplace, in contrast to the findings of Kleiber, Enzmann and Gusy (1995), who found no field of care effects on support in the workplace between oncology and HIV/AIDS. Given this concern for how support-seeking would appear in the eyes of their immediate colleagues, it was not surprising that this same group wanted individual support significantly more than the HIV/AIDS group. Additionally, given the apparently lower concern among HIV/AIDS staff for revealing personal emotional susceptibility in the workplace in the MOMS study, the greater social cohesion among HIV/AIDS workers than oncology workers, and the finding of independently significant associations between personal stress symptoms and burnout and GHQ-28 scores in this group, it was not surprising that they were significantly more likely to cite discussion of personal feelings and issues as their preferred topics for staff support than were oncology staff. Having said that, the study of HIV/AIDS facilities only revealed how specific organisational dynamics can influence staff morale, and perceptions of the safety with which personal issues can be raised. Of course, in the MOMS study, all sites were statutory hospital or community facilities, whereas the second UK study included two non-statutory services. The differing perceptions of safety over personal issues may reflect the separate realities herein.

The type of difference found in the MOMS study may lie in HIV/AIDS having a greater level of overt engagement on emotional issues in treatment than is found in oncology, although this seems unlikely. While the focus on counselling for emotional adjustment and care is certainly very prominent in HIV/AIDS management (Green and McCreaner, 1989), such emphasis is equally apparent in the current ethos of oncology care (Temoshok and Dreher, 1992). Perhaps differences lie in the degrees to which different institutions put such emphases into practice. Context and institutional dynamics may result in considerable variations in clinical management of emotional disturbance associated with this work. Where there is insufficient time to see all the patients and engage in discussion of their emotional concerns, emotion as a staff issue may also be subjugated to management of acute service provision issues. As noted earlier, the non-statutory services in the second UK study appeared to more overtly and actively acknowledge the necessity for personal vulnerability to be admitted, whereas for staff in statutory services generally, the opposite appeared to be the case.

The imperative to target support for staff is also reinforced by the findings that level of professional experience confers differences in perception of the capacity to use such a facility. Those with less professional experience were significantly more likely in this study to report that lack of resources was the most important obstacle to their using staff support, a sentiment reminiscent of the findings by Horstman and McKusick (1986) that pressure of work resulted in AIDS GPs never being able to escape from their work. The less experienced staff members were also significantly more likely than their more experienced colleagues to want to discuss personal feelings and issues arising from their work.

These findings reflect the practical realities of health care and hence are not unexpected: These studies demonstrate that the less experienced were younger and more junior staff who had less authority to manipulate their clinical resources, such as cover for those times when they might wish to have a support session. Additionally, it can be argued that having less experience may be reflected in having less practice at coping with the emotional complexities that can emerge in management of patients and their families. Being less experienced practically translates into knowing less about how to do things well, and where clinical demands frequently offer opportunities for doing important things only once, such as breaking bad news, and managing the deaths of patients, it is not unexpected that particular stresses may result. Cherniss (1980), and Leiter (1991) have emphasised that the discrepancies that grow between personal ideals and aspirations, and organisational conditions that allow such ideals to flourish, can be central to the development of burnout. The MOMS and other studies have demonstrated that junior staff are significantly more vulnerable to work stress as measured on the MBI subscales of depersonalisation and reduced personal accomplishment (Maslach and Jackson, 1982; Bennett, Michie and Kippax, 1991; Leiter, 1991; Cordes and Dougherty, 1993).

These results would therefore suggest it is appropriate to include direct emphasis on such clinical topics, and training about organising staff coverage, development of emotional expression and emotional de-briefing, for less experienced staff in both HIV/AIDS and oncology. It also suggests that working on the context of care to ensure that less experienced staff do have reliable access to staff support and clinical supervision may pay dividends in terms of their having an increased capacity for managing difficult clinical issues, such as the involvement of patients' loved-ones, breaking bad news, and relationships with patients and colleagues. The findings of the second UK study indicate that these are primary issues of concern that staff support needs to address.

Similarly, the MOMS study also found that those with more experience were more interested in discussing professional issues and coping with them, and that more experienced staff were less likely to show distress about work-related issues, suggesting that service management and professional coping would be targets for support in these populations.

The difficulty in attempting to satisfy the apparent support needs and traditions of all stratifiable groups of staff and organisations is that targeting staff support can then become too complex. For example, the MOMS study found that males are more likely to use stress prevention and relaxation strategies than females in order to reduce workplace stress, whereas females are more likely to rely on communication and active distraction strategies. Physicians and HIV/AIDS staff were each found to use more work-focused approaches for reducing work stress, that is, coping with stress at work by doing more work. Paramedics and oncology groups each use stress prevention and relaxation, and nurses and oncology staff groups each use active distraction. These findings are slightly at odds with the stress management strategies found by Kleiber, Enzmann and Gusy (1995). Physicians and nursing staff in their study were found to employ more social support and have less withdrawal in the workplace than psychosocial staff, although there were no professional group differences found in use of social support strategies outside the workplaces surveyed. These researchers found no effects for field of care, that is, no differences between oncology and HIV/AIDS workers in strategies employed. Once again, it might be the case that in the MOMS study the focus on prevention and relaxation in HIV/AIDS staff reflects the emphasis laid upon such approaches in the patient communities with which they work (Miller, 1987; Kleiber, Enzmann and Gusy, 1995), although psychological work has long been a part of oncology care also (Greer, Morris and Pettingale, 1979; Ader, 1982; Greer and Watson, 1985).

It is, of course, possible to ignore generalisation of staff support interventions, and to emphasise targeting to the extent that no single staff subpopulation would be without their own tailor-made support service, although this is probably uneconomic and would not have as many benefits as may be gained from more generalisable approaches (such as standardisation of clinical care, as mentioned by staff in the second UK study). Having said this, individual staff support can be construed as a type of clinical intervention, where individual issues are discussed as individuals require. Elsewhere, Miller (1995b) has argued for the importance of recognising that burnout and/or entrenched work stress are *chronic processes* that may well require *chronic interventions*, as do other clinical processes, particularly where depression has taken hold. Similarly, Handy (1988) has confirmed the value of placing burnout in a clinical context, where clinical exactness may be applied to treatment discussions and interventions, where concepts of burnout may be modified to admit temporal evolution (as process models do), and where interventions may then move away from the primarily educational (Gallop *et al.*, 1992; Bennett, Kelaher and Ross, 1994; Reynolds and Briner, 1994).

Generic possibilities and preferences in future staff support design

Many research reports, including that by Bennett (1995), van Servellen and Leake (1993), Constable and Russell (1986) and Leiter (1991), suggest that providing staff support and improving social cohesion in staff groups would be of major benefit in reducing stress in the workplace. It follows that targeting staff support to specific subgroups may therefore actually reinforce divisions in staff groups by keeping them apart rather than reinforcing means for working together. This is an untested empirical question. However, it may be assumed that staff support focusing on generic issues, while observing the specifics of individuals and professional subgroups, could also help considerably in reducing staff tensions by breaking down barriers and encouraging mutual understanding (Bennett, 1995).

We know from the MOMS and UK Burnout Prevention and Preferences studies that there are elements of staff support programmes that may be generalisable, that would help ensure the more confident engagement of staff, irrespective of field of care, age, seniority, profession, experience, or site of work. Bennett (1992a) asked group participants to identify personal burnout-prevention strategies that might be incorporated into intervention groups, and they identified strategies that were work-related, strategies separating work and personal lives, and strategies focusing on individual needs.

Bearing in mind that the people being asked their views in Shinn *et al.*'s (1984) study had no prior experience of staff support activities, the answers show an encouraging consistency with findings of the present studies. The suggestions from Shinn *et al.* (1984) focus on the areas of (a) training to improve clinical confidence; (b) reducing or altering work demands to reduce acute work pressures and increase organisational recognition of the individual; and (c) encouraging flexibility to allow non-work time to be constructively used. These findings are contextually focused – they are interesting because they make suggestions against the grain of traditional stress management in occupational settings that require the individual, not the organisation, to adjust to perceived workplace stressor (Reynolds and Briner, 1994). The present studies add weight to this emphasis, by highlighting the many important contextual areas that need attention if staff are going to feel sufficiently confident to engage supportive offerings in the first place.

The first concerns the atmosphere of professionalism that institutions may generate or perpetuate. Overall, in the MOMS study three-quarters of those questioned said there were factors making emotional support-seeking difficult in the workplace, and over two-thirds of these identified a lack of trust about how their colleagues would handle information about their expressed vulnerability as the main obstacle. These issues were echoed in the second UK study. In particular, many respondents reported that in their workplace there was an unstated but nonetheless concrete awareness that demonstrating emotional vulnerability was considered evidence of being unfit to do their job, or a sign of professional and personal weakness. It is this 'tyranny of professional invulnerability' (Miller, 1991) that has also been identified in populations of hospice and other oncology health workers in other studies (Lunt and Yardley, 1988).

Concern for individual, and perhaps collective, image and confidentiality has also prompted a large minority of responses in related areas in the MOMS and Prevention studies. For example, in the MOMS study two-thirds overall stated they wanted staff support to be provided from outside their organisation, and over one-third of these stated this was because outside facilitators were regarded as probably being more trustworthy, more impartial and non-judgemental of staff showing their emotional vulnerability. Indeed, facilitator issues were critical for just over half of those surveyed, with participants listing essential facilitator qualities that matched very closely those identified as important by Grossman and Silverstein (1993) – confidentiality, impartiality, awareness and safety.

Confidentiality was a recurring theme in staff designs for ideal staff support programmes, and was cited by half those surveyed as a primary prerequisite for feeling confident about using staff support. In addition, just under one-third of MOMS participants stated that structural and process issues, such as having ease of access to staff support, having clearly stated expectations of the support process, and having no feedback to service management, were necessary determinants for confident usage of staff support. Indeed, the role of a supportive service management in endorsing the support provision, without wanting details in each case of what the support process throws up, was emphasised in the second UK study.

Perhaps one of the greatest challenges for health service managers lies in the challenge the findings of this study make to traditional notions of what form staff support should be provided in. While levels of preference varied across the studies described, overall a minority only wanted *group* staff support alone, and over half in the MOMS stated *individual* support as their first choice, with a further quarter stating they wanted group support only in combination with opportunities for individual support. The consistently reported feature of these stated preferences was the feeling that individual support would ensure that individual concerns could be confidentially heard, and group support was held to be valuable where it could facilitate common goals and allow sharing of common experiences and team-building among team members. Studies in Sydney (Bennett, 1995) and Toronto (Gallop and Taerk, 1995) suggest that for educationally based staff support strategies, group interventions are well-accepted and judged by participants as successful. However, the value of groups for emotional and professional support appears more equivocal, with staff resistance being applied because of concern about appearing unprofessional in front of peers, difficulties in changing from care-giver to care-receiver, and status, among other issues (Bair and Greenspan, 1986; Frost *et al.*, 1991; Garside, 1993; Grossman and Silverstein, 1993).

A further common theme emerging both from the results of the present studies, regarding communication difficulties with colleagues, and from other research reports by Leiter (1991), Shinn *et al.* (1984) and Cordes and Dougherty (1993), is the implication that by improving opportunities for social support among colleagues at work, workplace morbidity may be reduced. There is a need identified by these studies for trust among colleagues to be increased, as evidenced by the reported lack of trust in how colleagues will handle personal vulnerability, the desire for confidentiality as the basis for engagement in staff support, and the reported difficulties in showing work-related distress to colleagues in the workplace. As the social support buffer hypothesis would predict, increasing a sense of social support among colleagues would help to reduce the impact of workplace stressors both at work and at home. Although staff in the MOMS study did not want groups as their primary form of staff support, Bennett (1995) reported that a regime of three weekly, 2-hour multidisciplinary discussion and relaxation groups actually acted to improve staff cohesion and understanding. This finding was endorsed by the second UK study.

The relationship between the provision of staff support, of a social nature or not, and the impact of work stress on home and social life is a topic for future research. It was clear from the Sydney HIV/AIDS workers burnout study of Bennett (1995), however, and from the MOMS study demonstrating the reported impact of work stress on domestic relationship morbidity (Miller and Gillies, 1996), that strategies that both acknowledge and address the impact of work stress on home life must be recognised and implemented. The fact that work stress has 'fallout' in the non-work arenas cannot be ignored in future staff support designs. Bennett (1995) actively encouraged burnout prevention group members to consider how to minimise work stress in the home arena, and admitted this issue into group discussion. While some staff may have difficulties in exposing domestic circumstances to colleagues of whom they are initially suspicious, the principle is an important first step. Kleiber, Enzmann and Gusy (1995) found no effects associated with field of care or profession, and social support and/or withdrawal effects outside the workplace. In the MOMS study, the finding of there being no significant differences between home- and work-based strategies employed for managing work-related stress, points to the necessity for assessing the impact of work stress outside work as part of individual stress management routines.

Implications for models of staff support

On balance, the results of these studies suggest that the optimal approach to staff support provision, incorporating individual and contextual issues, lies within the schema suggested in Chapter 10. Given the breadth of diversity identified throughout the MOMS study regarding self-reported stresses, reactions to them, and consequences of them, a model of staff support that can incorporate elements of individual emotional and professional support, group learning, stress management through information, social bonding and skills development, and contextual re-arrangement, would stand the greatest chance of making a meaningful impact on staff stress, and of engaging staff best. The second UK study reinforced the desirability of having a 'multi-layered' approach to staff support. In accord with the suggestions of Shinn *et al.* (1984), the findings of these studies suggest that while observing the majority preferences for confidentiality, impartial though experienced facilitation, social support-generating, and ease of access, an ideal and generic staff support programme would have distinct components, including:

- Stress management training.
- Symptom recognition and intervention.
- Environmental (context) management.

Training for stress reduction and management has been identified by junior and less experienced staff as particularly necessary in managing death and dying, and breaking bad news. Additionally, results of the present studies, and of studies by Kleiber, Enzmann and Gusy (1995), Ullrich and FitzGerald (1990), Constable and Russell (1986), van Servellen and Leake (1993), Cordes and Dougherty

(1993), Bennett (1995), and as reported by Schaufeli, Maslach and Marek (1993), indicate that training is important in managing the emotional consequences of relationships with patients, their loved-ones, and colleagues, stress associated with perceived dangers linked with HIV/AIDS care, and with watching the slow decline of paitents. As such, these aspects could form the basis, agenda or curriculum of a generic programme of support for staff in HV/AIDS (and in oncology – see Chapter 10). Training also appears necessary in managing staff shortages, and judging from the self-reported stress associated with structural changes in the NHS, training in the altering structures and functions of health systems may also help clarify staff perceptions of how they are placed in evolving organisations.

By instituting such training, the context of work would be altered, although staffs' imperatives for contextual change go much deeper than this. Staff were asking for their organisational environments to be less judgemental and less likely to make negative conclusions about demonstrations of staff vulnerability. For this to occur, it may be necessary for many levels of staff to be enrolled in training and organisational awareness. There is a great deal of work to do in this almost untapped realm of staff support research, and developing trials implementing the suggestions for context management identified and explicated in Chapter 10 would make a very useful beginning.

An additional empirical question is whether providing just a part of such approaches, rather than the full possible spectrum, could have real and sustained benefit, and what impact such work-based interventions and modifications would have on quality of care for patients. For example, in the modern NHS Trust culture in the UK, would managers and patients find extending waiting lists for new referrals acceptable if this meant their staff were happier and providing a better quality of service? This is one of many brave and difficult questions for possible future research.

However, the results of these studies also suggest ways forward for direct implementation of staff support activities now. It is clear that a sense of identity has some importance for staff, and that this can be constructively directed by the organisations in which they work. Perhaps after consulting with staff about the true aims and direction of health care teams, staff in different professions and at different levels of experience, for example, can be asked about their preferences for staff support. At the same time, managers can explicitly offer endorsement for improved staff care, and both of these can foster recognition that as experiences of staff support change for them, needs for staff support may alter also. The finding in these studies that generic elements do exist in staff support means that generic responses, such as training in breaking bad news, and infection control, can be developed and implemented on a rolling basis. Involving discussion of and with staffs' loved-ones may also be a useful first step in propagating the fragile bloom of staff cohesion. These are suggestions, but it is only by a further committment to empirical investigations in this area that we will be able to move confidently to assert our humanity vocationally, by vocationally asserting our human vulnerability.

A further discussion of management of occupational stress and burnout is given in Chapter 10.

9 Volunteers and burnout in HIV/AIDS

A context of care

Worldwide, it is a fact that the edifice of community-based care for people with HIV/AIDS would collapse without the support of volunteers. Indeed, the scope and ubiquity of counselling and support services for people affected by HIV is due to the work of volunteers, with peer-led community initiatives often becoming the template for later, government-sponsored services in HIV care and support (Miller, 1989). Additionally, studies of volunteer services in San Francisco have shown that they reduce the cost of care per patient with symptomatic HIV disease from $150,000 to $40,000 per year (Omoto and Snyder, 1990). Claxton, Burgess and Catalan (1993) reported that the estimated value of 'Buddy' volunteer services for people with HIV/AIDS in central London was £2,000,000 in 1991. Given the importance of such an army of carers, it seems astonishing that there is a relative lack of documentation about their efforts, and certainly about their personal experiences of the burdens of HIV/AIDS care.

Yet, in considering the range of issues already highlighted as possible correlates of work stress and burnout in formal health workers in HIV/AIDS, it would seem as likely that the informal sector would also be as vulnerable. Indeed, Maslach and Ozer (1995) identify may good reasons for being concerned about how volunteers might respond to their involvement:

- The breadth of care given, the demands being magnified by a lack of specific training for often complicated and significant tasks in personal care.
- The absence of established work day or time boundaries for many informal care-givers.
- The anxieties about possible personal (re)exposure to HIV through care-giving.
- The relative youth of patients, and of volunteer care-givers, leaving both with major adjustment issues at a time when they have little prior exposure to the need for them.
- Close identification with the patient may preclude the possibility of emotional distance or personal boundaries that may be necessary for personal coping.
- Close proximity to an ailing loved-one may also give cause for reflection with concern about their own lives after that person dies.

- Guilt and/or anger – about being healthy, about possibly having passed the infection to the patient, about the changes forced on their lives, about working harder than the patient at this time.
- Loss and role conflict – the power shifts in loving relationships that go with one being the carer and one being the patient, and the loss of mutual emotional support as caregiving becomes more focused on the patient. Also, losing the ability to plan ahead, and losing energy (and possibly increasing conflicts when attempting) to live life 'outside'.

Thus, the volunteer is at risk for burnout, because of the sheer physical and psychological demands of the role, vulnerability to feelings of helplessness when they are affected often as much by the patient's illness, but at a remove from their suffering, the unpredictability of the disease and the constant reactivity to it, leaving little possibility for forward planning or a manageable routine (Miller, 1987). Also, the closeness of carer and patient can mean a dilution or loss of prior roles on both sides, and of boundaries that may be necessary for adequate coping.

Maslach and Ozer's (1995) considerations raise some key points that will be considered in this chapter, not least that of definition. For what is a volunteer? Are their roles all the same? Where do the real tensions and opportunities arise, and what can be done to most effectively support volunteers against the possibility of burnout?

Definitions: what is a volunteer?

Volunteers are described in many different ways. An early clarification of roles in HIV/AIDS care was drawn by Pearlin, Semple and Turner (1988), when they described 'informal' and 'formal' carers:

- *Informal* – lovers, friends, neighbours and family – care is given as an expression of love or community committment (solidarity), and therefore is associated with a great emotional stake in the care-receiver;
- *Formal* – trained, contractually engaged workers – they may be drawn to their role by compassion and/or a sense of mission, or professional expression.

This distinction may not be entirely satisfactory, because it glosses over some important distinctions within the volunteer spectrum. For example, many of the tensions suggested by Maslach and Ozer (1995) relate more to volunteer caregivers who live with, and have a primary emotional link to, the patient for whom they care. For many volunteers, however, their HIV/AIDS activity is part time, an extension of their working day in which they give their *time and skill*, or a substitute for paid employment (Kalibala, 1995). Indeed, a crucial element in volunteering appears to be the *absence of material reward*, and of the expectation of any such (Blinkhoff *et al.*, 1999). This is not to deny the pressures associated with specifically domestic and external volunteering, however, or the burdens of volunteering not as a carer, but as an advocate for care, or for revision of social and legal conditions associated with the growing recognition of HIV in the community. The discussion below will also consider some of the anecdotal pressures associated with 'facing the barricades', armed only with experience and an ability skilfully to convey it meaningfully to others.

Basing a definition of volunteers on the lack of monetary or material payment also avoids the suggestion that volunteers are somehow a lower quality of carer, for whom the appropriate role is as the untrained assistant to formally trained health staff. Because the reality is that volunteers frequently are reported to provide expert quality assistance, whether it be in counselling (face-to-face or by telephone), in providing front-line community education about HIV/AIDS and prevention of infection, or in provision of specialised home-care for people and their families facing HIV/AIDS and TB, and other chronic, life-threatening diseases (Blinkhoff *et al.*, 1999). As Maslanka (1995) notes:

> 'It is only during periods of illness or crisis that the services of medical or social service specialists may be needed. Volunteers or other unpaid helpers, such as family and friends, have become critical for providing help of a more general and consistent nature. Increasingly, volunteers have become the specialists themselves, both in their knowledge of HIV, as well as in the sort of care they provide. Volunteers may be called upon to educate professional service providers about the latest research on HIV for the clients, or they may be called upon to deliver counselling when an individual first finds out they are HIV positive and are in a psychological crisis' (p. 152).

In addition, it is the case that with the increasing linkage between voluntary and statutory initiatives in HIV/AIDS caregiving, volunteers do have formal relationships – often contractually defined – with the organisations under whose umbrella they give HIV/AIDS care, and so by extension they have formally defined relationships with collaborative care organisations.

In considering the small literature on volunteering, burnout and HIV, it is clear that many tensions repeatedly emerge. Yet, opportunities for addressing those tensions also emerge, and the rest of this chapter will address some of these, and their significance for management and prevention of burnout.

Tensions associated with volunteers in HIV/AIDS

Stressors associated with volunteer work in families

For volunteer care-givers who are family members of the patient – whether of birth or of affiliation – the stresses have been well documented. Maj (1991) described many of the issues alluded to by Maslach and Ozer (1995) – challenges to roles within families, the corrosive impact of repeated disappointments in planning, the fears of infection control (Lovejoy, 1988), the anxieties about stigma. Miller (1987) has documented how the family care-giver finds themselves taking on multiple domestic responsibilities that previously may have been shared

– running the household, providing nursing care, managing finances and legal matters, participating in medical decisions, and acting as an intermediary between the patient and their social network. The tensions of these roles and responsibilities can result in a 'bonding or splitting' within the couple, where they become closer, or are pushed apart by the intrusions such experiences can generate (Miller, 1987). Much of the psychological pressure in concordant couples with HIV is presumed to be associated with thoughts for the future – the issues of 'what to do when my partner dies?', and the potential for mirroring the patient's reactions to illness that may have been so tragically modelled for the patient-to-be.

Using semi-structured interviews, Church, Kocsis and Green (1988) interviewed the partners of people with HIV. In a context of high anxiety overall, 25 per cent of those interviewed were more anxious and depressed than the people they cared for. Most carers reported that their work, social life, recreation and sexual relationships were greatly affected by the illness. Overall, 57 per cent reported high levels of stress, and this was linked to perceptions of support – when the patient had more support, carers had higher levels of stress; when the carers perceived themselves to be receiving more social support than the patients, their reported stress levels were low. The case for ensuring appropriate levels of support for 'family' carers seems clear from this study.

Additionally, the notion of *stigma* associated with volunteering – particularly its *isolating* impact on family members of people with HIV – has been documented in relation to families in many countries, including in some African countries, where the majority of care comes from family members (Ankrah, 1991; Seeley *et al.*, 1993). And these and related findings are extremely relevant to decisions about reinforcing sustainability in home carers, as they are such very important colleagues in provision of care, support and education: A UK survey suggested that 87 per cent of men with AIDS identified their partner or close friend as their primary care-giver (McCann and Wadsworth, 1992), and this circumstance appears to be shared with US urban centres (Folkman, Chesney and Christopher-Richards, 1994; Turner, Catania and Gagnon, 1994).

In HIV/AIDS volunteers, additional tensions can be discerned in considering the simple breadth and importance of the work of volunteers, the broad relationships between staff groups in the same agencies, and staff in statutory agencies, and between individual motivations, and the realities of organisations and the disease. As with so many of the relevant issues in this field, there appears to be relatively little data to base good strategies on, but what there is will be briefly considered.

Considering the breadth and importance of the volunteers' work . . .

A recent report on volunteers recruited from religious organisations in Zambia's copperbelt (Blinkhoff *et al.*, 1999) describes how volunteers have developed and maintain a comprehensive home care programme in a rural community in which over 19 per cent of the adult population has HIV infection. An important element in the HIV epidemic there is tuberculosis (TB), and the volunteer programme –

involving approximately 500 people reaching 23 townships with a total population of 400,000 – is playing a leading role in providing HIV/AIDS home care, and an effective entry point for community-based TB control. The clearly-defined responsibilities of the volunteers include:

- Identifying people in their neighbourhoods who are chronically ill, and putting them in touch with a TB nurse.
- Daily and weekly visits to patients to check on patients, and to ensure they are taking their TB medication in the correct way.
- Giving basic medical and nursing care, and explaining to family members how to provide home-based HIV/AIDS and TB nursing care.
- Arranging for patients to receive welfare support.
- Providing practical help, such as basic housework, washing and cooking.
- Providing emotional, social and spiritual support to patients and family members (including giving support counselling to people before and after HIV testing).
- Undertaking HIV awareness-raising and education to address stigma against those with HIV, and to promote HIV prevention.

Some home care programmes also provide small amounts of food and other material support, and pay for schooling and clothing of orphans.

For such substantial activities, volunteers receive two weeks' initial training in basic hygiene, HIV/AIDS and other sexually transmitted diseases (STDs), home nursing, nutrition and first aid. They receive a World Health Organization (WHO) home care handbook, and a bag containing a towel, soap, disinfectant, scissors, two small basins, rubber gloves, gauze, strapping and oral rehydration salts. Some volunteers receive subsequent training in support counselling, and all develop their skills 'on the job', often to a specialised degree.

The burden of these duties for the volunteer can be very considerable. One of them, Jacqueline, sums up the pressures, and the rewards, of her work:

'. . . sometimes I do think about giving up, like during the rainy season, when my roof is leaking. And sometimes the work is very unpleasant. Once I went to a house, and as I opened the door there was an overpowering smell like a decaying corpse. There on a mat in front of me was this poor bundle of humanity, like a lamb waiting to be slaughtered. I opened the window and saw that the man's body was covered in sores and maggots. And the pain in his eyes . . . There I was, alone with this burden. I thought 'Doctor, where are you? Sister, where are you? This is unbearable. O God, how can I go on? Isn't there someone out there who cares about me, a volunteer with limited knowledge, left to do this work?'

'What keeps me going is my religious faith, and the support of the nurses and my fellow volunteers. And I do appreciate the support I get from the project for the orphans I look after. I like the meetings we have with volunteers from other places, where we exchange gifts. But the volunteers need some kind of project to earn some money together'.

'Sometimes the situation seems hopeless, because the number of people with AIDS keeps increasing. But people here are becoming more concerned about AIDS and more helpful to one another. Those who were afraid of people with AIDS are being educated and are gradually accepting them'.

'Sometimes I wish there was some kind of reward for what we do. But I can't stop now. I'm too deeply involved. My finger is woven into the basket.' (Blinkhoff *et al.*, 1999)

Relationships between individual motivations, and the realities of organisations and the disease

Research on the 'Buddy' volunteers at the Terrence Higgins Trust (THT) in London has shed valuable light on motivations and difficulties associated with 'external' volunteering – i.e., volunteering on a part-time basis with non-loved-ones. Claxton, Burgess and Catalan (1993) analysed self-report information from 267 Buddies and found that 26 per cent scored as 'probably' cases of burnout on the MBI. Similarly, higher than expected mean scores for anxiety were found on the HAD scale. Nevertheless, Claxton concludes that these rates compare favourably with findings in cohorts of volunteers elsewhere. For example, in studies of volunteer HIV/AIDS counsellors in Australia, Raphael *et al.* (1990) and Guinan *et al.* (1991) found 37 per cent showed evidence of psychological morbidity in GHQ scores (a level generally similar to those found in statutory health workers in this field – see Chapters 5 and 7). In Claxton's study, stepwise multiple regressions based on the HAD and MBI scales against Buddy demographic variables yielded models that accounted for only small amounts of the variance. However, factors that occurred in more than one model as positive associates of burnout included dissatisfaction with training, wanting to feel needed, feeling close to the person Buddied, and that person becoming ill. Importantly, age was a factor also – younger Buddies showed greater levels of MBI-measured burnout.

Claxton, Burgess and Catalan (1993) found that poor outcome in being a Buddy included *motivational* issues, such as 'wanting to help others', and 'wanting to feel needed'. These have similarities to some of the motivations identified in Maslanka's New York GMHC study, in which she also showed that relative youth implied a vulnerability to negative outcomes in volunteering through its relationship with motivations and rewards. Increased motivation leads to increased rewards from volunteering, and absence of volunteer support was associated with lowered boundaries. Another London volunteer study by Calvert (1993) aimed to identify motivational factors that might influence retention or drop-out of volunteers. They found that volunteer retention was predicted where motivations for volunteering included a high need for personal support, a need for personal control, and not being angry about HIV (those expressing anger at social injustices around HIV were significantly less likely to be volunteering after three years). However, these motivations are equivocal – they may also make for needy volunteers and draw concern for the maintenance of boundaries between volunteers and patients (Maslanka, 1996). They also rely upon mechanisms for social support to sustain them.

Motivations for volunteering were also centre-stage in a study by Williams (1988):

> 'For [those] . . . who may be contemplating the possibility that they may well be infected themselves, the knowledge that there will be someone there to support them should they ever get sick is reassuring. For these men, the contribution that they are making might be viewed by them as an investment or an insurance policy that they hope they will never have to draw on . . .' (p. 49).

Williams also found that the *length* of time spent as a Buddy was not associated with psychological morbidity, whereas the *number* of times volunteers acted as a Buddy was related to risk of psychiatric symptomatology.

The issue of motivations thus throws up some concerns, particularly where the needs of the volunteer appear to be driving their involvement. Is this healthy? Paradis, Miller and Runion (1987) have reflected on how over-identification with the terminally ill can lead to obsessional information-seeking in the volunteer, which then impacts negatively upon both colleagues and patients. Is this any different from the motivations of paid health staff which, however much they are driven by personal need instead become enshrined in the temple of vocational commitment and self-sacrifice and are consequently rewarded by the public whom they serve? This is not an issue yet sustained by empirical clarity and, as Claxton, Burgess and Catalan (1993) point out, the range of volunteers' motivations can be so large as to defy attempts at staff de-selection of inappropriate candidates at times of interview for volunteering positions. Age gets in the way, too, with results consistently showing that the inexperienced and enthusiastic may become over-stretched and withdraw for want of the appropriate guidance.

A further study on THT Buddies, by Fraser *et al.* (1996), asked Buddies to identify what they found *most difficult* in their volunteer work. The three most-cited problems included lack of role clarity and maintenance of boundaries, having insufficient time to do the job, and the intensity and draining pressure of the emotions raised in themselves and their clients in their work. These mirror the presumed and reported tensions found within family-based volunteer carers also (see above), and similar prime sources of volunteer distress have been found in studies by Raphael *et al.* (1990) and Coyle and Soodin (1992). Fraser *et al.* (1996) also found that 33 per cent of new volunteer Buddies felt 'overwhelmed' by their tasks and wanted support in doing them, whereas this was the case for only 12 per cent of experienced volunteers – again, the heightened vulnerabilities of inexperienced colleagues appear to mirror those of inexperienced and junior paid staff (see Chapters 5 and 7).

In a study on volunteers in Australia, Guinan *et al.* (1991) developed the 'HIV Volunteer Inventory' to identify levels of stress in HIV/AIDS volunteers. Using factor analysis, they found that the four primary stress factors included emotional overload, client problems for which they felt inadequately prepared, lack of support, and lack of training. Additionally, rewards associated with volunteer work were identified as personal effectiveness, emotional support, social support, and empathy/self-knowing. Similarly, in an analysis of data on religious volunteers in the United States, Bennett, Ross and Sunderland(1996) found that MBI-measured burnout was associated with a felt lack of adequate training, and an absence of personal effectiveness (the presence of stress and the absence of reward).

Relationships between staff groups, and between voluntary and statutory staff

Avoidable perils in meshing voluntary and statutory services have been suggested in a study from Rome (Bove *et al.*, 1993), which examined the needs of 30 volunteers working with hospitalised people with AIDS. Over 65 per cent reported difficulties in communication with hospital staff, or even a lack of linkage at all with the hospital. A qualitative study from New Orleans (Webb *et al.*, 1993) assessed how local council officials felt they were perceived by community-based AIDS service organisations (ASOs). The results revealed many frustrations, suspicions and obstructive feelings, dealt with by both sides in the ways many have observed in those with life-threatening diagnoses – with anger, denial, blaming, withdrawal and depression.

The tensions between paid and voluntary staff, especially where an 'us and them' atmosphere comes to characterise intra-organisational relationships, can lead to profoundly damaging organisational responses and generate much stress for volunteers (Patton, 1989), not least when arguments and decisions become personalised and communications break down both internally and – ultimately – externally (Moreland and Legg, 1991). Responses to such tensions have been documented in the Ndola Diocese Home Care Programme (Blinkhoff *et al.*, 1999), discussed further below.

A further issue that arises particularly in settings of high stigma and low reported HIV prevalence is that of the lone HIV advocate, who becomes the 'voice' of people living with HIV/AIDS in communities struggling to accept the reality of the epidemic and of the need for a response to it. Consider the courage of such persons – facing their own process of adjustment to an illness for which they may have real problems in obtaining reliable, informed care, while also:

- Recognising and coming to terms with the fears of their loved-ones.
- Trying to maintain their livelihood.
- Being judged stereotypically as something they may not be (e.g., as gay, an IDU, a sex worker, morally inferior).
- Experiencing the powerful and isolating pain of stigma and discrimination, and possibly violence.

- Fighting illness.
- Attempting to educate their community in rational and supportive responses to HIV.
- Trying to mobilise support for themselves and others whose needs have no formal and/or political acknowledgement.
- Trying to stay focused, sane, and constructive.
- Trying to save lives and care for their fellow citizens.

Where these ambitions do get recognised and endorsed, the person involved may lose their identity under the consuming tide of HIV-related activity – they may become 'the HIV/AIDS person', rather than the person who also lives with HIV/AIDS. Effective advocates in low- and high-prevalence settings can become easily overwhelmed, so that what was initially affirming becomes a constant struggle against the increasingly growing (and possibly disappointed) expectations of a needy constituency. As the training studies by Gallop and co-workers (1992, 1995) showed, there is nothing quite so powerful as the personal story told first hand by the identifiable person with HIV/AIDS. But at what price to the person whose experience matters so much to those around them? How can personal limits be set against the demands of a social catastrophe *that remains preventable*?

Suggestions for management and prevention of burnout in volunteers

At least the findings reviewed above, sparse as they are, confer some predictability and enable a clearer discussion of appropriate support mechanisms for volunteers. For example, it seems consistently the case that younger and less experienced volunteers – as with paid health workers – need extra support to help them develop confident coping strategies, and supervision in ensuring that the desire to care is not translated into a loss of distance and an unhealthy dilution of boundaries that will ultimately work against their and their patients' interests. A reason that motivations appear to be such a complex issue here is that altruism is desparately needed and, with appropriate channelling and guidance, motivations of need can also be translated into extremely valuable collective action for others. Opportunities for burnout prevention arising from what we empirically know can be found in the often overlapping contexts of:

- A shared ethos.
- Emotional support and supervision.
- Training.
- Provision of appropriate logistical support.

Having a shared ethos

A key element in support and retention of documented volunteer populations has been the affirmation of a shared ethos – a shared committment to a cause, a philosophy or faith, and to a shared process or way of doing things. In a substantial and well-organised programme of 61 volunteer care teams involving 1,300 HIV/AIDS volunteers in Houston religious organisations, Sunderland and Shelp (1993) reported minimal rates of volunteer burnout, attributed to careful self-selection and de-selection of volunteers, particular attention being given to volunteers' grieving when their teams suffered bereavements, psychosocial support arising from regular team meetings, and the underlying ethos of compassionate support arising from the religious faith represented. The affirming and bonding that comes from a shared ethos was also found in a study of similar populations by Nesbitt *et al.* (1996), and of Christian home care volunteers in Zambia (Blinkhoff *et al.*, 1999).

For an ethos and an organisational aim or cause to be binding for members, it must be clearly articulated (and, of course, members must agree with it). The need for greater role clarity in Buddies of the Terrence Higgins Trust was answered by focus groups of service users, volunteers and service planners agreeing a document that clearly defined the Buddy role, and which is presently given to both Buddies and their clients at the start of Buddying relationships. In this way, expectations on both sides can be appropriate and activities undertaken in such relationships remain both appropriate and focussed. This links with provision of training about organisational expectations of staff and volunteers, and of what they may realistically achieve (see p. 189).

The importance of agreement about the aims and ethos of volunteering is highlighted in results of a study of religious volunteers by Nesbitt *et al.* (1996). They found that volunteer vulnerability is reduced where *volunteers are given a choice* over where to volunteer, over the amount of time they spend in volunteer work, and their ability to withdraw from such work. This is also mediated by the quality and level of supervision and support they have in volunteering.

Emotional support and supervision

As Chapter 10 describes, support and supervision may frequently be confused in the minds of support-giver and support-receiver. However, all researchers cited agree on the central importance of support in volunteer work – for retention, for quality of care, and for volunteers' psychological health. For some, social support is a major motivation for starting volunteering (Claxton, Burgess and Catalan, 1993; Maslanka, 1995), for others it is a binding element in the realisation of their committment to care for others (Sunderland and Shelp, 1993; Nesbitt *et al.*, 1996; Blinkhoff *et al.*, 1999), and for others, it is simply a necessary means for coping (Church, Kocsis and Green, 1988). As Maslanka (1996) showed, the more volunteers are supported by (paid) staff and volunteer colleagues, the more effective they feel, and greater levels of social support leads to increased rewards from volunteering. This fits naturally with the positive benefits of volunteering within a shared ethos of care and committment, but appropriate supervision is necessary in addition if appropriate boundaries are to be maintained and volunteer roles are not to become blurred with roles in the rest of life.

Boundary clarification was found to be a constructive outcome from a programme of relationship reviews set up for Buddies and their clients in London
(Fraser *et al.*, 1996). These reviews were created as an appraisal of Buddy
relationships – to give positive feedback to the Buddy from the service-user and
from the organisation, while also monitoring the acceptability and benefits of
having the Buddy to the needs of each individual service user. Reviews happen
after six months, then 12 months, then annually thereafter, with trained teams
interviewing both parties and then giving feedback. By so doing, the boundaries
of the relationship are re-assessed and reaffirmed, problems are addressed before
they become serious, and service-users' views of the parent organisation and its
activities can also be obtained.

This approach of formalising the role of volunteers has also been undertaken in
other community-based ASOs in the UK (including those described in Chapter 8
– see Table 8.5), where supervision is contracted at the start of volunteering. In
other words, as well as clarifying what the volunteer role is, and the expectations
the organisation places on the volunteer, their commitment to supervision –
including discussing client issues, monitoring of work quality, even having targets
for work and training – is also clarified and agreed to. It is subsequently reviewed
and updated.

Maslanka (1996) found that the only reward in volunteering that operated to
decrease burnout was having a sense of efficacy – those volunteers feeling more
effective feel less of a desire to withdraw from the agency. The role of clear,
realistic contracting and of staff support is clear here, particularly when volunteers
are relatively inexperienced. For those unable to withdraw, such as loved-ones and
family members, social support from the community is both a vital connection
and affirmation, and a way to learn and feel effective.

Empirically un-tested suggestions for management of volunteer stress in HIV/
AIDS management have been made by Lopez and Getzel (1987), including
group orientation and on-going supervision with a constant team, employing
closely supportive group dynamics in a modified crisis-intervention approach to
volunteer monitoring and support. The cross-over from care to management of
personal issues – sexuality, commitments, intimate relations – within the team and
often with team meetings in individuals' homes, suggests a family-style cohesion
that offers intense support, but which may run the risk of overwhelming the
individual team member. The authors do state, however, that volunteers must be
limited by their teams in the amount of client contact they experience, especially
where there have been multiple (i.e., more than two) bereavements within a six-
month period, because of the emotional toll this has on volunteer staff. One can
only wonder what these authors would suggest about the appropriateness of paid
health staff experiencing multiple bereavements *continually* with colleagues and
patients they have come to know very well over long periods of time.

For those working as volunteers alone, whether as advocates, teachers, or
neighbourhood care-givers, their supervision and support may come only from
within, or from those for whom they care. Quality of care is a function of quality
of health in the care-giver, both physical and psychological, and so the giving

of care requires also the discipline of self-assessment. Do the actions of the volunteer demonstrate the necessary discipline that goes with caring for others? Are they providing a good model for advocacy in their overlapping communities? Are all the actions of the care-giver aimed at the patient's or the community's improved health? Is there a reliable referent to whom the care-giver can turn to ensure their knowledge is accurate and up-to-date? Is there someone who can tell them how they are really doing? Do they dare ask the question? If not, it is time to review why they do what they do, and for whom! The skills and courage of high-profile advocates in low-prevalence or low-recognition settings are needed now more than ever. Teaming up with like-minded people is a good idea for their benefit, and the benefit of those for whom they work so hard. By doing so, they may change and enrich their worlds (e.g., Kaleeba, Ray and Wilmore, 1992).

Training

It is a curious and ironic fact that while experience of decline and deaths in patients may be a feature of hospital training and work for many medical and nursing and other paramedical staff, community volunteers with similar or less experiences may have *far better training and support* in managing their own and others' responses to such circumstances. Largely, this is because in many Western countries and communities, the emotional cost of working in such situations has explicitly been regarded *outside* statutory hospitals and clinics as a reality and worthy of care, not indicative of some flaw or shortcoming in the worker concerned (Miller and Gillies, 1993). Within some traditional statutory settings, on the other hand, emotional vulnerability in response to care and loss of patients may be defined in terms of a lack of ability or professionalism, rather than as an expected and healthy response to a vital part of the HIV/AIDS treatment cycle (Miller, 1991, 1995a). Training plays a big part in the quality of the individual health worker's and volunteer's response to the stresses of loss and bereavement, and to the other tensions associated with HIV/AIDS care (Brimlow, 1995). The quality and content of training in HIV/AIDS care offered by an organisation can act as a billboard that advertises its culture (its ethos) and its expectations or demands of staff.

While the importance of training is discussed more in Chapter 10, it makes sense to consider the organisational ethos as a central aspect of training, and also how to use the support on offer. As Chapter 10 shows, many staff don't use their support options appropriately, or even know how to use them. Fraser *et al.* (1996) describes Buddy services providing further training for volunteers in facilitation skills, in group dynamics and in basic counselling as a means of developing the skills of Buddies, but crucially also as a way of giving them and their role *due recognition*. Maslanka (1996) suggests that volunteers should be given early training in recognising signs of stress and burnout, and in identifying stressful situations so they can take remedial action before stresses become chronic or unmanageable.

Logistical support and the rewards of volunteering

A vital tension anecdotally reported in many settings occurs where volunteers work alongside paid staff, often doing the same level of work, but *without* the same reward (Patton, 1989). For example, in the Zambian township of Nkwazi where 52 volunteers participate in the home care programme, TB patients are identified by community volunteers through routine home visits, and then receive medication from a nurse as appropriate. Volunteers collect sputum from patients at key points in their treatment (over an eight-month period), and transport both the sample and the results each way. During the first two months of treatment for TB, volunteers visit the patients every morning to observe the medication being taken, and to educate and encourage the family members. Volunteers also keep records of medication taken. The degree of collaboration with qualified health staff is therefore vitally close, and results in an impressive 69 per cent completion/cure rate (Blinkhoff *et al.*, 1999). It also has positive benefits for volunteers, as a volunteer named Dominic described:

'The people in the neighbourhood appreciate our work. Other men used to laugh at me and say I was wasting my time. 'These people have got relatives to look after them,' they would say. I could only reply that I liked the work and found it interesting. Now some other men are interested too, and one wants to become a volunteer. I'm still discussing a few things with him, and the other volunteers in our section also have to agree'.

'What do I get out of this work? Well, I've learned a lot that can help other people and my own family. Now I know how to tend my children if they're sick. At Christmas the Sisters arrange a small party and they give us parcels of gifts that we can share with our families. And once a month we can buy a bag of mealie meal from the programme at a cheap price. . . . But the work has made me known in the community. People recognise me. They know I work in home care.' (Blinkhoff *et al.*, 1999)

Overall, about 70 per cent of volunteers trained between 1991–4 were still working as volunteers in 1998. Key factors in retention of this vital, unpaid community health resource appear to include:

- Religious conviction – particularly their Christian faith.
- Feelings of 'neighbourly love'.
- Seeing the health of their patients improve.
- Group solidarity.
- A sense of pride in what they achieve together.
- Social events ('secret friends' meetings) at which experiences and ideas can be exchanged.

In addition, the home care programme offers support by:

- Showing appreciation to each individual volunteer.
- An annual Christmas party, where volunteers receive gifts for themselves and their families.
- Weekly or fortnightly 'professional' supportive supervision from the programme nurses.
- Technical and logistic support, to assist with implementing appropriate regimes of treatment and intervention.
- 'Incentives' – volunteers can purchase mealie meal at 50 per cent of market price for their own families, and some have received grants or loans for development of income-generation activities.
- Reviews to obtain volunteers' views of how the programme could be improved.

Examples of the latter concerned complaints that nurses failed to consult with volunteers when planning future community activities, and volunteers would 'bottle-up' their resentments, which then led to tensions in the programme. The AIDS department responded by giving volunteers a voice in the selection of their community nurse. Another concern was about the variation in programme policies and activities across townships, leaving some communities relatively disadvantaged in the implementation of their activities (e.g., transport, and loans/grants). The AIDS department response has been to consider developing clearer policy guidelines that also respect the need for local autonomy and ownership.

Summary

Throughout this book, there are numerous hints for turning problems with work stress and burnout into opportunities for improving adherence, commitment, skills, morale and quality of care. Many apply equally to volunteers and to paid health workers, and they all amount to the following – improving recognition of what is done, of its difficulty, and of those who do it. The need to, and importance of, investing in volunteer and paid health and social service staff by giving them time, attention and on-going preparation is overwhelming.

To summarise, this brief review of volunteer HIV/AIDS workers enables the following basic suggestions for avoiding burnout:

- For every volunteer, clarify what is expected of them, and why, and agree on it.
- Provide a contract that clarifies expectations of their participation in supervision.
- Provide social support opportunities, and re-affirm the ethos of care and commitment their organisation embraces.
- Ensure that supervision includes examination of volunteers' stresses and difficulties – and rewards and successes – and review how their responses impact on appropriate boundaries between them and their patients/clients.
- Provide appropriate training to improve volunteers' sense of efficacy.
- Say 'thank you' whenever possible, for volunteers keep us all in a position to hope.

10 Management of occupational stress and burnout

'There is an attitude problem that we have perpetuated, and still help to foster throughout society and especially in the helping professions, that leads us to be proud of the fact that we strive to meet unrealistic expectations. In the health care system . . . we traditionally put ourselves and our patients at unnecessary risk by trying to accomplish too much, and we are so proud of our exhaustion that we make no serious effort to remedy the situation' (Lyall, 1989, p. 27).

This chapter will consider a number of issues relevant to the design of burnout prevention and management, and of the evaluation of its impact. First, the lack of good outcome studies will be discussed, along with a critique of approaches to intervention from the non-HIV/AIDS (and non-health services) arena – the issues raised may well inform future thinking on the conduct of stress interventions at an organisational level in HIV/AIDS and elsewhere. Then, models for stress and burnout management and prevention are discussed, based on what we know so far in HIV/AIDS and other fields of health staff care. The last part of the chapter concerns the range of additional issues to consider when investing in staff support. The overall aim is to be practical and relevant to the known needs of health workers in HIV/AIDS.

Staff stress intervention outcome studies

A surprising fact of the literature on burnout and occupational stress is the relative dearth of empirically tested suggestions for management and prevention of these conditions (Kahill, 1988; Briner, 1997). Many papers and studies offer *suggestions* for burnout prevention, but there is very little empirical evidence to support their speculations. Additionally, Reynolds and Briner (1994) have noted that beliefs about the value of occupational interventions to reduce stress in the workforce have gone unchallenged, and that they are based on simplistic views of organisations and individuals that simply do not match the complexities of causes and consequences identified in the burnout literature. Indeed, Briner (1997) has questioned the rationality of assumptions that stress management interventions (SMIs) could be effective at all:

- It is likely that all employees do not react similarly to the same conditions; therefore, changes in conditions may not produce uniform or expected – or even desirable – changes in responses of all staff.
- Such approaches assume that coping skills are more important than, say, personality in minimising stress effects.
- They also assume that coping skills can be taught effectively in a stress management training (SMT) format – or that they can be taught at all! However, the complexity of coping skills, particularly within complex organisations, suggests that even intensive training may not transfer into appropriate or useful workplace behaviour (consider the case of infection control practices!).

Such gloomy considerations aside, models of SMIs presented by Briner (1997) conform to the typology shown in Table 10.1, and he discusses two studies which come under the category of 'Context Management' (specifically, procedural/ structural initiatives – see Table 10.2) which do provide some evidence of outcome (Wall *et al.*, 1986; Cordery *et al.*, 1991). These studies each involved a 'job redesign intervention' in which employees were given greater autonomy or control over how their work was arranged and scheduled. The evaluation revealed that while some feelings, attitudes, job satisfaction and commitment improved as a result of the intervention, motivation and mental health indices did not alter, and absence and turnover actually increased. Briner and Reynolds (1998) have argued that this pattern of results is found in all evaluations of job redesign – context management may create as many (though different) problems as they remedy!

Pines and Maslach (1978) reported a case study of an active organisational intervention involving the reorganisation of a daycare centre from a structure-less organisation, to one in which structure was defined and implemented. After six months the results were 'extremely positive' in terms of reduced burnout and improved relationships within the centre. Stevens and Pfost (1983) reported on a burnout prevention group in terminal care staff showing improved engagement in problem-solving and team solution-finding. Findings reported are, however, impressionistic only – a common problem for the reader attempting to judge the relative merits of possible strategies for change.

Stress associated with organisational structure and atmosphere may, as we have considered earlier, be mediated by the worker's response to office politics, degree of participation in decision-making, imposition of limits and restrictions on appropriate autonomy, and being admitted to 'inside' information on company/ organisational issues (Cooper and Marshall, 1978). French and Kaplan (1972), and Margolis (1974) found that greater participation in organisational processes led to higher productivity, improved performance, lower staff turnover, and lower levels of physical and mental disorder, including stress-related activities such as escapist drinking and smoking.

Outcome efficacy has been demonstrated in the context of 'Emotional Support/ Therapeutic Counselling' as an SMI, a notable example being the Post Office study (Cooper *et al.*, 1990; Cooper and Sadri, 1991). This study examined the

Table 10.1 Models for staff stress management and prevention

	Professional supervision	Emotional support/ therapeutic counselling	Stress reduction/ management	Context management
Facilitator	External or Internal	External or Internal	External or Internal	Management
Nature	Individual or Group ('Team') (on demand)	Individual or Group ('Team') (on demand)	Individual or Group ('Team') (on demand)	See Table 10.2
Regularity	Regular or Irregular (on demand)	Regular or Irregular (on demand)	Regular or Irregular (on demand)	Continuous
Duration	On-going	On-going or limited duration (e.g., crisis management)	On-going or limited duration (e.g., crisis management)	Continuous
Frequency	Weekly, fortnightly or monthly	Weekly, fortnightly or monthly, or on request	Weekly, fortnightly or monthly, or on request	Following regular review
Composition	Same or mixed professions	Same or mixed professions for groups	Same or mixed professions for groups	Applies to all staff
Content	Case review, professional monitoring, skills assessment	Ventilation, emotional support, team-building and restoration	Relaxation strategies, including meditation, visualisation, massage, shiatsu and exercise, seminars and classes in, e.g., time management, team-building, etc.	See Table 10.2

Source: Miller and Gillies, 1993.

costs and benefits of providing staff support in the form of individual, open-access, specialist psychological counselling, based within the occupational health service of the Post Office. Twenty-two months after publicising the service through letters to employees, in-house magazine articles, and seminars to management, 40 per cent of referrals came from occupational health, 31.5 per cent came from self-referrals, 19 per cent came from welfare services within the organisation, and 9.5 per cent came from management, personnel and the trade unions. Mental health and stress issues (mainly anxiety and/or depression) represented 46 per cent of the caseload, while 24 per cent concerned relationship problems, especially marital difficulties. Other referrals concerned substance abuse, bereavement, assault and physical illness and disability. One of the more impressive findings of this study was that in addition to counselling resulting in significantly lowered levels of anxiety, depression, and psychosomatic illness, and higher levels of self-esteem, less substance abuse, and increased use of relaxation techniques and exercise, £100,000 in prevented absenteeism was saved for every 175 personnel

Table 10.2 Context management for prevention of staff stress

Procedural/structural initiatives	Environmental initiatives
Limiting working hours	Normalising the experience and expression of work stress
Providing pre-work orientation and training	Recognising the impact of (multiple) loss
Enabling expression of work successes	Providing opportunities for skills development
Training in stress recognition and management	Providing quiet staff areas
Enabling expression of initiative and work variation	Providing a pleasant work environment
Discouraging working alone	Actively encouraging that holidays be taken
Give increased control and autonomy over work tasks	
Planning time away from work	

Source: Miller and Gillies, 1993.

provided with counselling and supportive services in the workplace (Cooper and Cartwright, 1994). On the other hand, the counselling was found to have little impact on staffs' job satisfaction or organisational commitment – staff here, as elsewhere, appeared to be 'non-linear functional systems'! This latter finding alone points to the need for comprehensive measurement of outcomes – relying on simplistic measures is not enough (see Chapter 6).

Interventions to prevent burnout have been recommended to address specific aspects of care, rather than providing general and passive content (Bennett, Kelaher and Ross, 1994; Miller, 1995b; Miller, Gillies and Elliott, 1996). It is, of course, the application of a problem-solving focus that has been found effective for HIV patients undergoing counselling and psychosocial care (Green, 1986; Miller, 1987). This points again to the potential benefit to be gained from approaching staff stress and burnout management as a *clinical* issue, to be dealt with by a clinical approach (Handy, 1988). A difficulty with evaluations of SMIs, however, particularly the non-counselling activities such as professional monitoring, stress management, and context management, is that they are often approached as though they were clinical treatments, when in fact they embody *preventive* strategies – using psychological mood outcome measures in these instances is therefore usually inappropriate and will inevitably yield disappointing results (Briner, 1997). The lesson, then, is to be clear about what is being evaluated, so the measures of appropriate scope and breadth are put in place. This issue has been discussed in detail in Chapter 6.

Lessons and paradoxes from the literature

In addition to problems with reliably and usefully measuring work stress, burn-out, and responses to managing or preventing them, the literature has generated a number of paradoxes that possibly serve to perpetuate the absence of relevant and tested schemes for constructive change in the workplace:

1   Burnout and work stress appear to be rooted so much in organisational conditions, yet the majority of suggestions for change appear to be aimed at *individuals*, not organisations – individual workers are targetted as units of change to reduce the effects of work stresses, instead of the organisational conditions that are demonstrated to generate the stress (Leiter, 1991; Shinn *et al.*, 1984; Cooper and Cartwright, 1994; Reynolds and Briner, 1994).

2   Burnout is a consequence of *chronic* processes, yet the solutions often proposed are acute, perhaps involving exposure to workshops, seminars or training lasting no longer than a few days (Leiter, 1991; Gallop *et al.*, 1992; Bennett, Kelaher and Ross, 1994; Reynolds and Briner, 1994).

3   Additionally, proposed solutions are frequently *simplistic and formulaic* abstractions of clinical programmes designed for clinical audiences and primarily for use with individuals, and to be used in the context of multi-faceted treatment programmes. They are then applied uncritically to group approaches to management of chronic occupational distress that fail to recognise the inherent *complexity* of the interactional circumstantial and cognitive processes resulting in burnout (this also has implications for the appropriate measurement of change as a result of exposure to such pro-grammes, as discussed in Chapter 6) (Cooper and Cartwright, 1994; Reynolds and Briner, 1994);

4   Proposed solutions and approaches to management of burnout are logically for the benefit of workers at whom they are targetted (and therefore for the benefit of the organisations they work for), yet it is very unusual in the literature to see any attempts to ask staff what they want and need from such interventions – interventions appear routinely to be *imposed* on staff, and may therefore perpetuate rather than reduce the stresses they aim to address (see Chapter 8).

Because chronic processes will frequently require chronic interventions, the paradox of acute interventions has significance for the definitions being used in planning and implementing preventive and ameliorative strategies. As any psychology clinician will attest – particularly when managing the consequences of a chronic stress-related process – recovery management similarly takes time. Burnout can not be expected to be meaningfully dealt with in a 'one-off' session, although stress prevention – a very different issue – might. The need to avoid confusing stress and burnout, and educational and clinical interventions, is therefore paramount if management and preventive design are to be appropriate and effective.

A related concern is that many proposed solutions or interventions for staff stress and occupational morbidity are too often sweeping in their design, promising or recommending far more than can be achieved even through a medium- or long-term intervention, as might be the case with individual clinical approaches. If we consider recommendations to enhance self-esteem, social and clinical psychologists recognise that the concept of self-esteem is a multi-layered, often fragile entity that arises usually from years of experience. No-one would argue that strategic targetting of interventions for individuals to help manage specific issues impacting on self-esteem would probably be beneficial – as seen, for example, in the literature on assertion-training (e.g., Lange and Jakubowski, 1976). But to suggest that group membership and a psychometric score will somehow confirm the likelihood of lasting beneficial impact when so many other work, social, personality and other issues similarly affect the construct is naive and may ultimately undermine the potential of more focused, realistic efforts.

An important although usually unstated element in reports from the literature is that staff care, stress and distress management and/or prevention actually is a *clinical* process, deserving and demanding the same degree of rigour and seriousness – irrespective of the clinical seriousness of presenting issues – as the management of any other physical and psychological presenting process. As a clinical process, it should also be recognised that recovery processes are so often not linear, but follow many winding and often illusory paths (Kesler, 1990).

Suggestions and models for staff support and prevention of burnout

Although most cited studies of work stress and burnout in HIV/AIDS – and other fields of health care – offer suggestions for implementing staff support, the need for effective models of staff stress management and prevention is more pressing than ever. Such models are generally absent or have yet to be clearly characterised in this arena. As we have seen, a result is that suggestions for interventions very rarely have outcome data upon which to assess their efficacy or value (and/or their potential for making things worse!). The following schema is an attempt to co-ordinate suggestions for implementation of staff support in a manner consistent with characterisations of *individualised* (professional supervision, emotional support, stress reduction) versus *organisational* (context management) approaches to reducing burnout and staff stress, as proposed by, for example, Cooper and Davidson (1987), Leiter (1991) and Reynolds and Briner (1994).

As a precursor to suggested models for staff support, The National Association for Staff Support (NASS) has issued general policy principles which they describe as:

'. . . an essential part of any national or local policy [on staff support]:

• Staff in health care services have individual rights to be valued and respected, just as any other citizens have.

- Staff who are cared for provide the best quality of service; where there is inadequate care and support, staff will show high sickness, absenteeism and wastage rates.
- Staff are a valued and expensive resource. It makes good sense to maintain their fitness and capacity to give a good service in the interests of their personal job satisfaction and of maintaining the quality of patient care.
- A range of integrated services together with a general ethos of care is an essential provision. Also recognition of the nature of stress and of the need for emotional support in the workplace at all times is important.
- Identifying who is responsible for providing a stated policy, both nationally and locally, is necessary for coordination in all workplaces.' (NASS, 1992, pp. 4–5)

Staff support may be characterised according to four different modalities: (a) professional supervision; (b) emotional support/therapeutic counselling; (c) stress reduction/management programmes; and (d) context management (Miller and Gillies, 1993). Each of these is explicated in Table 10.1, and in the text that follows. This schema has many similarities and points of overlap with the three-level classification system of SMIs described by Briner (1998):

- *Primary interventions* – those which change job conditions such as the level or nature of work demands or stressors (what are here referred to as forms of 'context management').
- *Secondary interventions* – those giving people coping skills in the face of such stressors (here referred to as forms of 'stress reduction/management').
- *Tertiary interventions* – those which aim to directly treat individuals experiencing high levels of distress (here referred to as forms of 'emotional support/therapeutic counselling').

Perhaps a problem with each classification system is that the elements appear frequently to be confused in practice, with ultimately undermining consequences for the staff involved. It is pertinent to recall the paradox mentioned above, that it appears so often to be individuals who are targetted for change in stress management, rather than the organisations generating the stresses.

This point has been made with some emphasis by Shinn *et al.* (1984), Reynolds and Briner (1994), and Leiter (1991). Leiter suggests that the gap between professionals' expectations and the realities of their working circumstances may be closed by: (a) lowering expectations – a strategy implicit in self-help and other approaches to individual stress management, that also deflects the need for (perhaps expensive) organisational change; (b) bringing work settings more into line with expectations, implying organisational and cultural change – context management; and (c) doing some of both. In arguing for option (b), Leiter (1991) states:

'The organisational structure and management practices in human service agencies are incompatible with the needs of all but a few of their stake-holders [mainly administrators]. It is time to change the emphasis in applied work on burnout' (p. 549).

The room for manoeuvre in preventive approaches with respect to individuals is relatively narrow, when compared with options for organisations. This was illustrated in suggestions for burnout prevention by Miller (1991), and themes from this earlier schema have been incorporated into the four models proposed below. As Cooper and Cartwright (1994) concur, many of these strategies for institutional or organisational change are directed at, and could only happen with, employee participation (option (c) of Leiter, 1991). It is the potentially disruptive and organisationally expensive prospect of implementation that directs attention for change back to individuals, however (Cooper and Cartwright, 1994; Reynolds and Briner, 1994). Nevertheless, if we maintain the tendency to pathologise individual reactions to unreasonable and largely preventable work stresses, this will merely serve to perpetuate the conditions in which stress will flourish, and in which staff are increasingly lost. Focusing alone on individuals for change may therefore be more expensive for organisations, and costly in other ways for the patients using them, than working to alter fundamentally destructive organisational conditions – and similarly corrosive political conditions and imperatives that maintain them. In addition to the four general models in Table 10.1, achieveable *organisational* options for stress prevention are also described in Table 10.2.

Professional supervision

This is the intervention provided to monitor and enhance the clinical and professional activities of health care workers. It may be provided to teams, such as ward staffs or community care units, or to individual health professionals. It may be provided by supervisors from either within or outside the setting in which people are being supervised, and where groups or teams are being supervised they may be of either the same or mixed professions. Such intervention may also be regular (e.g., weekly, fortnightly, or monthly) or irregular (e.g., when need is identified). As the intention of professional supervision is usually to maintain standards of professional care, it will most commonly involve reviewing case or patient management, monitoring of professional understanding and practices, evaluation of professional procedures and skills. In voluntary contexts where codes of professionalism cannot be necessarily enforced, professional supervision may more appropriately be thought of as 'supervision of appropriate standards of intervention', perhaps by a professionally qualified and experienced health professional. Conventional examples of this type of intervention in ward settings include ward rounds and case-conferences. A problem with such monitoring is that while it may aim to maintain and even increase the confidence of health staff in their skills and interventions, it may often be competitive and stress-inducing because it exposes the staff member to professional and peer criticism and performance pressure in circumstances where time for constructive discussion is very limited.

Leach *et al.* (1999) have refined the notion of clinical supervision, which describes:

> '. . . formal, planned and regular discussions between an expert practitioner and one or more supervisees which has the purpose of facilitating reflecting practice so as to support the practitioner(s) in their role, encourage the development of practice skills, and maintain professional and ethical standards in the context of on-going professional development' (Leach *et al.*, 1999).

Clinical supervision may be thought of as distinct but necessarily complementary to professional supervision and monitoring – it may be supportive, but the focus is primarily on the work with the client or patient, and the support is given to the supervisee in their working role. Procter (undated) describes clinical supervision as having three basic functions:

1   *Formative* – developing the skills, understanding and abilities of the clinician/ health worker, by reflecting on and exploration of work with clients.
2   *Restorative* – responding to the health worker's feelings associated with the patient/client's distress, pain and fragmentation, and examining how this has affected the health worker.
3   *Normative* – ensuring the health worker remains appropriate and is working within defined ethical standards.

The importance of clinical supervision for managing the issues of boundaries is discussed in detail below.

Emotional support/therapeutic counselling

As illustrated in Table 10.1, the format of emotional supervision/theraputic counselling for health workers contains many similarities to those for professional supervision. There are important differences, however, in the aims and therefore content of each. In providing emotional support or therapeutic counselling to health staff, the intention is to *relieve* or *support* the health worker facing the stresses of their job. It goes without saying that this implies an acceptance, first that their work contains stresses that may need to be addressed or ventilated, and second that expression of emotional vulnerability associated with work is seen as a *legitimate* circumstance, rather than a sign of weakness or unprofessionalism. The intention, therefore, includes ensuring that stresses do not become issues of crisis or, if they do, that crises can be localised and managed effectively for all concerned. Interventions under this general heading thus can contribute effectively yet indirectly to team-building or restoration, even when health workers are seen individually.

Some examples of the types of interventions that may come within this model include that reported by Kesler (1990), in which Lazarus's BASIC ID schema for formulating psychological distress and interventions formed a useful basis for understanding and resolving self-reported burnout. Maynard (1985) has suggested that crisis interveners seldom stop and identify their own feelings – they will mask them to maintain effectiveness with clients, but this will make it more difficult to stay attuned to their own feelings. Maynard describes the use of support groups to enable regular and free ventilation of suppressed/masked feelings to avoid build-up and burnout in these populations. In a similar vein, Friedman (1985) reported working with family therapists, giving attention to expectations, role definition, sharing of feelings, and theraputic ambition (and patients' versus therapists responsibilities in this) to ease strain on the therapist.

In a multi-disciplinary qualitative study of AIDS health care workers' responses to the novel pressures of HIV/AIDS care, Wade, Perlman and Simon (1993) described a phenomenon of therapeutic alliance they termed 'survival bonding': in a qualitative study of only ten persons (five pairs), the pairs of health workers would form intense informal relationships that acted as a buffer against self-reported stress, isolation and emotional exhaustion. These bonds were characterised by trust, respect, shared decision-making, and peer support. These survival bonds would dissolve as they shared less work together.

Stress reduction/management

Once again, the format of such interventions is relatively similar to those for professional supervision and emotional support/theraputic counselling, yet the aims determine substantial differences in content. This mode of health worker care aims to directly reduce or prevent the experience of work-related stress, and usually employs *active* relaxation and stress-reduction techniques, and/or development of skills to prevent stress arising. These may be facilitated either within or outside work time, and to groups or individuals. Approaches to stress reduction, management and prevention have been described by Strassmeier (1986), using a systems theory perspective to develop an ecosystem approach toward social networks, social development, crisis intervention and help-seeking behaviour. Bair and Greenspan (1986) describe Training in Effectiveness through Assertiveness in a Medical Setting (TEAMS) – a programme of workshops for multi-disciplinary communication building and restoring. The aims are to increase collaborative practice, leadership skills, and knowledge of team-building and stress management. Piercy and Wetchler (1987) have reported on a didactic-experiential workshop programme to examine and unclog issues from family therapists' own families and relationships, to enable them to avoid burnout which may otherwise result.

An example of an attempt at staff stress reduction through a knowledge-based intervention study has recently been reported by Gallop and Taerk (1995). These authors surveyed staff from three AIDS management sites who had participated in a random allocation study to one of four conditions: (1) 20-minute knowledge video about HIV/AIDS, followed by 30-minute discussion with an AIDS expert; (2) Video followed within two weeks by a 60-minute group discussion of attitudes and concerns about AIDS; (3) As for (2) plus a video of a homosexual person with AIDS discussing his illness and experience of hospitalisation; (4) As for (3) with the discussion in the presence of a person with AIDS. Following the inerventions, participants were surveyed on their knowledge, attitudes and fears about HIV/AIDS. The researchers found that the knowledge package alone was enough to increase knowledge about HIV/AIDS. However, this alone was *not* enough to change attitudes and fears, and emotional responses to HIV and AIDS – this required focused group discussions. Additionally, to reduce significantly the fear of risk of infection and homophobia required the presence of a person with AIDS sharing their personal story – either on video or in person. The authors suggest that this approach with staff could be strengthened with multiple group sessions.

Reynolds and Briner (1994) have made a series of important criticisms of approaches to staff stress management, particularly stress management training (SMT) based usually on cognitive behaviour therapy (CBT), and applied to groups of staff. They point to key differences between these two approaches which suggest that logically, we could not expect outcomes in industry from SMT as favourable as clinical outcomes with CBT:

1   SMT is not designed to meet needs of individual participants, in the way that individual CBT is – SMT is usually offered as a package, meaning individual needs are met to varying degrees, and organisational problems raised may not be amenable to a package approach based on CBT.
2   The two approaches are brought to bear on very different levels of distress – most SMT participants are voluntary, with non-clinical levels of psychological indices, such as anxiety and depression, whereas CBT recipients usually present with clinically significant levels of psychological distress (in which beneficial change is also easier to measure).
3   The general aims of the two differ, with SMT usually having a preventive focus, thus making measurement of its efficacy in 'normal' populations very difficult to assess. CBT is by definition applied to clinical populations in whom theraputic change is far quicker and more easily quantifiable.

The authors suggest that an important reason for focusing on changing individual employees rather than improving features of the working environment is the increasing threat of employee litigation. Reynolds and Briner (1994) also challenge the notion that self-worth is dependent upon success at work and that interventions must prevent staff loss – where counselling positively identifies that a worker would be better off working elsewhere, an organisational outcome of stress prevention could be actually to increase staff turnover.

Some studies of the impact of SMT have borne out their doubts. For example, Sallis *et al.* (1987) randomly allocated 76 staff to either multi-component SMT, relaxation training, or an education support group. Psychological well-being, job satisfaction, work stress and blood pressure were measured at the start and at the end of the eight-week interventions, and three months subsequently. Each resulted in significant reductions in depression and hostility – maintained at follow-up – but not in work stress, blood pressure or job satisfaction measures. This manifestation of equivalent outcomes – familiar in clinical psychological and psychophysiological intervention research – suggests that enabling staff to discuss important issues in a supportive atmosphere was the critical common element, but also emphasises the difficulty in finding meaningful beneficial change in non-clinical populations.

Similarly, when attempting to assess the value of such interventions for organisations, SMT outcomes give equivocal results (Reynolds and Briner, 1994). The Post-Office study cited above by Cooper and colleagues found no evidence that improved attendance was accompanied by improved performance, despite the significant individual gains in the clinical populations. A complex study involving identifying and tackling sources of work stress, providing SMT and employee assistance programmes for all staff in 22 hospitals, with another 22 hospitals as matched controls, showed highly significant reductions in malpractice claims against the experimental group, and no changes in the controls (Jones *et al.*, 1988). However, the very complexity of the interventions made isolating the instrumental aspects of the interventions difficult to identify. Longer-term benefits in this and other studies have not been tested.

Context management

This mode of stress management or prevention involves environmental or contextual initiatives that assist in raising staff appreciation, and reducing staff stress. They may involve procedural/structural initiatives, such as limiting allowable working hours for health staff, or environmental initiatives, such as the provision of quiet rest areas for staff, or refurbishment of facilities to make working environs more pleasant. Interventions for context management have been suggested by Miller and Gillies (1993) (see Table 10.2).

In this context it is interesting to speculate on the possible value of institutional structure and hierarchy in helping to reduce stress on health workers. Wilcoxon (1989) found that agencies with administrators with high 'initiative structure' and consideration had reduced reported therapist burnout in rural community health centres. High structure was seen to be associated with reduced deterioration of therapist–client relations – presumably everyone knew clearly where they stood. This notion of high institutional and/or professional structure resulting in lowered role ambiguity and therefore lowered occupational and role-related stress is certainly deserving of closer study in future, perhaps by comparing health workers in the armed or religious services with those in the outside worlds (although these populations may not be strictly comparable for other reasons). A study assessing the value of a clear institutional ideology would also shed important light on the potential for avoidance of occupational morbidity associated with health care in religious contexts, for example. Such lessons would be of particular value in those settings – such as many developing countries – where significant proportions of health care are provided by mission hospitals. And research discussed in Chapters 5 and 8 revealed the importance of a clear organisational ethos and sense of affiliation with that ethos (e.g., the AIDS cause, gay community and gay rights, christian principles) in reducing burnout and increasing volunteer retention and satisfaction in HIV/AIDS care.

A valuable form of context management involves providing a contract for health worker supervision and support. This has been implemented in some peer-led community support agencies in the UK and, although the results have not been quantified, anecdotally the provision of such structural endorsement of staff support appears to be associated with low staff turnover, low levels of service-user complaint, and rational use of support that is provided.

A recent approach to context management has been to enable the expression of psychosocial successes in AIDS care to boost clinical confidence and balance the negative aspects of working in this field (Bennett, Kelaher and Ross, 1994). This approach is based on work by Clark (1989), who suggests that deaths of patients may at times be seen by workers as a personal failure, and that workers should be encouraged to accumulate a personal record of identifiable, significant and positive events that have contributed to the emotional well-being and quality of life of patients and their loved-ones. Clark's hypothesis is that staff focusing on positive achievements – and whose psychosocial achievements are professionally recognised – may be less prone to burnout.

Cooper and Cartwright (1994) suggest that context management may most usefully be optomised by regular and detailed 'stress audits', involving sampling of workers from all levels of staff, which may act as a baseline measure of staff stress, and may also provide information about good issues for change, and a measure of the impact and effectiveness of interventions for burnout prevention and amelioration. A similar approach of needs assessment for all workplace stress-reduction interventions has been advocated by Ivanecevich and Matteson (1987).

Some implications of such models for planning of staff support

Perhaps the main point to be made about this division of staff support modalities is that they are often confused in practice, precisely because the different aims of each – and the true needs for them – are not clearly considered in stress prevention planning. This is particularly so in observing the differences between professional supervision and emotional support. For example, where professional supervision is being given by a higher-ranking colleague (who themselves may be responsible for much of the stresses experienced by the junior colleague – especially where clinical and management responsibilities overlap), it may often be simply unrealistic to expect that emotional vulnerability will be admitted by the junior colleague. As such, emotional stresses will not be expressed, and may thus be seriously compounded and lead to greater stresses and pressures on the institution.

Similarly, it is reasonable to assume that each of the modalities presented will only be effectively taken up if they are seen to have the active support of management. In this way, health professionals may lose the fear that using such facilities exposes them to the charge of being professionally suspect, or weak, or vulnerable. Such institutional and managerial endorsement may also help to reduce staff fears that their use of staff support facilities to express any occupationally derived emotional vulnerability will result in their 'professional exposure' because of a lack of confidentiality or an institutional condition that all details be made known to managers. From this it follows that any such enterprise will only usually succeed when culturally accepted confidentiality can be guaranteed.

It is also clear that these models for staff stress management and prevention are not mutually exclusive and can be employed in any combination. Although there are so few empirical data on efficacy of any approach, it seems likely that where more strategies are available to the individual health worker, one or some will be more likely to be taken up, and the likelihood of effective beneficial outcome will be greater. The UK burnout studies (see Chapters 7 and 8) revealed the preferences of staff for access to more than one modality of staff support.

In preparing HIV staff for the stresses associated with their work, Sherr and George (1989) suggested a combination of professional and structural/organisational elements, such as stress innoculation training, assuring adequate staff levels and staff communications, and ensuring a pleasant work environment and adequate consideration of individual interpersonal factors. Rugg *et al.* (1989) found varying tasks performed and limiting hours spent in direct counselling of people with HIV to be important for reducing burnout in HIV counsellors. Dinoi and Brettler (1991) described a programme for a haemophilia treatment team involving an initial individual staff psychological consultation, then referral to staff support groups to help reduce isolation, develop perspectives on patients' issues, enable sharing of coping styles and develop staff support networks. Corcoran and Bryce (1983) reported using interpersonal skills training in groups of social service workers to reduce burnout scores on the MBI. After four sessions over one month, empathy increased, and MBI burnout decreased, while increasing significantly in the non-intervention control group. Such activities presume that there is a trusting work milieu in which sharing of vulnerability is possible without fear of reprisal.

Finally, each of these general models conveys responsibilities both for the institution and the individuals involved. For the institution, a main responsibility is to make such models available, singly or in combination. For the individual, a main responsibility is to make use of the models or, where they are not available, to argue coherently and appropriately for their establishment.

In their comprehensive review of available research, anecdotal reports and findings from the UK burnout studies, Miller, Gillies and Elliott (1994) suggested a summary of key features of successful staff support activities. It suggests a broad wish-list of suggestions which need much more empirical investigation before their true importance can be agreed. However, it provides a useful starting guide, and is presented in Table 8.6.

Further issues to consider in planning staff support

What obstacles exist to implementation of effective health staff care?

In addition to the burdens listed above, experience and research suggests that major obstacles exist to implementation and usage of appropriate staff support programmes. For example, as noted by Miller and Gillies (1993):

- Staff may not often know precisely *what* they want when they say they want staff support, or when they are offering it.
- Many assumptions are being made about the degree of trust colleagues may have for each other – frequently it seems staff refuse to disclose their emotional vulnerability to others because they do not trust how that information will be perceived or subsequently be used.
- Many staff interviewed suggest there remains a prevailing view in the health services in the UK that disclosure of vulnerability is dangerous because it will be seen as indicative of non-professionalism or unsuitability to do the job they are doing.
- Staff may feel unable to move from the supportive role to being supported in the workplace, even for brief periods.
- There may be insufficient time or staff cover to enable regular or reliable support sessions.
- Health professionals in HIV/AIDS are working within a culture of secrecy while facing the acute and complex needs of their patients.
- There may be assumptions made about the appropriate development and maintenance of interventions designed to improve staff morale, but which may actually be counter-productive – e.g., support groups may have very limited effective durations, yet may be carried on to the point of adding to staff tensions, rather than reducing them.

Being realistic about the impact of stigma

A further critical challenge is to get rid of the *stigma* surrounding work stress. No research to date has addressed this directly, although occasional reports (e.g., Bair and Greenspan, 1986) make reference to it indirectly, e.g., by reporting interns being reluctant to acknowledge to their colleagues outside support groups that they were spending group time away from other elements of their work for this. The MOMS study on staff groups in the fields of HIV/AIDS and oncology indicated that stigma about professional vulnerability was an issue that could directly be influenced beneficially by managerial modelling of non-discriminatory views towards staff who sought help for stress (Miller, Gillies and Elliott, 1996). The issue of absence of mutual trust having an important and negative impact on social services personnel has been explored by O'Driscoll and Schubert (1988). Their findings match earlier observations of the critical role of support and trust at all levels within human service agencies (Pines, 1982; Shinn *et al.*, 1984).

Instructional groups for staff about recognising, understanding and managing work stress may be a vital concurrent element in generating trust and openness about the trials of health care, at all levels. Explicit training in HIV treatment issues and roles may also dispel the professional 'contagion' mentioned as a potential contributor to work stress and burnout, in Chapter 5.

Clinical supervision, boundaries and burnout

The relationships between burnout and boundary issues – and violations – have rarely been explicated in the context of HIV/AIDS, apart from within research examining impact of HIV/AIDS work on volunteers (e.g., Maslanka, 1995, 1996). Yet, as researchers and commentators have frequently pointed out, boundary violations are regularly documented in contexts addressing psychological vulnerabilities (Edelwich and Brodsky, 1980) as psychotherapeutic relationships tend to be isolated (i.e., priveleged and confidential), have significant length and intensity, have elements of transference and sometimes high dependency (Gabbard, 1994), and patients have high emotional vulnerability (Plaut, 1997). Gartrell *et al.* (1992) showed that 5–10 per cent of licensed psychotherapists in North America admitted to at least one relationship with a client in their career, and 9 per cent of non-psychiatrist physicians have admitted to at least one sexual relationship with a patient. Boundary violations are exploitative and are known in many instances to cause very serious harm to vulnerable patients (Gabbard, 1994). Given the documented heightened risk of burnout associated with emotional issues raised in HIV work, particularly in junior and less-experienced health staff, and the difficulties reported in discussing emotional consequences of work, the important possibilities of boundary problems in HIV/AIDS staff, and the need to address them, becomes clear.

Boundary violations do not have to be sexual, of course – they may emerge in any power relationship where potential harm to the patient may arise because of pressures arising from a 'dual relationship' – where either the provider serves two professional roles, or where the professional relationship includes certain personal elements (Plaut, 1997). One of the difficulties of therapeutic relationships is that, especially where intimacy and chronicity are involved, dual elements almost inevitably become admitted. Indeed, Gessler *et al.* (1996) have suggested that the context of HIV and STDs has *encouraged* boundary tensions by actively blurring boundaries on an organisational and structural level – at least in the UK – in order to counteract the stigma and increase the attractiveness of statutory services to those at risk for HIV who may otherwise be disinclined to attend (Gessler *et al.*, 1996). If such models exist in statutory settings, it should be no surprise to see boundary blurring, and the enhanced likelihood of boundary problems, also in voluntary care initiatives.

Much more research is needed to identify the nature and avoidance of boundary problems in contemporary health care, not least because where reliable information is lacking, doubt, innuendo and prejudice may take the place of appropriate respect and willingness to collaborate in responding to a health emergency.

Plaut (1997) suggests that the best approach in addressing boundary issues – whether as a consequence of burnout or not – is by raising such tensions in professional education and training, including the use of case scenarios in which staff must make decisions about ethical and appropriate, humane interventions, and by setting organisational guidelines on appropriate responses to potential boundary violations. For example, in regarding the specific demand character- istics associated with HIV/AIDS, Plaut acknowledges:

> Specific situations may also suggest a reconsideration of appropriate boundaries. Whereas a psychotherapist may normally restrict the extent of touch to a handshake, a more supportive touch given by that same therapist may be considered quite appropriate when offered to a person with AIDS who may feel 'untouchable', a patient in grief, or a patient who is terminally ill in an institutional setting, where human touch is often minimal (Gutheil and Gabbard, 1993; Offit, 1994). (pp. 87–8)

To facilitate this process of transparency, Plaut (1997) suggests the following guidelines for individual health workers, and for the on-going content of super- vision:

- Be aware of ethical standards for the conduct of care.
- Be prepared to refer onwards where appropriate.
- Know the risk factors and warning signs in therapeutic relationships that could lead to sexual intimacy.
- Know risk factors for vulnerable clients.
- Know risk factors for vulnerable health workers.
- Know how to respond to inappropriate advances by clients.
- Be honest with yourself about whose needs are being met.
- Know how to address a questionable boundary crossing.

Content of staff support – developing an agenda

The case for formalising staff support and supervision was made in the context of volunteers (see Chapter 9), and it applies with equal merit to clinical and pro- fessional supervision for HIV/AIDS workers, not least because it helps to avoid the boundary issues that may easily emerge (above). Structuring the supervision process helps to clarify its aims, its processes – and hence its accessibility. Given the potentially difficult, problematic, sensitive and embarrassing nature of much that may emerge, a further aid may be in formalising an agenda for supervision in advance. If the agenda is mutually predetermined and agreed, later hesitancy and awkwardness may be diminished and avoided – and the reality of the issues for the individual is legitimised.

For example, simply based on findings and suggestions reviewed in this book, a clinical supervision agenda may include:

- Difficulties in keeping up-to-date with clinical developments.

- Monitoring emotional exhaustion and emotional de-briefing.
- Difficulties with working in isolation.
- Issues arising from current (or anticipated) organisational conditions.
- Identification with patients, and relationships with their loved-ones.
- Feeling de-skilled over the chronic decline of patients.
- Difficulties associated with sexuality stereotyping, gender and peer issues.
- Issues arising from being a junior/less-experienced staff member.
- Fears/concerns associated with possible HIV exposure.
- Issues of interaction and communication with colleagues.
- Organisational and team dynamics, and relations with other health workers.
- Coping with breaking bad news, and with patient bereavements.
- Work–home overlap and consequences.
- Ethos and direction of the organisation.
- Motivations for work – current and previous.
- Participation in decision-making.
- Boundary concerns and dilemmas.

As with recommendations for management of other aspects of HIV/AIDS stress and burnout, the viability and appropriateness of any agreed agenda would have to be regularly evaluated by both sides, as in the manner described by Fraser *et al.* (1996) in the context of Buddy relationships.

The role of service managers

The longitudinal survey of four models of staff support in HIV/AIDS facilities in England (Miller, Gillies and Elliott, 1996; see also Chapter 8) has highlighted the crucial role of managers in staff support provision. Interventions for treatment or prevention of staff psychosocial stress will succeed only where there is active, supportive, consistent and explicit management endorsement of them, to the extent that supportive engagement by skilled and trained professionals is recognised as an appropriate part of work for every worker with the same occupational status and institutional recognition and importance as paid holidays. A major problem for managers highlighted in recent research in the radically altering context and political ethos surrounding health care in England, however, was that staff appeared to not trust managers' perceptions of staff vulnerability, so they would not disclose the need for support, i.e., they feared being sacked if they showed signs of the stress they felt (Miller, 1993). Macks and Abrams (1992) suggest that managers openly should be involved in additional skills training to make them more accessible to staff whom they might direct elsewhere for help.

The role of groups in staff support

Groups may frequently be the first recourse for worried health service and staff managers, because of the generalised and possibly erroneous perception that group sessions will enable cementing of staff relations following open sharing of distressing or difficult issues (Grossman and Silverstein, 1993). They are also presumed to be cheaper than individual interventions.

Important elements for effective support groups have recently been identified by a number of authors. For example, Frost *et al.* (1991) describe five elements based on the experience of a multidisciplinary staff support group for those caring with AIDS patients meeting weekly over a three-month period:

1   Consistency – a set time and pace, and regular attendance.
2   Format based on case presentations – to make discussion more relevant to case management issues.
3   Open membership – self-selected, and a maximum of 15 participants.
4   The use of diaries – about feelings raised by, and experiences of, case management, but without diaries being read by other group members.
5   A group facilitator – from outside the hospital but with group management skills, who can observe the differences between being a therapist and being a facilitator in the group.

Frost *et al.* (1991) noted that physicians were considerably under-represented in their group meetings, but that those who did participate found the group sessions helpful. In anecdotally describing a physicians' 'mutual aid' support group for HIV, Garside (1993) suggests that physicians are reluctant to join such activities because of their strong need to be as in control and professionally autonomous, and a disinclination to share feelings, particuarly with professional peers. Garside cites a study by Pruyser (1984) suggesting that physicians feel a moral obligation to be self-sufficient, even though survey populations of physicians have cited peer support as their third greatest need in relation to the stress of AIDS care (Federal Centre for AIDS, 1992). Where there are possibilities that any staff populations may need yet feel unable to access support, clearly it is important to identify why, and what can be done to increase uptake of such services where they are needed.

For groups to work effectively, they need clear and authoritative (but not necessarily intrusive or directive) facilitation by a leader or facilitator. As Kanas (1986) notes, effectiveness relies to a large extent also on having clear goals that are agreed and endorsed by group members, active flexible leadership, and informed leadership well versed in general systems theory and task differentiation. Salt (1997) has proposed employing a systemic approach to staff stress management that uses groups in a team-oriented and task-focused fashion.

The importance of good facilitation for staff groups has been emphasised in an outcome evaluation study of multi-disciplinary staff support groups for health professionals working directly with people with AIDS in New York (Grossman and Silverstein, 1993). Their groups typically have 10–15 weekly sessions with a maximum of 15 participants, and a minimum of eight. Grossman and Silverstein suggest that appropriate facilitators must meet the following criteria:

1   Have working experience with people with HIV/AIDS.
2   Be knowledgeable about group processes.

3   Be open to the feelings of others.
4   Be aware of non-verbal communication.
5   Have experience of dealing with their own feelings about death and dying, sexuality, homophobia, substance abuse, and minority issues.
6   Observe the distinctions between a support group and group therapy.

Key features contributing to the success of staff support groups have been identified in the UK burnout prevention study (Miller, Gillies and Elliott, 1994; see also Table 8.6).

The study of New York support groups by Grossman and Silverstein (1993) identified the six most prominent problems brought by HIV/AIDS staff to the groups as follows:

• Coping with death and dying of patients.
• Work overload and burnout associated with extra time demands of terminal AIDS care.
• Identification with patients and maintaining professional distance.
• Depression associated with witnessing the decline and deaths of patients.
• Dealing with patients' suicidal ideation.
• Feeling angry becuase staffs' families' negative reactions to their working in this field.

On the other hand, open-ended statements concerning the value of the support groups revealed that greatest value was placed by group members on the groups lessening of a sense of professional isolation, being able to ventilate feelings of grief, helplessness and anger, being able to raise uncomfortable issues 'safely', and reducing fears associated with AIDS care-giving.

Groups do have a number of potential problems, however. There are often on-going dilemmas about whether groups should be open to all-comers at each meeting, or with closed membership and a requirement for strictly observed attendance. While group sessions may last on average for 60–90 minutes, some may need longer. It is not often easy for all appropriate group members (e.g., ward nursing staff from all shifts) to convene at the same time. The content of group discussions may become controversial, especially if individual members are in a position to dominate, or have pressing personal agendas that they bring to group discussions. In some settings, this actually appears to be encouraged, as group discussion then maintains a focus, rather than degenerating into a vauge 'gripe session' against the organisation (Macks and Abrams, 1992). The appropriateness of on-going versus crisis-management groups has not been empirically explored or even clearly articulated.

The importance of targetted education

While the finding in the London MOMS study – that a general lack of trust among staff hinders display of emotional needs – suggests that groups may not always be the best way of achieving this in that culture (Miller, 1995a), increasing studies are reporting that *educational* groups are judged by participants as successful (Bennett, 1995; Gallop and Taerk, 1995). What is clear, however, is that staff find groups important and acceptable in facilitating communication and training for staff skills development. Suggestions for training to reduce and prevent staff stress from recent studies include:

- Orienting volunteers to have realistic expectations of what they can achieve, and to what the organisation wants (Maslanka, 1995).
- Stress management, handling stigma, and developing social support through group interventions (Bennett, 1995).
- Managing psychological aspects of clinical relationships (Visintini *et al.*, 1995).
- Providing clinical management updates, and training in multi-disciplinary management of psychosocial difficulties and counselling for patients (Miller, 1995a).
- Managing interpersonal relationships, and group situations (Bellani *et al.*, 1996).

In describing the content of training courses in HIV management for physicians and dentists in Texas, Brimlow (1995) identified the essential components of a core curriculum as infection fear and avoidance, homophobia, spouse/partner fear or reluctance, identification with patients, anger, helplessness, grief and burnout, clinical skill development, patient issues of disability, disfigurement, dementia and death, and sexual history-taking. Gallop *et al.* (1992) summarised the results of a well-controlled study assessing the inclusion of testimony from people with HIV in training, and found that having either a video or a person present was equally helpful.

Facilitating social support in the workplace

These suggestions for training concern facilitating communication and sharing of experience. Social support in the workplace is possibly boosted through such interventions also (Cordes and Dougherty, 1993), although this needs testing.

Social support has long been considered as a potential buffer of work stress and burnout. The buffering hypothesis states that social support does not necessarily lower the stress experienced by the worker, but acts as an aid to coping with work stress, although empirical results concerning this hypothesis have been inconsistent (Constable and Russell, 1986). These authors examined the impact (beneficial or otherwise) of social support on the effects of perceived work stress by administering the MBI, the Work Environment Scale (Moos and Insel, 1974), and a social support measure by House and Wells (1978), to 310 US Army nurses. As they expected from the buffering hypothesis of social support, their results indicated that as supervisory support increased, emotional exhaustion decreased – indeed supervisor support interacted with job enhancement to predict emotional exhaustion. However, Constable and Russell (1986) found that there was no significant relationship between burnout and support from colleagues, spouses, and/or family and friends. A similar result has been found in a study of factory workers by House (1981), which revealed that support from supervisors – and not from co-workers – was the most significant source of support in buffering and reducing the effects of stress on workers' health.

Leiter and Maslach (1988) examined the effects of different sources of inter-personal contact on MBI subscale scores in mental health settings. In making a distinction between pleasant and unpleasant co-worker and supervisor contacts in a group of nurses, they found that unpleasant supervisor contact was related to emotional exhaustion, whereas pleasant supervisor contact was negatively related to depersonalisation, and pleasant co-worker contact was positively related to personal accomplishment.

In a study of 266 formal, trained volunteers who had been working at Gay Mens' Health Crisis in New York City for six months or more, Maslanka (1992) employed path analyses to assess the role of social support in influencing the degree of stress experienced as a volunteer. She found staff support was more important than peer support in reducing negative outcomes of volunteering. Maslanka found that staff support (emotional support through listening, being helpful and reliable) directly decreases levels of (MBI-defined) burnout and indirectly increases the levels of reward experienced by volunteers. However, she also found that the characteristics volunteers themselves bring to their work – such as the need for companionship or for a new career – also play a major role in experienced burnout. Further, those volunteers with high levels of reward from their volunteer work were also those experiencing high levels of burnout on the measure employed, especially if they were younger. Having said this, Maslanka found that overall MBI burnout levels for volunteers after six months were generally low, and rewards felt were generally high.

Social support and the role of families and friends

The most significant research studies considering the buffering effects of support on burnout have been performed by Leiter (1988, 1990, 1991). Leiter makes an empirical distinction between personal (i.e., having family resources), informal and professional support. Leiter (1988) identified that having informal contacts and support mechanisms was significantly related to higher levels of MBI-measured personal accomplishment, while professional support was related to higher levels of personal accomplishment *and* emotional exhaustion. In a later report, Leiter (1990) further defined organisational support as the opportunity to constructively implement and develop work skills, and found negative correlations between personal support and emotional exhaustion and depersonalisation, and organisational support was negatively related to depersonalisation and reduced sense of personal accomplishment. He hypothesised that family coping resources would take some time to appear as influences on the experience of burnout, and in a study of 122 hospital workers, conducted over two time points six months apart, found that family resources complement professionally based resources to alleviate burnout or prevent its development. He found that family coping resources were largely independent of work-related coping resources, and extended the individual's capacity for coping with work stress – people with more resources for coping with family problems were more able to overcome work-related exhaustion, either by not having family issues adding to work stress, and/or by having family supports adding to actions to reduce work stress. Family coping resources were not related to diminished personal accomplishment in this study. A third report by Leiter (1991) found that *co-worker* support was positively related to personal accomplishment, and that support by supervisors was not significantly related to any of the MBI subscales (in contrast to the findings by Constable and Russell, 1986).

Reports investigating the links between HIV/AIDS work and non-work responses have been provided by Baggaley *et al.* (1996), and Miller and Gillies (1996). Baggaley found that of 101 HIV/AIDS counsellors, 70 had a relative who had died of AIDS, but few of those surveyed could discuss the illness with the relative. Seventy-two of those surveyed worried about their own HIV status, yet 53 did not want to know their own HIV status, and only 24 had been tested for HIV. Additionally, only 27 had ever used a condom in their own sexual lives and, as might be expected in settings where sexual negotiation by women is still unusual, the female counsellors surveyed revealed they could not discuss sex with their partners or with their clients.

Miller and Gillies (1996) studied the impact of working in HIV/AIDS or oncology on the social and domestic lives of 203 health staff, and found that friends appear more likely than families of HIV/AIDS staff to be supportive of their work, that HIV/AIDS staff discuss work significantly more often than oncology staff in social settings, and that colleagues are the main source of social contact for staff from both settings. Overall, 44 per cent of staff reported work issues causing active conflict with domestic partners, mainly centring on the domestically intrusive demands and commitments work in these fields caused. Those interviewed reported that work was responsible for domestic distress up to 90 per cent of the time, just under one-quarter had reported serious relationship difficulties because of work, and one in three had experienced a broken serious relationship or marriage, the demise of which they attributed directly to work. Such findings are not routine, even where they are researched – no correlations between work-based stresses and subsequent social or domestic adjustment were found by Kleiber, Enzmann and Gusy (1995).

To summarise, it appears that professional and personal sources of support are indeed different and may have independent effects. The need to admit non-work life into work support programmes has recently been both demonstrated (Miller and Gillies, 1996) and undertaken (Bennett and Kelaher, 1993).

The importance of asking staff what they want from staff support

Although it may seem obvious as a means to improving compliance with staff support, there is surprisingly little evidence in the literature that *staff are asked what they want from staff support.* In her Sydney study, asking staff led Bennett (1995) to characterise personal burnout-prevention strategies as being either work-related, as those separating work and home lives, and/or as those focusing on individual needs. The UK burnout studies described in Chapters 7 and 8 also asked HIV/ AIDS health workers about their preferences for staff support. These studies found that staff required support to be *accessible* when they needed it, a facilitator whose *neutrality and expertise* they could trust (usually preferring an 'outsider'), a *mixture of individual and group support*, complete *confidentiality* with support *unlinked to management*, management *endorsement* of support-receiving, and agreed, clear *ground-rules* to clarify the aims of staff support. As to content, Miller, Gillies and Elliott (1994) also found that those who scored as 'cases' on the GHQ-28, and as having high personal accomplishment in their work, were significantly more likely to want to discuss personal feelings and issues, as opposed to 'external' topics such as resource inadequacies.

Asking the right questions

Findings from the recent longitudinal survey of four UK models of staff support (Miller, Gillies and Elliott, 1996; see also Chapter 8) suggest that a number of critical questions need to be asked to ensure design and implementation of support programmes that are considered relevant and useful by potential users (Table 10.3).

Table 10.3 Questions to ask in staff support planning

- Has the form(s) of staff support been *negotiated* with those for whom it is being provided?
- Is there more than one *format* for staff support (e.g., individual and group support) available for staff?
- Have *ground rules* – including the motives for and aims of staff support – been *clarified* with those who will receive it?
- Has there been a clear statement about the *confidentiality* of staff support, in particular, that the content of support to identified individuals will not be reported directly to *management*?
- Is there an *impartial facilitator* who understands the area of work involved?
- Is the support easily *accessible*, both geographically and logistically?
- Are there appropriate, confidential mechanisms to *feed back* pertinent and not individually attributable issues from staff support to management?
- Has there been *agreement* between staff and managers about the importance of staff support within the team, and have all team members been 'heard' in planning the content and processes of support?
- Have *feedback* opportunities between staff and management been allowed for, so that issues raised in support can be discussed in a practical sense?
- Is the support matched to the issues currently affecting the organisation?
- Is there scope for the *organisation* to accommodate appropriate suggestions for change to reduce stress in future, and has this been communicated to staff?
- Have mechanisms for *evaluation* of staff support impact been agreed and put in place?

Finally, it seems worth investigating the relative importance of issues that have emerged in recent reviews of staff stress and burnout literature (Horsman and Sheeran, 1995; Miller, 1996), to assess their utility in preventative design. Such issues may include:

- Reviewing the motivations of potential employes at the staff selection stage, especially regarding the degree of identification they may show with patients.
- Ensuring clear communication within and between communities of carers, and institutions providing care, to enable assessment of the degree to which collegiate support is a buffer to stress at work.
- Organising the work setting to reflect the interests and welfare of staff, particularly in ensuring confidentiality when it is appropriate.
- Ensuring that overt recognition and validation is given to workers' efforts and investment in their work, particularly at times of bereavement and loss.
- Nurturing the ethos and principles that may have brought caring communities together in the first place, and which may sustain communities and individuals when loss is experienced.

Distinguishing between a crisis and a chronic problem

As critical reports on the sometimes inappropriate content of staff stress prevention regimes have suggested (Reynolds and Briner, 1994), the nature of support given may not always reflect adequately the nature of the problem. Anecdotally, it seems especially important to recognise the difference between acute crises and chronic difficulties in work stress, and to target short-term or long-term interventions accordingly (Miller, Gillies and Elliott, 1996). Figure 10.1 suggests an algorithm by which action may be instituted for staff support following emotional crises.

In order to enable clearer *strategic* management in preventing work stress and minimising the possibility of it arising, Table 10.4 identifies appropriate staff support actions at evolving stages of HIV service implementation.

Concluding remarks

The area of staff stress and its management in HIV/AIDS is still in its infancy. To protect ourselves, we have little option but to research ways in which we can manage ourselves – and hence serve our patients and communities – better. For this, we need more models of burnout management and prevention, and they need to be more rigorously researched and tested, so that we know how to adapt them without losing their most useful aspects. A vital part of this lies in working against the view that support-seeking is a sign of weakness in health staff working in traditionally hierarchical professions. An organisation that ignores or encourages pride in the exhaustion of its staff can only expect *negative* outcomes – in staff morale, in organisational atmosphere, and in *quality of care*. It is to

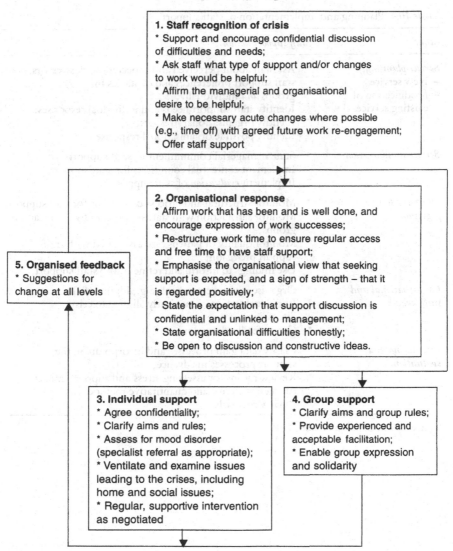

Figure 10.1 Algorithm for emotional support of staff in crisis.

be hoped that with the growing emphasis put on rational expectations of organisations and the staff working within them, a more mature approach will eventually
affirm that pride in – or tolerant maintenance of – staff exhaustion is evidence of
mismanagement, of professional incompetence, and adult immaturity. If we are
honest with ourselves as clinicians and as people, we have to recognise that
acknowledging vulnerability to stress is evidence of professional and adult
maturity, and that to do so is a sign of strength.

Table 10.4 Planning and implementation of staff support

Stage	Staff support action
Service planning: – New service – Modification of existing service	* Ask staff about perceived and expected work stressors, staff support preferences and obstacles in groups *and* individually; * Identify staff support needs and individual responses; * Identify organisational stressors; * Identify possible organisational responses.
Service inauguration:	* State managerial commitment to staff support; * Implement contextual conditions for staff support; * Implement *evaluation* of staff support.
On-going service provision:	* Monitor structural and process conditions for staff support; * Monitor satisfaction with staff support, individually and in groups; * Monitor quality of patient care associated with staff support provision; * Use findings to inform and refine future staff support.
Organisational and staff 'crises':	* Organise response protocol (e.g., Figure 10.1) * Individual staff sessions clearly aligned to crisis discussion; * Group feedback sessions.
Monitoring and evaluation:	* Clarify data gain processes and incorporate in the support processes in advance; * Review means for assessing stress and support impact (using qualitative and quantitative methods); * Review regularly.

Source: Miller, Gillies and Elliott, 1996

11 Conclusion

This book has attempted to show where burnout comes from, conceptually, practically and empirically. It has also shown how research findings are moving towards a unity that provides an increasingly solid base for the development of coherent models of intervention. However, there is still much that needs to be understood. The next phase of empiricism in burnout *must* test models of intervention. In doing so, intervention research in burnout needs to reflect the wider contexts of HIV/AIDS health care if it is to legitimise them, and the stresses to which they give rise.

Initially, the book identified characteristics of work stressors, such as the nature and topography of jobs, employee roles, work relationships and the available workplace supports. The need to clarify job demographics in burnout research was clarified. Chapter 3 showed how operational definitions of burnout have had enduring relevance, and have provided a conceptual base enabling the development of empirical and theoretical understanding through the recent process models of burnout. Subsequently, the case was made that we must expand our notions of the carer to include loved-ones, families, volunteers, and the communities in which they live. All are organisms that suffer the stresses and rewards of caring, both directly through their being witnesses to and instruments of the needs of those for whom they care, and indirectly through the acidic outrages of stigma and discrimination. Nowhere is this more apparent than in the developing worlds where the shock of recognition of the sheer extent of the HIV/AIDS crisis is alone sufficient to induce helplessness – unless we also take care to see the inspiration and opportunities that exist at the most basic levels of intervention. Support of the community agents in place is vital and must be further documented, characterised and tested.

Chapter 5 showed that knowing something like the value of infection control procedures does not necessarily change our behaviour as health care workers. It also showed how knowing something too well can change our behaviour adversely, as with over-identification with patients. The evidence also suggests that our roles as health workers in HIV/AIDS really are expanding, yet we don't seem to account for this rationally. When we use new procedures with our patients we monitor, assess and evaluate the outcomes. Yet when we initiate major changes in the conduct of our health staff, we don't. Why? Is this perhaps an extension of the political denial that has existed for years in so many areas of health development? Do we have to wait for major mistakes and litigation to become the norm before we take the needs of staff seriously enough to put appropriate resources into staff care as part of our investment in patient care? As long as we do not address this circumstance, health politicians content to point at flagship facilities will not realise that merely doing so is different to addressing the fundamental needs of human professionals doing serious, intense, sophisticated and difficult work for the benefit of their communities. It is rather like spending billions on the development of a new car, only to then refuse it the appropriate level of servicing and maintenance and watch it slowly come to a halt – and blame the car for stopping!

Many methodological issues have been raised in this book, not least the need to expand our bases of measurement in burnout research. And in view of the evidence about the importance of social support, we need to look outwards – to characterise the impact of work in domestic and social networks (particularly in high prevalence settings) and invest in longitudinal studies. We particularly need to examine the outcomes of models of intervention. The UK MOMS study showed the real and serious extent of workplace morbidity in HIV/AIDS, and that it was shared with oncology staff. This study also revealed many ideas that might inform interventions. Further, the UK burnout prevention study showed how staff have many ideas for the interventions that would reflect their realities. We need to ask staff in each site about this. We also have so little information about the support needs of staff and carers in developing countries, yet the evidence we do have indicates that in resource-poor settings, the needs may be even greater. What is clear from the two UK studies described in detail is that staff support needs to be multi-modal if it is to address the complexities of the issues staff face, and the needs that then emerge. The chapter on volunteers also reveals that volunteer issues are as relevant and as pressing as for statutory colleagues.

Finally, the chapter on management of burnout describes modes of staff support, along with clear suggestions from staff in the field about what would make staff support options for them both relevant and usable. Practical suggestions are made about agendas for supervision, questions to consider in setting up staff support, and for responding to staff crises. Critically, the relative lack of empirical data also points to the need for good outcome studies that can help us shape and refine what we know into something that serves a useful purpose.

If we are to maintain the conceit that we are providing the best possible care for our patients, we must start showing – and testing – that we really do also care for staff. Staff support programmes should start reflecting the complexities of the situation and of the individuals within them, rather than being based on the simplistic assumption that by working on the stressed individual, the organisation that generates the stress will feel and be better. This book points clearly to such assumptions being misleading and wasteful and, perhaps more importantly in view of what has been revealed throughout this book, dishonest. In an age where work-related stress and distress are treated as expressions of individual pathology, we need to shift the burden of responsibility back on to working structures that actually generate the stress, rather than blaming the individual for experiencing the stress that workplaces create. In future years, failing to do so, and failing to invest in quality health care by also investing in staff welfare, may be seen as actionable. Rather than insinuations of lapsed professionalism being the reward of the self-identifying burnout sufferer, the response may hopefully become one of greater respect for having the professionalism to make such an admission. Organisations that do not make such a shift may be seen as working against the patients' interest, because they foster atmospsheres of blaming and denial that should not today be tolerated outside their walls.

Options for a future research agenda have been identified particularly in Chapters 6 and 10, and will not be repeated. However, what does need to be repeated is the importance of investing in staff as a means to improving care for all. Let us have the wisdom to acknowledge the shortcomings of the organisations in and for whom we work. The fear that such acknowledgement will cost money to the organisations concerned – by requiring necessary investment in change – is a simple reality that will not go away or lessen by ignoring it. We have seen worldwide how such logic has added to the catastrophe of our age. All of us in the HIV/AIDS field – and most of those outside it – will have our professional lifetimes dominated by this tragedy. Yet it remains so preventable. By investing in our colleagues, we invest in our communities and our futures. Is there anything more worthwhile?

Appendix
Data tables from the UK Multi-centre
Occupational Morbidity Study (MOMS)

Table 1 Differences between HIV/AIDS and oncology staff regarding self-reported and psychometric measures of work-related stress: univariate and multi-variate analyses

Variable	Category	HIV/AIDS (n = 103)	Oncology (n = 100)	Unadjusted χ^2, d.f., P-value	χ^2 d.f., P-value adjusted by sex, age, professional group
46. Material resources at work are adequate	Poor	21	7	6.56, 1 d.f., P = 0.01	5.82, 1 d.f., P = 0.016
	Adequate	82	93		
107. Cigarettes smoked daily	0	65	78	7.79, 2 d.f., P = 0.005 (Tr)	11.04, 2 d.f., P<0.001 (Tr)
	1–9	8	10		
	10+	30	12		
143.4. Skin complaints	No	49	68	7.85, 1 d.f., P = 0.005	10.02, 1 d.f., P = 0.002
	Yes	54	32		
39. Work premises are adequate	No	72	50	7.57, 1 d.f., P = 0.006	8.50, 1 d.f., P = 0.004
	Yes	31	50		
141.4. Appearance of new infections a work stress	Yes	55	31	9.18, 1 d.f., P = 0.002	8.59, 1 d.f., P = 0.003
	No	48	68		
111. Ever seriously disagree with colleagues	No	60	77	6.38, 1 d.f., P = 0.011	5.67, 1 d.f., P = 0.017
	Yes	41	23		
114. Any professional concern about overlap with other professions' work	Yes	60	35	10.10, 1 d.f., P = 0.001	4.58, 1 d.f., P = 0.032
	No	43	65		
116. Is concern about overlap resolved	Up to half the time	40	11	9.67, 1 d.f., P = 0.001	6.43, 1 d.f., P = 0.011
	Often/always	20	24		
154. Participating in decisions over professional conditions and future	Not at all	8	22	6.77, 1 d.f., P = 0.0092	3.02, 1 d.f.; P = 0.082
	Sometimes or more	93*	78		
97.6. 'Shut off' by sport activities	Yes	12	31	10.25, 1 d.f., P = 0.001	7.64, 1 d.f., P = 0.006
	No	91	69		

*Two missing values. Further analyses were done to adjust for length of professional experience and title, but numbers became too small to be reliable in many instances. Also, the only variables where such adjustments produced overall change in significance (i.e., all were no longer significant) were as follows: 'Concerned about work overlapping with other professions' (χ^2 = 3.33, 1 d.f., P = 0.068); 'Participating in decisions over professional conditions and future' (χ^2 = 3.02, 1 d.f., P = 0.082); 'Shutting off work by socialising' (χ^2 = 2.91, 1 d.f., P = 0.088).

Table 2 Differences between sexes regarding self-reported and psychometric measures of work stress: univariate and multi-variate analyses

Variable	Category	Male (n = 42)	Female (n = 161)	Unadjusted χ^2, d.f., P-value	χ^2, d.f., P-value adjusted by HIV/oncology, age, professional group
105. Weekly units of alcohol consumed	0	1	12	8.17, 2 d.f., P = 0.016	5.29, 2 d.f., P = 0.021
	1–14	27	125		
	15+	14	24		
145.2. Hypersensitivity as a stress symptom	Never	15	30	4.68, 1 d.f., P = 0.03	3.13, 1 d.f., P = 0.077
	Yes	27	131		
93. Percentage of colleagues who are stressed	<51	14	28	4.23, 1 d.f., P = 0.039	3.01, 1 d.f., P = 0.083
	51+	28	133		
114. Concerned at professional overlap	Yes	29	66	9.43, 1 d.f., P = 0.002	5.02, 1 d.f., P = 0.025
	No	13	95		
151. Have difficulties showing distress to colleagues	Yes	27*	136	7.11, 1 d.f., P = 0.007	5.63, 1 d.f., P = 0.018
	No	14	23		

*One missing value.

Further analyses were done to adjust for length of professional experience and title (i.e., rank), but numbers usually became insufficient for meaningful interpretation. Where they were sufficient, the results were little changed, mainly because length and title correlate so closely with age in the populations interviewed. The only change related to the variable 'Units of alcohol consumed weekly' ($\chi^2 = 2.71$, 17 d.f., P = 0.099).

Table 3 Differences between age groups (<30 and 30+ years) regarding self-reported and psychometric measures of work stress

Variable	Category	<30 (n = 72)	30+ (n = 131)	Unadjusted χ^2, d.f., P-value	χ^2, d.f., P-value adjusted by HIV/oncology, sex, professional group
144.4. Prone to anger and prejudice	Yes	32	94	13.58, 1 d.f., P<0.001	16.45, 1 d.f., P<0.001
	No	40	37		
145.3. Overidentification with patients' needs	Yes	36	93	7.95, 1 d.f., P = 0.004	8.53, 1 d.f., P = 0.003
	No	36	38		
117. How many colleagues have experienced burnout	0	13	30	9.72, 2 d.f., P = 0.008	10.20, 2 d.f., P = 0.006
	1–5	45	54		
	6+	13	46		
118. How many colleagues have burned out in HIV/oncology since working in their present field	0	34	45	12.01, 2 d.f., P = 0.002	13.44, 2 d.f., P = 0.001
	1–2	28	37		
	3+	10	48		

As with Table 2, adjustments were not made for months of professional experience or title, due to numbers becoming too small. There were no significant changes, however, for any of the variables above after such adjustments.

Table 4 Differences between physicians and nurses regarding self-reported and psychometrically measured work stress

Variable	Category	Physicians (n = 27)	Nurses (n = 126)	Unadjusted χ^2, d.f., P-value	χ^2, d.f., P-value adjusted by HIV/oncology, age, sex
108. Seen a GP in the past 6 months	Yes	9	79	6.69, 1 d.f., P = 0.009	6.31, 1 d.f., P = 0.012
	No	18	47		
26. What needs to be done to reduce work stress (1 missing value from each group)	More resources/stress	6	72	10.28, 2 d.f., P = 0.006	11.14, 2 d.f., P = 0.004
	Better management	10	27		
	Less patient work	10	26		

Once again, further analyses conducted to adjust for length of professional experience and seniority involved numbers becoming too small for meaningful interpretation of results. Where numbers were adequate, the only alteration involved having 'Seen a GP in the past 6 months' which was no longer significant ($\chi^2 = 3.58$, 1 d.f., P = 0.058).

Table 5 Differences between nurses and paramedics regarding self-reported and psychometric measures of work stress

Variable	Category	Nurses (n = 126)	Paramedics (n = 50)	Unadjusted χ^2, d.f., P-value	χ^2, d.f., P-value adjusted by HIV/oncology, age, professional group
141.21. Breaking bad news is a work stress	Yes	93	18	21.08, 1 d.f., P<0.001	19.30, 1 d.f., P<0.001
	No	32	32		
155.11. Breaking bad news to loved-ones is problematic in relations with patients	Agree	75	11*	15.69, 1 d.f., P<0.001	16.68, 1 d.f., P<0.001
	Disagree	51	35		
150. Are you professionally obstructed by colleagues?	Yes	92	46**	9.15, 1 d.f., P = 0.002 (Tr)	7.50, 1 d.f., P = 0.006
	No	34	3		
26. What needs to be done to reduce work stress?	More resources/stress	72	13***	12.87, 2 d.f., P = 0.001	Numbers too small
	Better management	27	20		
	Less patient work	26	14		

*Four missing values; ** one missing value; ***three missing values.
After further adjusting for months of professional experience and seniority, all variables remained significant.

Table 6 Differences between senior and junior staff concerning self-reported and psychometric measures of work stress: univariate and multi-variate analyses

Variable	Category	Nurses (n = 83)	Paramedics (n = 120)	Unadjusted χ^2, d.f., P-value	χ^2, d.f., P-value adjusted by HIV/oncology, age, sex, professional group
20. Overtime hours per week	0 1 - 10 11+	10 * 53 18	39 * 74 5	20.75, 1 d.f., P <0.001 (Tr)	19.4, 1 d.f., P <0.001
145.1. Emotional numbness/indifference	Yes No	42 41	86 34	8.46, 1 d.f., P = 0.003	8.91, 1 d.f., P = 0.003
45. Rating of the work atmosphere	Poor Good	8 75	36 84	10.81, 1 d.f., P = 0.001	11.64, 1 d.f., P <0.001
141.3. Deaths of patients a work stress	Yes No	55 28	102 17	9.59, 1 d.f., P = 0.002	6.55, 1 d.f., P = 0.010
141.8. Involvements of families a stress	Yes No	40 43	80 39	6.58, 1 d.f., P = 0.010	7.85, 1 d.f., P = 0.005
155.5. Close relationships with patients is problematic	Agree Disagree	20 61	55 65	8.36, 1 d.f., P = 0.004	7.70, 1 d.f., P = 0.006
155.11. Breaking bad news to relatives is a problem	Agree Disagree	29 51	67 52	6.92, 1 d.f., P = 0.008	3.09, 1 d.f., P = 0.079
141.20. Lack of training in death and dying a stress	Yes No	30 53	68 51	7.81, 1 d.f., P = 0.005	6.98, 1 d.f., P = 0.008
151. Difficulties in showing distress to colleagues	Yes No	56 24	107 13	10.46, 1 d.f., P = 0.001	9.71, 1 d.f., P = 0.002
MBI PA Category score	High/moderate Low	38 44	84 35	10.97, 1 d.f., P <0.001	8.67, 1 d.f., P = 0.003

*Two missing values.

As numbers become too small to be reliable after further adjustments for months of professional experience, these are not tabulated. The only change in significance involved loss of significance after these adjustments, on 'Difficulties in showing distress to colleagues' (χ^2 = 3.55, 1 d.f., P = 0.059).

Table 7 Differences associated with months of professional experience regarding self-reported and psychometric measures of work stress: univariate and multi-variate analyses

Variable	Category	0–95 months	96+ months	Unadjusted χ^2, d.f., P-value	χ^2, d.f., P-value adjusted by HIV/oncology, age, sex, professional group
145.1. Emotional numbness/indifference	Yes	72	56	10.20, 1 d.f., P = 0.001	8.88, 1 d.f., P = 0.003
	Never	24	51		
38. Do you have enough time to do your work	No	54	80	6.93, 1 d.f., P = 0.008	8.60, 1 d.f., P = 0.003
	Yes	42	27		
141.20. Lack training in death and dying	Yes	58	40	10.36, 1 d.f., P = 0.001	5.52, 1 d.f., P = 0.019
	No	37	67		
151. Have difficulties showing distress to colleagues	Yes	85	78	8.28, 1 d.f., P = 0.004	10.04, 1 d.f., P = 0.002
	No	9	28		
MBI DP Category Score	High/moderate	46	26	12.16, 1 d.f., P <0.001	5.19, 1 d.f., P = 0.023
	Low	48	81		
97.4. Shut off from work by socialising	Yes	55	39	8.02, 1 d.f., P = 0.004	4.30, 1 d.f., P = 0.038
	No	41	68		
97.8. Shut off from work in other ways	Yes	45	78	13.28, 1 d.f., P <0.001	4.25, 1 d.f., P = 0.039
	No	51	29		

For the purposes of this analysis, months of professional experience were split at the median of 95/96 months. Because of numbers becoming too small, further adjustments for seniority were not tabulated. Changes were noted, however, with 'Emotional numbness/indifference' ($\chi^2 = 3.57$, 1 d.f., $P = 0.059$), 'Lack training in death and dying' ($\chi^2 = 2.67$, 1 d.f., $P = 0.10$), and 'Shut off from work by socialising' ($\chi^2 = 2.0$, 1 d.f., $P = 0.16$) all losing significance. 'MBI DP Category score' ($\chi^2 = 3.49$, 1 d.f., $P = 0.062$).

Table 8a Odds ratios (OR)* and chi-square values of associations with Question 25 ('Is your work stressful?') for HIV/AIDS staff where P <0.01

Question no. + variable	Category	Cases (Work is stressful; n = 85)	Controls (Work not stressful; n = 18)	OR	95% Confidence limits	χ^2	d.f	P
MBI Emotional exhaustion subscale category score	High/moderate	66**	7	6.10	1.83–20.92	10.24	1	0.001
	Low	17	11	1.00				
Q.117. How many colleagues have experienced burnout	1+	72	9	5.54	1.63–19.15	8.69	1	0.003
	0	13	9	1.00				
Q.141. Deaths of patients is a work stress	Yes	69	8	5.39	1.63–18.20	8.76	1	0.002
	No	16	10	1.00				

*Unadjusted analysis; **Two missing values.

Table 8b Multi-variate logistic model for HIV/AIDS staff: Outcome 'Is your work stressful?'

Co-variate	Category	OR Unadjusted	OR Adjusted	95% confidence interval for adjusted OR	P
MBI FE Subscale Category score:	High/moderate	6.10	3.82	1.10–13.21	0.034
	Low	1.00	1.00		
117. How many colleagues have experienced burnout:	1+	5.54	9.72	2.19–43.16	0.003
	0	1.00	1.00		
141. Deaths of patients a work stress	Yes	5.39	8.59	2.01–36.62	0.004
	No	1.00	1.00		

Table 9a Odds ratios (OR)* and chi-square values of associations with Question 25 ('Is your work stressful?') for oncology staff where $P < 0.01$

Question no. + variable	Category	Cases (Work is stressful; $n = 68$)	Controls (Work not stressful; $n = 32$)	OR	95% Confidence limits	x^2	d.f.	P
Q.87. Currently experiencing stress with work	Yes No	66 2	25 7	9.24 1.00	2.25–37.93	7.35	1	0.006
Q.103. Self-reported health state	Vulnerable/exhausted/miserable Fine/okay	33 35	3 29	9.11 1.00	2.33–41.63	12.83	1	0.000
Q.GHQ total score (conventional scoring)	5+ 0–4	37 31	5 27	6.45 1.00	2.03–21.79	11.89	1	0.000
Q.93. Percentage of stressed colleagues from own profess-on	51–100% 0–50%	62 6	21 11	5.41 1.00	1.91–15.36	8.34	1	0.003
Q.37. The work environment is stressful	Yes No	51 17	12 20	5.00 1.00	1.86–13.70	11.57	1	0.000
Q.38. I have enough time for my work	No Yes	53 15	14 18	4.54 1.00	1.68–12.46	10.01	1	0.001
Q.145. Experiencing depression as a stress symptom	Yes No	46 22	11 21	3.99 1.00	1.68–9.48	8.52	1	0.003
Q.143. Experiencing sleeplessness as a stress symptom	Yes No	55 13	17 15	3.73 1.00	1.52–9.14	7.00	1	0.008
Q.95. Time feeling overworked	51–100% 0–50%	48 20	13 19	3.51 1.00	1.49–8.28	7.00	1	0.008
Q.96. Shutting off from work	Difficult Easy	39 29	9 23	3.44 1.00	1.27–9.46	7.45	1	0.006

* Unadjusted analysis.

Table 9b Multi-variate logistic model for oncology staff: Outcome 'Is your work stressful?'

Co-variate	Category	OR Unadjusted	OR Adjusted	95% confidence interval for adjusted OR	P
Q.103. 'Self-reported health state'	Vulnerable/exhausted/ miserable	9.11	6.02	1.45–25.00	0.013
	Fine/okay	1.00	1.00		
Q. 'GHQ-28 total score'	5+	6.45	3.61	1.05–12.37	0.041
	0–4	1.00	1.00		
Q.37. 'The work environment is stressful'	Yes	5.00	4.53	1.52–13.49	0.007
	No	1.00	1.00		
Q.38. 'I have enough time for my work'	Yes	4.54	1.96	0.66–5.84	0.225
	No	1.00	1.00		

Table 10a Odds ratios (OR)* and chi-square values of associations with Question 87 ('Do you currently experience stress associated with your work?') for HIV/AIDS staff where P <0.01

Question no. + variable	Category	Cases (Work is stressful; n = 83)	Controls (Work not stressful; n = 20)	OR	95% Confidence limits	χ^2	d.f.	P
Q.9. Potential exposure to HIV since 1980	Yes	59	5	7.38	2.19–28.30	12.65	1	<0.001
	No	24	15	1.00				
Q.144. Prone to anger and prejudice	Yes	57	7	3.85	1.25–12.23	6.40	1	0.01
	No	26	13	1.00				
Q.145. Have inattention and distractability as stress symptoms	Yes	67	10	4.19	1.33–13.34	6.51	1	0.01
	No	16	10	1.00				

*Unadjusted analysis

Table 10b Multi-variate logistic model for HIV/AIDS staff: Outcome 'Do you currently experience stress associated with your work?'

Co-variate	Category	OR Unadjusted	OR Adjusted	95% confidence interval for adjusted OR	P
Q.9. Potential exposure to HIV since 1980	Yes	7.38	12.42	1.40–109.7	0.023
	No	1.00	1.00		
Q.144. Proneness to anger and prejudice	Yes	3.85	4.50	0.78–26.05	0.093
	No	1.00	1.00		
Q.145. Inattention and distractability as stress symptoms	Yes	4.19	3.10	0.62–15.56	0.169
	No	1.00	1.00		

Table 11a Odds ratios (OR)* and chi-square values of associations with Question 87 ('Would you say that you currently experience stress associated with your work?') for oncology staff where P <0.01

Question no. + variable	Category	Cases (Work is stressful; n = 73)	Controls (Work not stressful; n = 27)	OR	95% Confidence limits	x^2	d.f.	P
Q.144.6. Have problems in communication with colleagues	Yes No	65 8	15 12	6.50 1.00	1.99–21.50	11.80	1	<0.001
Q.143.7. Have gastro-intestinal disturbances	Yes No	38 35	4 23	6.24 1.00	1.84–26.35	9.74	1	0.001
Q.145.9. Have depression as a stress symptom	Yes No	50 23	7 20	6.21 1.00	2.11–19.59	12.88	1	<0.001
Q.141.16. Confidence in clinical skills makes work stressful	Yes No	39** 33	5 22	5.20 1.00	1.65–19.24	8.71	1	0.003
Q.143.2. Have lingering minor illnesses as stress symptoms	Yes No	42 31	6 21	4.74 1.00	1.58–15.87	8.48	1	0.003
Q.143.6. Have sleeplessness as a stress symptom	Yes No	59 14	13 14	4.54 1.00	1.57–13.08	8.88	1	0.002
Q. GHQ total scores (conventional scoring).	5+ 0–4	37 36	5 22	4.52 1.00	1.44–16.73	7.10	1	0.007
Q.143.3. Have muscle pains as stress symptoms	Yes No	52 21	10 17	4.21 1.00	1.51–11.97	8.38	1	0.003
Q.145.12. Have inattention and distractibility	Yes No	53 20	11 16	3.85 1.00	1.39–10.01	7.36	1	0.006
Q.103. Self-reported health state	Vulnerable/ miserable Fine/okay	36 37	0 27	Undefined	Undefined	18.72	1	<0.001

*Unadjusted analysis; **one missing value.

Table 11b Multi-variate logistic model for oncology staff: Outcome 'Would you say you currently experience stress associated with your work?'

Co-variate		OR Unadjusted	OR Adjusted	95% confidence interval for adjusted OR	P
Q.144.6. 'Problems in communicating with colleagues'					
	Yes	6.50	4.70	1.52–14.99	0.007
	No	1.00	1.00		
Q.145.9. 'Depression as a stress symptom'	Yes	6.21	4.88	1.73–13.76	0.003
	No	1.00	1.00		

Table 12a Odds ratios (OR)* and chi-square values of associations with Question 103 ('How do you generally feel?') for HIV/AIDS staff where P = 0.01

Question no. + variable	Category	Cases: Vulnerable/miserable (n = 41)	Controls: Fine/OK (n = 62)	OR	95% Confidence limits	χ^2	d.f.	P
Q.123. Primary emotional relationship has suffered as a result of work**	Yes	13	5	7.06	1.87–29.24	9.74	1	0.001
	No	14	38	1.00				
Q. GHQ total scores (conventional scoring)	5+	25	15	5.11	1.98–13.32	12.97	1	<0.001
	0–4	15	46	1.00				
Q.143.8. Malaise as a stress symptom	Yes	32	26	4.92	1.87–13.61	11.65	1	<0.001
	No	9	36	1.00				
Q.143.2. Lingering minor illnesses as stress symptoms	Yes	33	30	4.40	1.63–12.67	9.40	1	0.002
	No	8	32	1.00				
Q.143.4. Skin complaints as stress symptoms	Yes	30	24	4.32	1.70–11.30	10.41	1	0.001
	No	11	38	1.00				
Q.143.5. Palpitations as stress symptoms	Yes	19	11	4.00	1.50–10.88	8.44	1	0.003
	No	22	51	1.00				
Q.144.3. Anxiety/anxiety attacks as stress symptoms	Yes	29	24	3.83	1.53–9.81	8.89	1	0.002
	No	12	38	1.00				
Q.144.10. Withdrawal from non-involved others as a stress symptom	Yes	27	23	3.27	1.33–8.15	7.06	1	0.007
	No	14	39	1.00				

*Unadjusted analysis; **Missing values where not in a primary emotional relationship.

Table 12b Multi-variate logistic model for HIV/AIDS staff: Outcome 'How do you generally feel?'

Co-variate	Category	OR Unadjusted	OR Adjusted	95% confidence interval for adjusted OR	P
Q. GHQ total scores (conventional scoring)	5+	5.11	3.42	1.35–8.62	0.009
	0–4	1.00	1.00		
Q.143.8. Malaise as a stress symptom	Yes	4.92	3.95	1.48–10.56	0.006
	No	1.00	1.00		

Table 13a Odds ratios (OR)* and chi-square values of associations with Question 103 ('How do you generally feel?') for oncology staff where $P = 0.01$

Question no. + variable	Category	Cases: Vulnerable/ miserable (n = 36)	Controls: Fine/OK (n = 64)	OR	95% Confidence limits	χ^2	d.f.	P
Q.144.2. Nervousness and agitation as stress symptoms	Yes / No	34 / 2	40 / 24	10.20 / 1.00	2.22–93.56	10.62	1	0.001
Q.143.2. Lingering minor illnesses as stress symptoms	Yes / No	28 / 8	20 / 44	7.70 / 1.00	2.75–22.70	18.16	1	<0.001
Q.143.6. Sleeplessness as a stress symptom	Yes / No	33 / 3	39 / 25	7.05 / 1.00	1.86–39.06	9.32	1	0.002
Q.145.6. Pessimism and hopelessness as stress symptoms	Yes / No	32 / 4	35 / 29	6.63 / 1.00	1.98–28.31	10.69	1	0.001
Q.143.3. Muscle pains as stress symptoms	Yes / No	31 / 5	31 / 33	6.60 / 1.00	2.13–24.09	12.32	1	<0.001
Q.143.7. Gastrointestinal disturbances as stress symptoms	Yes / No	25 / 11	17 / 47	6.28 / 1.00	2.35–17.17	15.68	1	<0.001
Q.GHQ total scores (conventional scoring)	5+ / 0–4	25 / 11	17 / 47	6.28 / 1.00	2.35–17.17	15.68	1	<0.001
Q.145.12. Inattention and distractability as stress symptoms	Yes / No	31 / 5	33 / 31	5.82 / 1.00	1.88–21.29	10.48	1	0.001
Q.143.8. Malaise as a stress symptom	Yes / No	27 / 9	24 / 40	5.00 / 1.00	1.87–14.01	11.51	1	<0.001
Q.141.16. Confidence in clinical skills is a work stress	Yes / No	24 / 12	20 / 43	4.30 / 1.00	1.66–11.35	9.94	1	0.001
Q.145.9. Depression as a stress symptom.	Yes / No	28 / 8	29 / 35	4.22 / 1.00	1.55–12.27	8.63	1	0.003
Q.144.3. Anxiety/anxiety attacks as stress symptoms	Yes / No	24 / 12	24 / 40	3.33 / 1.00	1.31–8.67	6.73	1	0.009
Q.154. Help make decisions about changes in professional activities and conditions	No / Yes	15 / 21	7 / 57	0.17 / 1.00	0.05–0.53	10.95	1	<0.001

*Unadjusted analysis.

Table 13b Multi-variate logistic model for oncology staff: Outcome 'How do you generally feel?'

Co-variate	Category	OR Unadjusted	OR Adjusted	95% confidence interval for adjusted OR	P
Q.143.2. 'Lingering minor illnesses as stress symptoms'	Yes No	7.70 1.00	4.22 1.00	1.32–13.48	0.015
Q.143.3. 'Muscle pains as stress symptoms'	Yes No	6.60 1.00	2.04 1.00	0.54–7.75	0.293
Q.143.7. 'Gastrointestinal disturbances as stress symptoms'	Yes No	6.28 1.00	2.64 1.00	0.81–8.63	0.109
Q. 'GHQ-28 total scores (conventional scoring)'	5+ 0–4	6.28 1.00	1.80 1.00	0.56–5.83	0.325
Q. 143.8. 'Malaise as a stress symptom'	Yes No	5.00 1.00	1.84 1.00	0.56–6.07	0.316
Q.154. 'Help make decisions about changes in professional activities and conditions'	No Yes	0.17 1.00	4.35 1.00	1.20–15.73	0.025

Table 13c Multi-variate logistic model for oncology staff: Outcome 'How do you generally feel?'

Co-variate	Category	OR Unadjusted	OR Adjusted	95% confidence interval for adjusted OR	P
Q.143.2. 'Lingering minor illnesses as stress symptoms'	Yes No	7.70 1.00	7.58 1.00	2.76–20.78	<0.001
Q.154. 'Help make decisions about changes in professional activities and conditions'	No Yes	0.17 1.00	5.68 1.00	1.79–18.05	0.003

Table 14a Odds ratios (OR)* and chi-square values of associations with GHQ-28 total scores for HIV/AIDS staff where P <0.01**

Question no. + variable	Category	Cases (GHQ >5; n = 40)	Controls (GHQ <4; n = 61)	OR	95% Confidence limits	χ^2	d.f.	P
Q.145.9. Experiencing depression as a stress symptom	Yes No	34 6	28 33	6.68 1.00	2.25–20.80	13.97	1	<0.001
Q.150. Feel professionally obstructed by colleagues	Yes No	37 3	42 19	5.58 1.00	1.40–25.89	6.60	1	0.010
Q.145.10. Experiencing a sense of failure as a stress symptom	Yes No	35 5	34 27	5.56 1.00	1.76–18.73	9.84	1	0.002
Q.145.6. Experience pessimism and hopelessness as stress symptoms	Yes No	34 6	32 29	5.14 1.00	1.73–15.96	9.91	1	0.002
Q.103. How you generally feel	Vulnerable/ miserable Fine/okay	25 15	15 46	5.11 1.00	1.98–13.41	12.97	1	<0.001
Q.94. Ability to distance self from patients' difficulties	Poor Good	18 22	11 49	3.64 1.00	1.35–9.97	7.04	1	0.008
Q.143.3. Experience muscle pains as a stress symptom	Yes No	32 8	32 29	3.63 1.00	1.33–10.18	6.75	1	0.009
Q.144.3. Experience anxiety/anxiety attacks as stress symptoms	Yes No	28 12	24 37	3.60 1.00	1.42–9.23	7.90	1	0.005
Q.37. The working environment is stressful	Yes No	31 9	30 31	3.56 1.00	1.34–9.66	6.96	1	0.008
Q.143.2. Experience lingering minor illnesses as stress symptoms	Yes No	31 9	30 31	3.56 1.00	1.34–9.66	6.96	1	0.008
Q.144.9. Experience self-righteousness ('heroism') as a stress symptom	Yes No	29 11	27 34	3.32 1.00	1.30–8.61	6.70	1	0.01

*Unadjusted analysis. **Two missing values from sample.

Table 14b Multi-variate logistic model for HIV/AIDS staff: Outcome 'GHQ-28 Total scores'

Co-variate	Category	OR Unadjusted	OR Adjusted	95% confidence interval for adjusted OR	P
Q.103. 'Self-reported health state'	Vulnerable/miserable	5.11	4.72	1.85–12.00	0.001
	Fine/okay	1.00	1.00		
Q.145.9. 'Depression is a stress symptom'	Yes	6.68	6.18	2.15–17.81	<0.001
	No	1.00	1.00		

Table 15a Odds ratios (OR)* and chi-square values of associations with GHQ-28 total scores for oncology staff where P <0.01

Question no. + variable	Category	Cases (GHQ >5; n = 42)	Controls (GHQ <4; n = 58)	OR	95% Confidence limits	χ^2	d.f.	P
Q.145.2. Experiencing hypersensitivity as a stress symptom	Yes	41	41	17.00	2.20–358.39	10.21	1	0.001
	No	1	17	1.00				
Q.143.6. Experiencing sleeplessness as a stress symptom	Yes	40	32	16.25	3.35–107.29	17.46	1	0.000
	No	2	26	1.00				
Q.141.16. Maintaining confidence in clinical skills is a work stress	Yes	29	15	6.93	2.60–18.85	17.81	1	0.000
	No	12	43	1.00				
Q.143.8. Experiencing malaise as a stress symptom	Yes	32	19	6.57	2.46–17.93	16.69	1	0.000
	No	10	39	1.00				
Q.103. How you generally feel	Vulnerable/miserable	25	11	6.28	2.34–17.22	15.68	1	0.000
	Fine/okay	17	47	1.00				
Q.154. Having control over future professional activities and conditions	No	16	6	5.33	1.69–17.51	9.37	1	0.002
	Yes	26	52	1.00				

Table 15a (Continued)

Question no. + variable	Category	Cases (GHQ >5; n = 42)	Controls (GHQ <4; n = 58)	OR	95% Confidence limits	χ^2	d.f.	P
Q.143.5. Experiencing palpitations as stress symptoms	Yes No	20 22	9 49	4.95 1.00	1.78–14.08	10.68	1	0.001
Q.144.3. Experiencing anxiety/anxiety attacks as stress symptoms	Yes No	29 13	19 39	4.58 1.00	1.80–11.83	11.44	1	0.001
Q.143.3. Experiencing muscle pains as stress symptoms	Yes No	34 8	28 30	4.55 1.00	1.66–12.85	9.70	1	0.002
Q.155.10. Patients challenging my work makes patient relations problematic	Agree Disagree	14 28	6 52	4.33 1.00	1.36–14.39	6.67	1	0.010
Q.144.10. Withdrawal as a stress symptom	Yes No	31 11	23 52	4.29 1.00	1.67–11.24	10.11	1	0.001
Q.145.9. Depression as a stress symptom	Yes No	32 10	25 33	4.22 1.00	1.62–11.26	9.57	1	0.002
Q.155.2. Knowing patients will die is problematic	Yes No	23 19	13 45	4.19 1.00	1.62–10.98	9.70	1	0.002
MBI Emotional exhaustion category score	High/moderate Low	35 7	32 26	4.06 1.00	1.42–11.98	7.51	1	0.006
Q.54. Times broken bad news in last 6 months	11+ 0–10	10 32	31 27	3.67 1.00	1.41–9.76	7.66	1	0.006
Q.141.27. Feeling professionally inadequate is a work stress	Yes No	24 17	17 41	3.40 1.00	1.36–8.64	7.29	1	0.007

*Unadjusted analysis.

Table 15b Multi-variate logistic model for oncology staff: Outcome 'GHQ-28 Total scores'

Co-variate	Category	OR Unadjusted	OR Adjusted	95% confidence interval for adjusted OR	P
Q.103. 'How do you generally feel'	Vulnerable/miserable	6.28	2.51	0.75–8.42	0.135
	Fine/okay	1.00	1.00		
Q.144.3. 'Anxiety/anxiety attacks as stress symptoms'	Yes	4.58	1.54	0.46–5.15	0.481
	No	1.00	1.00		
Q.144.10. 'Withdrawal as a stress symptom'	Yes	4.29	4.72	1.40–15.87	0.012
	No	1.00	1.00		
Q.143.8. 'Malaise as a stress symptom'	Yes	6.57	2.31	0.70–7.59	0.169
	No	1.00	1.00		
Q.143.6. 'Sleeplessness as a stress symptom'	Yes	16.25	9.88	1.57–62.28	0.015
	No	1.00	1.00		
Q.141.6. 'Confidence in clinical skills'	Yes	6.93	4.41	1.37–14.23	0.013
	No	1.00	1.00		
Q.145.2. 'Hypersensitivity as a stress symptom'	Yes	17.00	6.30	0.63–63.06	0.117
	No	1.00	1.00		

Table 16a Odds ratios (OR)* and chi-square values of associations with MBI 'Emotional exhaustion' category scores for HIV/AIDS staff where P <0.01*

Question no. + variable	Category	Cases (High–moderate; n = 73)	Controls (Low; n = 28)	OR	95% Confidence limits	χ^2	d.f.	P
Q.144.9. Self-righteousness ('heroism') a stress symptom	Yes	49	7	6.13	2.09–18.59	12.88	1	<0.001
	No	24	21	1.00				
Q.25. Finding work stressful	Yes	66	17	6.10	1.83–20.92	12.19	1	0.001
	No	7	11	1.00				
Q.145.4. Grief as a stress symptom	Yes	66	18	5.24	1.55–18.13	8.09	1	0.004
	No	7	10	1.00				
Q.145.10. A sense of failure as a stress symptom	Yes	57	12	4.75	1.70–13.47	10.03	1	0.001
	No	16	16	1.00				
Q.145.6. Pessimism and hopelessness as stress symptoms	Yes	55	11	4.72	1.71–13.31	10.08	1	0.001
	No	18	17	1.00				
Q.144.6. Communication problems with colleagues	Yes	63	16	4.72	1.56–14.58	8.46	1	0.003
	No	10	12	1.00				
Q.150. Feeling professionally obstructed	Yes	63	16	4.72	1.56–14.58	8.46	1	0.003
	No	10	12	1.00				
Q.37. Work environment is stressful	Yes	51	10	4.17	1.52–11.66	8.49	1	0.004
	No	22	18	1.00				
Q.144.5. Communication problems with patients	Yes	55	12	4.07	1.48–11.35	8.16	1	0.004
	No	18	16	1.00				
Q.144.10. Withdrawal as a stress symptom	Yes	41	7	3.84	1.33–11.46	6.68	1	0.009
	No	32	21	1.00				
Q.145.3. Over-identification with patients' needs as a stress symptom	Yes	54	12	3.79	1.39–10.48	7.33	1	0.006
	No	19	16	1.00				
Q.144.3. Anxiety attacks as stress symptoms	Yes	44	8	3.79	1.35–10.91	6.92	1	0.008
	No	29	20	1.00				
Q.145.9. Depression as a stress symptom	Yes	51	11	3.58	1.32–9.85	6.74	1	0.009
	No	22	17	1.00				

*Unadjusted analysis; **Two missing values.

Table 16b Multi-variate logistic model for HIV/AIDS staff: Outcome 'MBI EE subscale category scores'

Co-variate	Category	OR Unadjusted	OR Adjusted	95% confidence interval for adjusted OR	P
Q.144.9. Self-righteousness ('heroism') as a stress symptom	Yes	6.13	5.02	1.60–15.86	0.006
	No	1.00	1.00		
Q.25. Finding work stressful	Yes	6.10	6.88	1.81–26.16	0.005
	No	1.00	1.00		
Q.145.6. Pessimism and hopelessness as stress symptoms	Yes	4.72	3.70	1.07–7.51	0.039
	No	1.00	1.00		
Q.145.10. A sense of failure as a stress symptom	Yes	4.75	2.06	0.57–7.51	0.272
	No	1.00	1.00		

Table 17a Odds ratios (OR)* and chi-square values of associations with MBI 'Emotional exhaustion' category scores for oncology staff where P <0.01

Question no. + variable	Category	Cases (High–moderate; n = 67)	Controls (Low; n = 33)	OR	95% Confidence limits	χ^2	d.f.	P
Q.143.5. Palpitation as stress symptoms	Yes / No	27 / 40	2 / 31	10.46 / 1.00	2.16–66.99	10.98	1	<0.001
Q.93. Percentage of colleagues who are stressed	51–100% / 0–50%	62 / 5	21 / 12	7.09 / 1.00	1.99–26.55	11.12	1	<0.001
Q.141.17. Coping with technology is a work stressor	Yes / No	26 / 40	3 / 30	6.50 / 1.00	1.65–29.84	8.34	1	0.003
Q.141.20. Lack of training in death and dying is a work stress	Yes / No	39 / 27	7 / 26	5.37 / 1.00	1.87–15.95	11.21	1	<0.001
Q.141.18. Overwork is a work stressor	Yes / No	56 / 10	17 / 16	5.27 / 1.00	1.83–15.46	10.96	1	<0.001
Q.144.3. Anxiety attacks as stress symptoms	Yes / No	40 / 27	8 / 25	4.63 / 1.00	1.67–13.18	9.76	1	0.001
Q. GHQ total score	5+ / 0–4	35 / 32	7 / 26	4.06 / 1.00	1.42–11.98	7.51	1	0.006
Q.141.27. Feeling professionally inadequate is a work stress	Yes / No	34 / 32	7 / 26	3.95 / 1.00	1.38–11.66	7.12	1	0.007
Q.155.3. Seeing patients dying is problematic	Agree / Disagree	42 / 25	10 / 23	3.86 / 1.00	1.46–10.44	8.04	1	0.004
Q.141.16. Clinical confidence is a work stress	Yes / No	36 / 30	8 / 25	3.75 / 1.00	1.36–10.64	7.00	1	0.008
Q.155.2. Knowing patients will die is problematic	Agree / Disagree	30 / 37	6 / 27	3.65 / 1.00	1.22–11.38	5.68	1	0.003
Q.145.9. Depression is a stress symptom	Yes / No	45 / 22	12 / 21	3.58 / 1.00	1.37–9.45	7.35	1	0.006

*Unadjusted analysis.

Table 17b Multi-variate logistic model for oncology staff: Outcome 'MBI EE subscale category scores'

Co-variate	Category	OR Unadjusted	OR Adjusted	95% confidence interval for adjusted OR	P
Q.143.5. Palpitations as stress symptoms	Yes No	10.46 1.00	8.98 1.00	1.33–60.56	0.024
Q.93. Percentage of colleagues who are stressed	51–100% 0–50%	7.09 1.00	9.57 1.00	2.20–41.55	0.003
Q.141.20. Lack of training in death and dying as a work stress	Yes No	5.37 1.00	7.18 1.00	2.03–25.36	0.002
Q.141.18. Overwork is a work stress	Yes No	5.27 1.00	5.99 1.00	1.71–21.03	0.005
Q.144.3. Anxiety attacks as stress symptoms	Yes No	4.63 1.00	3.10 1.00	0.90–10.61	0.072

Table 18a Odds ratios (OR)* and chi-square values of associations with MBI 'Depersonalisation' category scores for HIV/AIDS staff where $P <0.01$**

Question no. + variable	Category	Cases (High–moderate; n = 41)	Controls (Low; n = 60)	OR	95% Confidence limits	χ^2	d.f.	P
Q.145.1. Emotional numbness/indifference as a stress symptom	Yes No	38 3	26 34	16.56 1.00	4.22–75.91	23.47	1	<0.001
Q.145.8. Cynicism as a stress symptom	Yes No	33 8	21 39	7.66 1.00	2.76–21.97	18.47	1	<0.001
Q.141.7. Relations with staff are a work stress	Yes No	33 8	26 34	5.39 1.00	1.97–15.22	12.35	1	<0.001
Q.141.12. Relations with patients are a work stress	Yes No	28 13	18 42	5.03 1.00	1.96–13.08	12.90	1	<0.001
Q.143.2. Lingering minor illnesses are stress symptoms	Yes No	33 8	28 32	4.71 1.00	1.72–13.26	10.27	1	0.001
Q.62. Difficulties in emotional support-seeking	Yes No	35 6	34 26	4.46 1.00	1.50–13.89	7.99	1	0.004
Q.144.10. Withdrawal as a stress symptom	Yes No	28 13	20 40	4.31 1.00	1.70–11.07	10.57	1	0.001
Q.143.7. Gastrointestinal disturbances as stress symptoms	Yes No	29 12	22 38	4.17 1.00	1.64–10.78	9.98	1	0.001
Q.143.5. Palpitations as stress symptoms	Yes No	19 22	11 49	3.85 1.00	1.44–10.45	7.86	1	0.005
Q.17. Professional seniority	Senior Junior	8 33	29 31	0.26 1.00	0.09–0.71	7.52	1	0.006

*Unadjusted analysis; **Two missing values.

Table 18b Multi-variate logistic model for HIV/AIDS staff: Outcome 'MBI DP subscale category score'

Co-variate	Category	OR Unadjusted	OR Adjusted	95% confidence interval for adjusted OR	P
Q.145.1. Emotional numbness/indifference a stress symptom	Yes	16.56	9.48	2.13–42.16	0.003
	No	1.00	1.00		
Q.145.8. Cynicism as a stress symptom	Yes	7.66	2.77	0.81–9.47	0.104
	No	1.00	1.00		
Q.141.7. Relations with staff are a work stress	Yes	5.39	2.82	0.81–9.85	0.104
	No	1.00	1.00		
Q.141.12. Relations with patients are a work stress	Yes	5.03	2.67	0.86–8.31	0.089
	No	1.00	1.00		
Q.143.2. Lingering minor illnesses are stress symptoms	Yes	4.71	1.69	0.47–6.09	0.420
	No		1.00	1.00	
Q.144.10. Withdrawal as a stress symptom	Yes	4.31	2.23	0.69–7.16	0.178
	No	1.00	1.00		
Q.143.7. Gastrointestinal disturbances as stress symptoms	Yes	4.17	2.68	0.85–8.48	0.093
	No	1.00	1.00		

Table 19a Odds ratios (OR)* and chi-square values of associations with MBI 'Depersonalisation' category scores for oncology staff where P <0.01

Question no. + variable	Category	Cases (High–moderate; n = 31)	Controls (Low; n = 69)	OR	95% Confidence limits	χ^2	d.f.	P
Q.145.8. Cynicism as a stress symptom	Yes	30	38	24.47	3.24–509.07	15.23	1	<0.001
	No	1	31	1.00				
Q.145.1. Emotional numbness/indifference as stress symptoms	Yes	28	34	9.61	2.45–43.92	13.60	1	<0.001
	No	3	35	1.00				
Q.144.3. Anxiety attacks as stress symptoms	Yes	23	25	5.06	1.81–14.56	10.87	1	<0.001
	No	8	44	1.00				
Q.145.6. Pessimism and hopelessness as stress symptoms	Yes	27	40	4.89	1.41–18.59	6.94	1	0.008
	No	4	29	1.00				
Q.143.7. Gastrointestinal disturbances as stress symptoms	Yes	21	21	4.80	1.77–13.29	10.74	1	0.001
	No	10	48	1.00				
Q.141.16. Clinical confidence is a work stress	Yes	21	23	4.67	1.69–13.17	9.95	1	0.001
	No	9	46	1.00				
Q.155.3. Seeing patients dying is problematic	Agree	23	29	3.97	1.43–11.30	7.62	1	0.005
	Disagree	8	40	1.00				
Q.155.2. Knowing patients will die is problematic	Agree	18	18	3.92	1.47–10.61	8.16	1	0.004
	Disagree	13	51	1.00				
Q.143.5. Palpitations as stress symptoms	Yes	15	14	3.68	1.34–10.23	6.89	1	0.008
	No	16	55	1.00				

*Unadjusted analysis.

Table 19b Multi-variate logistic model for oncology staff: Outcome 'MBI DP subscale category score'

Co-variate	Category	OR Unadjusted	OR Adjusted	95% confidence interval for adjusted OR	P
Q.145.8. Cynicism as a stress symptom	Yes	24.47	21.61	2.38–195.6	0.006
	No	1.00	1.00		
Q.145.1. Emotional numbness/indifference as stress symptoms	Yes	9.61	9.89	2.06–47.50	0.004
	No	1.00	1.00		
Q.144.3. Anxiety attacks as stress symptoms	Yes	5.06	4.48	0.98–20.57	0.054
	No	1.00	1.00		
Q.143.7. Gastrointestinal disturbances as stress symptoms	Yes	4.80	1.21	0.28–5.18	0.795
	No	1.00	1.00		
Q.141.16. Clinical confidence is a work stress	Yes	4.67	2.83	0.85–9.42	0.089
	No	1.00	1.00		

Table 20a Odds ratios (OR)* and chi-square values of associations with MBI 'Reduced sense of personal accomplishment' category scores for HIV/AIDS staff where $P < 0.01$

Question no. + variable	Category	Cases (High–moderate)	Controls (Low)	OR	95% Confidence limits	x^2	d.f.	P
Q.99. Number of days off work other than holidays	6 +	18	1	12.12	1.57–255.24	6.96	1	0.008
	0–5	49	33	1.00				
Q.83. Issues leading to seeking work elsewhere	Personal	21	20	0.28	0.10–0.76	6.68	1	0.009
	Work	41	11	1.00				

*Unadjusted analysis.

Table 20b Multi-variate logistic model for HIV/AIDS staff: Outcome 'MBI PA subscale category scores'

Co-variate	Category	OR Unadjusted	OR Adjusted	95% confidence interval for adjusted OR	P
Q.99. Days off work for reasons other than holidays	6+	12.12	1.02	0.35–2.98	0.963
	0–5	1.00	1.00		
Q.83. Issues leading to seeking work elsewhere	Personal	0.28	2.16	0.91–5.13	0.081
	Work	1.00	1.00		

Table 21a Odds ratios (OR)* and chi-square values of associations with MBI 'Reduced sense of personal accomplishment' category scores for oncology staff where $P < 0.01$

Question no. + variable	Category	Cases (High–moderate; $n = 64$)	Controls (Low; $n = 36$)	OR	95% Confidence limits	χ^2	d.f.	P
Q.155.6. Watching the physical decline of patients is problematic	Agree	51	17	4.38	1.64–11.88	9.72	1	0.001
	Disagree	13	19	1.00				
Q.17. Professional seniority	Senior	21	24	0.24	0.09–0.63	9.35	1	0.002
	Junior	43	12	1.00				

*Unadjusted analysis.

Table 21b Multi-variate logistic model for oncology staff: Outcome 'MBI PA subscale category scores'

Co-variate	Category	OR Unadjusted	OR Adjusted	95% confidence interval for adjusted OR	P
Q.155.6. Watching the physical decline of patients is problematic	Agree	4.38	4.05	1.58–10.36	0.004
	Disagree	1.00	1.00		
Q.17. Professional seniority	Senior	0.24	0.26	0.10–0.65	0.004
	Junior	1.00	1.00		

References

Ader, R. (ed.) (1982). *Psychoneuroimmunology*. New York: Academic Press.

Amchin, J., Polan, H. J. (1986). 'A longitudinal account of staff adaptation to AIDS patients on a psychiatric unit'. *Hospital and Community Psychiatry*, 37, 1235–8.

American Psychiatric Association (1994). *Diagnostic and Statistical Manual of the Mental Disorders* (4th edn). Washington, DC: APA.

Ancona, L., Di Giannantonio, M., Mattioni, T., *et al.* (1991). 'Health care personnel and AIDS: how many risks of burnout syndrome?' Poster presented at VII International Conference on AIDS, Florence, 16–21 June. (Unpublished)

Anderson, M. B. G., Iwanicki, E. F. (1984). 'Teacher motivation and its relationship to burnout'. *Educational Administration Quarterly*, 20, 109–32.

Ankrah, E. M. (1991). 'AIDS and the social side of health'. *Social Science and Medicine*, 32 (9), 967–80.

Ankrah, E. M. (1993). 'The impact of HIV/AIDS on the family and other significant relationships: the African clan revisited'. *AIDS Care*, 5, 5–22.

Ankrah, E. M., Lubega, M., Nkumbi, S. S. (1989). 'The family and care-giving in Uganda'. Paper presented at V International Conference on AIDS, Montreal, 4–9 June. (Unpublished)

Arnetz, B. B., Brenner, S. O., Hjelm, R., *et al.* (1988). 'Stress reactions in relation to threat of job loss and actual unemployment: physiological, psychological and economic effects of job loss and unemployment'. *Stressforkingsrapporter*, 1 – 206.

Arthur, N. (1990). 'The assessment of burnout: a review of three inventories useful for research and counselling'. *Journal of Counselling and Development*, 69, 186–9.

Baggaley, R., Sulwe, J., Kelly, M., Ndovi Macmillan, M., Godfrey-Faussett, P. (1996). 'HIV counsellors' knowledge, attitudes and vulnerabilities to HIV in Lusaka Zambia 1994'. *AIDS Care*, 8(2), 155–66.

Bailey, J. T., Steffen, N., Grout, J. W. (1980). 'The stress audit: identifying the stressors with ICU nursing'. *Journal of Nursing Education*, 19, 15–25.

Bair, J. P., Greenspan, B. K. (1986). 'TEAMS: teamwork training for interns, residents and nurses'. *Hospital and Community Psychiatry*, 37 (6), 633–5.

Baldwin, P. J., Dodd, M., Wrate, R. M. (1996). *Young Doctors: Work, Health and Welfare. A Class Cohort 1986–1996*. London: Department of Health, 1996.

Banham, J. (1992). 'The cost of mental ill health to business'. In: R. Jenkins, N. Coney (eds.), *Prevention of Mental Ill Health at Work*. London: HMSO, 24–9.

Barbour, R. S. (1994). 'The impact of working with people with HIV/AIDS: a review of the literature'. *Social Science and Medicine*, 39(2), 221–32.

Barbour, R. S. (1995). 'The implications of HIV/AIDS for a range of workers in the Scottish context'. *AIDS Care*, 7(4), 521–35.

Barley, S. R., Knight, D. B. (1992). 'Toward a cultural theory of stress complaints'. *Research in Organisational Behaviour*, 14, 1–48.

Bates, F. M., Moore, B. N. (1975). 'Stress in hospital personnel'. *Medical Journal of Australia*, 15, 765–7.

Bellani, M. L., Protti, E., Pezzotta, P., *et al.* 'Psychiatric disorders in health care personnel working in AIDS units'. Poster presented at IX International Conference on AIDS/IV STD World Congress, Berlin, 6–11 June 1993. (Unpublished)

Bellani, M. L., Furlani, F., Gnecchi, M., *et al.* (1996) 'Burnout and related factors among HIV/AIDS health care workers'. *AIDS Care*, 8(2), 207–21.

Bennett, L. (1992a). 'The experience of nurses working with hospitalised AIDS patients'. *Australian Journal of Social Issues*, 27 (2), 125–43.

Bennett, L. (1992b). 'The impact of HIV/AIDS on health care professionals: psychosocial aspects of care'. Unpublished Doctoral Thesis, Faculty of Medicine, University of Sydney.

Bennett, L. (1995). 'The Sydney study: interventions to assist responses of health care professionals in HIV/AIDS'. In: L. Bennett, D. Miller, M. W. Ross, (eds), *Health Workers and AIDS: Research, Intervention and Current Issues in Burnout and Response*. Reading: Harwood Academic Press, 191–212.

Bennett, L., Kelaher, M. (1993). 'Longitudinal determinance of patient care-related stress in HIV/AIDS health professionals'. Paper presented at IX International Conference on AIDS/IV STD World Congress, Berlin, 6–11 June. (Unpublished)

Bennett, L., Michie, P., Kippax, S. (1991). 'Quantitative analysis of burnout and its associated factors in AIDS nursing'. *AIDS Care*, 3 (2), 181–92.

Bennett, L., Kelaher, M., Ross, M. W. (1994). 'The impact of working with HIV/AIDS on health care professionals: development of the AIDS Impact Scale'. *Psychology and Health: An International Journal*, 9 (3), 221–32.

Bennett, L., Miller, D., Ross, M. W. (eds) (1995). *Health Workers and AIDS: Research, Intervention and Current Issues in Burnout and Response*. Reading: Harwood Academic Press.

Bennett, L., Ross, M. W., Sunderland, R. (1996). 'The relationship between recognition, rewards and burnout in AIDS caring'. *AIDS Care*, 8(2), 145–54.

Berkeley Planning Associates (1977). *Evaluation of Child Abuse and Neglect Demonstration Project 1974–1977, Vol IX: Project management and worker burnout – final report*. Berkeley: BPA.

Bibeau, G., Dussault, G., Larouche, L. M., *et al.* (1989). *Certains Aspects Culturals, Diagnostiques et Juridiques de Burnout*. Montreal: Confederation des Syndicats Nationaux.

Birch, M. (1975). *To Nurse or not to Nurse*. London: Royal College of Nursing Research Series.

Blinkhoff, P., Bukanga, E., Syamalevwe, B., Williams, G. (1999). *Under the Mupundu Tree (Strategies for Hope No. 14)*. Oxford: Actionaid.

Blumenfeld, M., Smith, P. J., Milazzo, J., *et al.* (1987). 'Survey of attitudes of nurses working with AIDS patients'. *General Hospital Psychiatry*, 9, 56–63.

Bolle, J. L. (1988). 'Supporting the deliverers of care: strategies to support nurses and prevent burnout'. *AIDS*, 23, 843–50.

Bove, G., Speranza, T., Pennacchi, D., *et al.* (1993). 'Needs of volunteer in hospitalised AIDS patients assistance'. Paper presented at IX International Conference on AIDS, Berlin, June 6–11 (POD 214061). (Unpublished)

Breault, A., Polifroni, E. (1992). 'Caring for people with AIDS: nurses' attitudes and feelings'. *Journal of Advanced Nursing*, 17, 21–27.

Bredfelt, R., Dardeau, F., Wesley, R., *et al.* (1991). 'AIDS: family physicians' attitudes and experiences'. *Journal of Family Practice*, 32(1), 71–5.

Breslow, L., Buell, P. (1960). 'Mortality from coronary heart disease and physical activity of work in California'. *Journal of Chronic Disease*, 11, 615–27.

Bresolin, L. B., Rinaldi, R. C., Henwig, J. J., *et al.* (1990). 'Attitudes of US primary care physicians about HIV disease and AIDS'. *AIDS Care*, 2, 117–25.

Brettle, R. P., Willocks, L., Hamilton, B. A., *et al.* (1994). 'Out-patient medical care in Edinburgh for IDU-related HIV'. *AIDS Care*, 6, 49–58.

Brimlow, D. (1995). 'Training to prevent burnout: HIV/AIDS programmes for physicians and dentists'. In: L. Bennett, D. Miller, M. W. Ross, (eds), *Health Workers and AIDS: Research, Intervention and Current Issues in Burnout and Response*. Reading: Harwood Academic Press, 247–58.

Briner, R. B. (1997). 'Improving stress assessment: towards an evidence-based approach to organisational stress interventions'. *Journal of Psychosomatic Research*, 43 (1), 61–71.

Bulkin, W., Brown, L., Fraoli, D., *et al.* (1988). 'Hospice care of the intravenous drug user AIDS patient in a skilled nurse facility'. *Journal of Acquired Immune Deficiency Syndromes*, 1, 375–80.

Burisch, M. (1989). *Das Burnout-Syndrom. Theorie der inneren Erschopfung [The Burnout Syndrome. A theory of Inner Exhaustion]*. Heidelberg: Springer.

Burisch, M. (1993). 'In search of theory: some ruminations on the nature and etiology of burnout'. In: W. B. Schaufeli, C. Maslach, T. Marek (eds), *Professional Burnout: Recent Developments in Theory and Research*. New York: Taylor & Francis, 75–94.

Burke, M. J., Brief, A. P., George, J. M. (1993). 'The role of negative affectivity in understanding relations between self-reports of stressors and strains: a comment on the applied psychology literature'. *Journal of Applied Psychology*, 78, 402–12.

Burke, R. J., Shearer, J., Deszca, G. (1984). 'Burnout among men and women in police work: an examination of the Cherniss model'. *Journal of Health and Human Resources Administration*, 7, 162–88.

Calvert, G. M., (1993). 'Volunteer motivation and retention in an voluntary AIDS service organisation'. Paper presented at IX International Conference on AIDS IV STD World Congress. Berlin, 6–11 June 1993. (Unpublished)

Caplan, R. D. (1971). 'Organisational stress and individual strain: a social-psychological study of risk factors in coronary heart disease among administrators, engineers and scientists'. Unpublished Doctoral Dissertation, University of Michigan.

Caplan, R. P. (1994). 'Stress, anxiety, and depression in hospital consultants, general practitioners, and senior health service managers'. *British Medical Journal*, 309, 1261–3.

Carballo, M., Miller, D. (1989). 'HIV/AIDS Counselling: a new agenda for the 1990s'. *AIDS Care*, 1(2), 117–24.

Carlestam, C. C., Karlsson, C. C., Levi, L. (1973). 'Stress and disease in response to exposure to noise: a review'. Reprinted from *Proceeding of the International Congress on Noise as a Public Hazard*, Dubrovnick, Yugoslavia, by US Environmental Protection Agency.

Carnwath, T., Miller, D. (1986). *Behavioral Psychotherapy in Primary Care: A Practice Manual*. London: Academic Press.

Cherniss, C. (1980). *Staff Burnout: Job Stress in the Human Services*. Beverley Hills, CA: Sage.

Cherniss, C. (1992). 'Long-term consequences of burnout: an exploratory study'. *Journal of Organisational Behaviour*, 13, 1–11.

Church, J., Kocsis, A. E., Green, J. (1988). 'Effects on lovers of caring for HIV infected individuals related to perceptions of cognitive, behavioral and personality changes in the sufferer'. Paper presented at IV International Conference on AIDS, Stockholm, June 1988. (Unpublished)

Clark, E. J. (1989). 'Offsetting burnout in the thanatologic setting: recognition and emphasis of "psychosocial successes" in social work intervention'. In: D. T. Wessells, Jr, A. H. Kutscher, I. B. Seeland, *et al.* (eds), *Professional Burnout in Medicine and the Helping Professions*. New York: The Haworth Press.

Claxton, R. P. R., Burgess, A. P., Catalan, J. (1993). 'Motivational factors and psychosocial stress in emotional support volunteers (buddies) for people living with AIDS'. Paper presented at IX International AIDS Conference and III World Congress, Amsterdam, 18–24 June. (Unpublished)

Cobb, S., Rose, R. M. (1973). 'Hypertension, peptic ulcer and diabetes in air traffic controllers'. *Journal of the American Medical Association*, **224**, 489–92.

Constable, J. F., Russell, D. W. (1986). 'The effect of social support and the work environment upon burnout among nurses'. *Journal of Human Stress*, **12**, 20–26.

Cooper, C. L. (1983). 'Identifying stressors at work: recent research developments'. *Journal of Psychosomatic Research*, **2**, 369–76.

Cooper, C. L. (1992). Cited in *BMA Press Release*, London, October 1992.

Cooper, C. L., Cartwright, S. (1994). 'Stress management interventions in the workplace: stress counselling and stress audits'. *British Journal of Guidance and Counselling*, **22**(1), 65–73.

Cooper, C. L., Davidson, M. (1987). 'Sources of stress at work and their relation to stressors in non-working environments'. In: R. Kalimo, M. A. el-Batawi, C. L. Cooper (eds). *Psychosocial Factors at Work and their Relation to Health*. Geneva: World Health Organization, 99–111.

Cooper, C. L., Marshall, J. (1976). 'Occupational sources of stress: a review of the literature relating to coronary heart disease and mental ill health'. *Journal of Occupational Psychology*, **49**, 11–28.

Cooper, C. L., Marshall, J. (1978). 'Sources of managerial and white collar stress'. In: C. L. Cooper, R. Payne (eds), *Stress at Work*. Chichester: Wiley, 81–105.

Cooper, C. L., Sadri, G. (1991). 'The impact of stress counselling a work'. *Journal of Social Behaviour and Personality*, **6**, 411–23.

Cooper, C. L., Sloan, S., Williams, S. (1988). *Occupational Stress Indicator: Management Guide*. Windsor: NFER-Nelson.

Cooper, C. L., Sadri, S., Allison, T. (1990). 'Stress counselling in the post office'. *Counselling Psychology Quarterly*, **3** (1), 3–12.

Corcoran, K. J., Bryce, A. K. (1983). 'Intervention in the experience of burnout: effects of skill development'. *Journal of Social Services Research*, **7**(1), 71–9.

Cordery, J. L., Mueller, W. S., Smith, L. M. (1991). 'Attitudinal and behavioural effects of autonomous group working: a longitudinal field study'. *Academy of Management Journal*, **34**, 464–76.

Cordes, C. L., Dougherty, T. W (1993). 'A review and integration of research on job burnout'. *Academy of Management Review*, **18** (4), 621–56.

Cox, T. (1981). *Stress* (2nd edn). London: MacMillan.

Cox, T., Mackay, C. J. (1981). 'A transactional approach to occupational stress'. In: E. Corlett, J. Richardson (eds), *Stress, Work Design, and Productivity*. Chichester: Wiley.

Cox, T., Kuk, G., Leiter, M. P. (1993). 'Burnout, health, work stress, and organisational healthiness'. In: W. B. Schaufeli, C. Maslach, T. Marek (eds) *Professional Burnout: Recent Developments in Theory and Research*. Washington, DC: Taylor & Francis, 177–99.

Coyle, A., Soodin, M. (1992). 'Training, workload and stress among HIV counsellors'. *AIDS Care*, **4**, 217–21.

Crump, J. H., *et al.* (1980). 'Investigating occupational stress: a methodological approach'. *Journal of Occupational Behaviour*, **1**, 191–202.

Davidson, G., Gillies, P. (1993). 'Safe working practices and HIV infection: knowledge, attitude, perception of risk, and policy in hospital'. *Quality in Health Care*, **2**, 21–6.

Davidson, P., Jackson, C. (1985). 'The nurse as survivor: delayed post-traumatic stress reaction and cumulative trauma in nursing'. *International Journal of Nursing Studies*, **22**, 1–13.

Delvaux, N., Razaki, D., Farvacques, C. (1988). 'Cancer care: a stress for health professionals'. *Social Science and Medicine*, **27**, 159–66.

Des Jarlais, D. C. (1990). 'Stages in the response of the Drug Abuse Treatment System to the AIDS epidemic in New York City'. *The Journal of Drug Issues*, **20** (2), 335–47.

Dickinson, E. (1995). 'Using marketing principles for healthcare development'. *Quality in Health Care*, **4** (1), 40–4.

Di Giannantonio, M., Favetta, S., Pozzi, G., *et al.* (1993). A psychosocial study of burn-out syndrome in a sample of 152 Italian health care workers dealing with AIDS patients. Poster presented to IX International Conference on AIDS/IV STD World Congress, Berlin, 6–11 June. (Unpublished)

Dinoi, R., Brettler, D. (1991). 'The group process in the consultation to a comprehensive haemophilia treatment team: reducing staff burnout relating to HIV'. Poster presented at VII International Conference on AIDS, Florence, 16–21 June. (Unpublished)

Eakin, J. M., Taylor, K. M. (1990). 'The psychosocial impact of AIDS on health workers'. *AIDS*, **4** (suppl. 1), S257–S262.

Edelwich, J., Brodsky, J. (1980). *Burnout: Stages of Disillusionment in the Helping Professions*. New York: Human Sciences Press.

Egan, M. (1993). 'Resilience at the frontlines: hospital social work with AIDS patients and burnout'. *Social Work in Heath Care*, **18** (2), 109–25.

Elkin, A. J., Rosch, P. J. (1990). 'Promoting mental health at work'. *Occupational Medicine State of the Art Review*, **5**, 739–54.

Federal Centre for AIDS (1992). *Ending the Isolation*. Ottowa: Ministry of Health and Welfare.

Fernandez, F., Holmes, V. E., Levy, J. K. (1989). 'Consultation-liaison psychiatry and HIV-related disorders'. *Hospital and Community Psychiatry*, **40**, 146–53.

Field, T. M., McCabe, P. M., Schneiderman, N. (eds) (1985). *Stress and Coping*. Hillsdale, NJ: Erlbaum.

Firth, H., McIntee, J., McKeown, P., Britton, P. G. (1986). 'Burnout and professional depression: related concepts ?'. *Journal of Advanced Nursing*, **11**, 633–41.

Firth-Cozens, J. (1987). 'Emotional distress in junior house officers'. *British Medical Journal*, **295**, 533–36.

Firth-Cozens, J., Morrison, L. (1989). 'Sources of stress and ways of coping in junior house officers'. *Stress Medicine*, **5**, 121–26.

Folkman, S., Chesney, M. A., Christopher-Richards, A. (1994). 'Stress and coping in caregiving partners of men with AIDS'. *Psychiatric Clinics of North America*, **17**, 35–53.

Fraser, P., Franklin, A., Kellow, E., Calvert, G. (1996). The myth of burnout. Paper presented at XI International Conference on AIDS, Vancouver, 7–12 July (Abstract no. We. D. 251).

Frazer, R. (1947). 'The incidence of neurosis among factory workers'. *Industrial Health Research Board of the Medical Research Council Report, no. 90*. London: HMSO.

French, J. R. P. Jr, Caplan, R. D. (1972). 'Organisational stress and individual strain'. In: A. J. Marrow (ed.), *The Failure of Success*. New York: AMACOM, 30–66.

Freudenberger, H. J. (1974). 'Staff burnout'. *Journal of Social Issues*, 30, 159–65.

Freudenberger, H. J. (1977). 'Burn-out: occupational hazard of the child care worker'. *Child Care Quarterly*, 6, 90–9.

Freudenberger, H. J. (1981). 'Burnout: contemporary issues and trends'. Paper presented at the National Conference on Stress and Burnout, New York. (Unpublished)

Friedman, R. (1985). 'Making family therapy easier for the therapist: burnout prevention'. *Family Process*, 24 (4), 549–553.

Frost, J. C., Makadon, H. J., Judd, D., *et al.* (1991). 'Care for care givers: a support group for staff caring for AIDS patients in a hospital-based primary care practice'. *Journal of General Internal Medicine*, 6, 162–67.

Gabbard, G. O. (1994) 'Reconsidering the American Psychological Association's policy on sex with former patients: is it justifiable?', *Professional Psychology: Research and Practice*, 25, 329–35.

Gaines, J., Jermier, J. M. (1983). 'Emotional exhaustion in a high-stress organisation'. *Academy of Management Journal*, 26, 567–86.

Gallop, R., Taerk, G. (1995). 'The Toronto intervention study'. In: L. Bennett, D. Miller, M. W. Ross (eds), *Health Workers and AIDS: Research, Intervention and Current Issues in Burnout and Response*. Reading: Harwood Academic Press, 229–46.

Gallop, R., Taerk, G., Lancee, W., *et al.* (1992). 'A randomised trial of group interventions for hospital staff caring for persons with AIDS'. *AIDS Care*, 4 (2), 177–85.

Garside, B. (1993). 'Physicians mutual aid group: a response to AIDS-related burnout'. *Health & Social Work*, 18 (4), 259–67.

Gartrell, N. K., Milliken, N., Goodson, W. H., Thiemann, S., Lo, B. (1992). 'Physician–patient sexual contact: prevalence and problems'. *The Western Journal of Medicine*, 157, 139–43.

Gerbert, B., Maguire, B., Badner, V., Altman, D., Stone, G. (1988). 'Why fear persists: health care professionals and AIDS'. *Journal of the American Medical Association*, 260, 3481–3.

Gessler, S., Alcorn, R., Miller, D. (1996) 'Borderline Personalities and HIV: The View from Britain'. Paper presented at II European Congress on Personality Disorders, Milan, 26–29 June 1996.

Gillies, P. (1991). 'Questionnaires and interviewers: notes on methodological considerations'. In: R. C. Fraser, M. L. M. Goeting, (eds), *Research Methods in General Practice*. Southampton: Duphar Laboratories Ltd, 39–49.

Gilmore, N., Somerville, M. A. (1995). 'Health care professionals responding to AIDS: Ethics, Law and Human Rights'. In: L. Bennett, D. Miller, M. Ross (eds), *Health Workers and AIDS: Research, Intervention and Current Issues in Burnout and Response*. Reading: Harwood Academic Press; 361–400.

Gladding, S. T. (1991). 'Counsellor self-abuse'. *Journal of Mental Health Counselling*, 13 (3), 414–19.

Gold, Y. (1985). 'Does teacher burnout begin with student teaching?' *Education*, 105, 254–57.

Goldberg, D. P. (1978). *Manual of the General Health Questionnaire*. Windsor, Berks: NFER-Nelson.

Goldberg, D. P. (1981). 'Estimating the Prevalence of a Disorder from the Results of a Screening Test'. In: J. K. Wing, P. Bebbington, L. Robins, *What is a Case?* London: Grant, McIntyre, 129–36.

Goldberg, D., Williams, P. (1988). *A Users Guide to the General Health Questionnaire*. Windsor, Berks. : NFER-Nelson.

Golembiewski, R. T., Scherb, K., Boudreau, R. A. (1993). 'Burnout in cross-national settings: generic and model-specific perspectives'. In: W. B. Schaufeli, C. Maslach, T. Marek (eds), *Professional Burnout: Recent Developments in Theory and Research*. Washington, DC: Taylor & Francis, 217–36.

Gordin, F. M., Willoughby, A. D., Levine, L. A., *et al.* (1987). 'Knowledge of AIDS among hospital workers: behavioral correlates and consequences'. *AIDS*, 1, 183–88.

Gray-Toft, P., Anderson, J. G. (1980). 'A nursing stress scale: development of an instrument'. *Journal of Behavioural Assessment*, 3, 11–23.

Gray-Toft, P., Anderson, J. G. (1981). 'Stress among hospital nursing staff: its causes and effects'. *Social Science and Medicine*, 15a, 639–47.

Green, J. (1986). 'Counselling HTLV-III sero positives'. In: D. Miller, J. Weber, J. Green (eds), *The Management of AIDS Patients*. London: MacMillan Press, 151–68.

Green, J., McCreaner, A. (eds) (1989). *Counselling in HIV Infection and AIDS*. Oxford: Blackwell Scientific Publications.

Green, J., Miller, D. (1987). 'The psychosocial impact of AIDS and human immunodeficiency virus'. In: M. S. Gottlieb, D. J. Jeffries, D. Mildvan, *et al.* (eds), *Current Topics in AIDS*: Vol. 1. New York: John Wiley & Sons, 287–302.

Greer, D. S., Mor, V. (1986). 'An overview of national hospice study findings'. *Journal of Chronic Diseases*, 39, 5–7.

Greer, S., Morris, T., Pettingale, K. W. (1979). 'Psychological response to breast cancer: effect on outcome'. *Lancet*, ii, 785–7.

Greer, S., Watson, M. (1985). 'Towards a psychobiological model of cancer: psychological considerations'. *Social Science and Medicine*, 20 (8), 773–7.

Grimshaw, J. (1995). 'The birth of body positive'. *Body Positive*, 182 (27 February), 1–2.

Grossman, A. H., Silverstein, C. (1993). 'Facilitating support groups for professionals working with people with AIDS'. *Social Work*, 38 (2), 144–51.

Gruber, M., Beavers, F., Johnson, B., *et al.* (1989). 'The relationship between knowledge about AIDS and the implementation of universal precautions by registered nurses'. *Clinical Nurse Specialist*, 3, 182–5.

Guinan, L., McCallum, W., Painter, L., *et al.* (1991). 'Stressors and rewards of being an AIDS emotional-support volunteer: a scale for use by care-givers for people with AIDS'. *AIDS Care*, 3 (2), 137–50.

Gutheil, T. G., Gabbard, G. O. (1993). 'The concept of boundaries in clinical practice: theoretical and risk management dimensions'. *American Journal of Psychiatry*, 150, 188–96.

Halton, W. (1995). 'Institutional stress on providers in health and education'. *Psychodynamic Counselling*, 1 (2), 187–98.

Handy, J. (1987). 'Understanding stress in psychiatric nursing'. Unpublished Doctoral thesis, University of Lancaster.

Handy, J. A. (1988). 'Theoretical and methodological problems within occupation stress and burnout research'. *Human Relations*, 41 (5), 351–69.

Harding, R. M., Mills, F. J. (1983). 'Is the crew fit to fly?' *British Medical Journal*, ii, 192–5.

Hayward, R., Shapiro, M. (1991). 'A national study of AIDS residency training: experiences, concerns and consequences'. *Annals of Internal Medicine*, 114, 23–31.

Hochschild, A. (1989). *The Second Shift*. New York: Avon Books.

Horsman, J. M., Sheeran, P. (1995). 'Health care workers and HIV/AIDS: a critical review of the literature'. *Social Science and Medicine*, 41(11), 1535–67.

Horstman, W., McKusick, L. (1986). 'The impact of AIDS on the physician'. In: L. McKusick (ed.), *What to do about AIDS?* Berkeley: University of California Press, 63–74.

House, J. S. (1981). *Workstress and Social Support*. Reading, MA: Addison-Wesley.

House, J. S., Wells, J. A. (1978). 'Occupational stress, social support, and health'. In: G. McLean, G. Black, M. Colligan (eds), *Reducing Occupational Stress*. Government Printing Office: US department of health, education, and welfare publication no. (NIOSH) 78–243, 8–29.

Hunter, C. E., Ross, M. W. (1991). 'Determinants of health care workers' attitudes toward people with AIDS'. *Journal of Applied Social Psychology*, 21, 947–56.

Ivancevich, J. M., Matteson, M. T. (1987). 'Organisational level stress management interventions: a review and recommendations'. *Journal of Organisational Behavioral Management*, 81, 229–48.

Jackson, S. E., Maslach, C. (1982). 'After-effects of job related stress: families as victims'. *Journal of Occupational Behaviour*, 3, 63–77.

Jackson, S. E., Schwab, R. L., Schuler, R. S. (1986). 'Toward an understanding of the burnout phenomenon'. *Journal of Applied Psychology*, 71, 630–40.

Jenkins, R. (1993). 'Mental health at work – why is it so under-researched?'. *Occupational Medicine*, 43, 65–7.

Johansson, G. (1975). 'Psychophysiological stress reaction in the saw mill: a pilot study'. In: B. Ager (ed.), *Ergonomics in Saw Mills and Woodworking Industries*. Stockholm: National Board of Occupational Safety and Health.

Johns, G. (1991). 'Substantive and methodological constraints on behaviour and attitudes in organisational research'. *Organisational Behaviour and Human Discussion Processes*, 49, 105–23.

Jones, J. W. (1981). 'Dishonesty, burnout, and unauthorised work break extensions'. *Personality and Social Psychology Bulletin*, 7 (3), 406–9.

Jones, J. W., Barge, B. N., Steffy, B. D., et al. (1988). 'Stress and medical malpractice: organisational risk assessment and intervention'. *Journal of Applied Psychology*, 73, 727–35.

Kagan, A., Levi, L. (1971). 'Adaptations of the psychosocial environment to man's abilities and needs'. In: L. Levi (ed.), *Society, Stress and Disease*, Vol. 1. London: Oxford University Press.

Kahill, S. (1988). 'Symptoms of professional burnout: a review of the empirical evidence'. *Canadian Psychology*, 29 (3), 284–97.

Kahn, R. L. (1974). 'Conflict, ambiguity, and overload: three elements in job stress'. In: A. MacLean (ed.), *Occupational Stress*. Springfield, IL: Charles C. Thomas.

Kahn, R. L., Wolfe, D. M., Quinn, R. P., et al. (1964). *Organisational Stress: Studies in Role Conflict and Ambiguity*. New York: Wiley.

Kaleeba, N., Ray, S., Willmore, B. (1991). *We Miss You All. Noerine Kaleeba: Aids in The Family*. Harare, Zimbabwe: Women and AIDS Support Network.

Kalibala, S. (1995). 'Impact of HIV/AIDS caregiving on health markers in Uganda and other parts of sub-Saharan Africa'. In: L. Bennett, D. Miller, M. W. Ross (eds), *Health Workers and AIDS: Research, Intervention and Current Issues in Burnout and Response*. Reading: Harwood Academic Press, 285–306.

Kanas, N. (1986). 'Support groups for mental health staff and trainees'. *International Journal of Group Psychotherapy*, 36 (2), 279–96.

Karger, H. J. (1981). 'Burnout as alienation'. *Social Science Review*, June, 270–83.

Kasl, S. V. (1978). 'Epidemiological contributions to the study of workstress'. In: Cooper, C. L., Payne, R. (eds), *Stress at Work*. Chichester: Wiley, 3–48.

Keinan, G., Melamed, S. (1987). 'Personality characteristics and proneness to burnout: a study among internists'. *Stress Medicine*, 3, 307–15.

Kelaher, M., Ross, M. W. (1995) 'Measurement issues in Burnout'. In: L. Bennett, D. Miller, M. W. Ross (eds), *Health Workers and AIDS: Research, Intervention and Current Issues in Burnout and Response*. Reading: Harwood Academic Press, 61–72.

Kesler, K. (1990). 'Burnout: a multi-model approach to assessment and resolution'. *Elementary School Guidance and Counselling*, 24, 303–11.

Kleiber, D., Gusy, B., Enzmann, D., Beerlage, I. (1992). 'Causes and prevalence of stress and burnout among health care personnel in the field of AIDS'. Paper presented at VIII International Conference on AIDS/III STD World Congress, Amsterdam, 19–24 July. (Unpublished)

Kleiber, D., Enzmann, D., Gusy, B. (1993). 'Stress and burnout among health care personnel in the field of AIDS: causes and prevalence'. In: H. van Dis, E. van Dongen (eds), *Burnout in HIV/AIDS Health Care and Support: Impact for Professionals and Volunteers*. Amsterdam: University of Amsterdam Press, 23–40.

Kleiber, D., Enzmann, D., Gusy, B. (1995). 'Stress and burnout in AIDS health care: are there special characteristics?' In: L. Bennett, D. Miller, M. W. Ross (eds), *Health Workers and AIDS: Research, Intervention and Current Issues in Burnout and Response*. Reading: Harwood Academic Press, 115–30.

Kornhauser, A. (1965). *Mental Health of the Industrial Worker*. New York: Wiley.

Kothari, P. (1989). *Orgasm: New Dimensions*. Bombay: VRP Publishers.

Kroes, W. H. (1976). *Society's Victim – the Policeman : an Analysis of Job Stress in Policing*. Springfield, IL: Charles C. Thomas.

Lange, A. J., Jakubowski, P. (1976). *Responsible Assertive Behaviour: Cognitive/Behavioral Procedures for Trainers*. Champaigne, IL: Research Press.

Leach, G., French, L., Miller, D. (1999). 'Clinical Supervision for Health Advisers: Supporting Professional Practice'. In: S. Chippindale (ed.), *The Health Advisers' Manual*. London: Blackwell (in press).

Leiter, M. P. (1988). 'Burnout as a function of communication patterns'. *Group Organisation Studies*, 13, 111–28.

Leiter M. P. (1989). 'The development of burnout among mental health workers: a longitudinal study'. In: M. P. Leiter, *Perspectives on the Development of Burnout and Job Stress*. Symposium presented at the Annual Convention of the Canadian Psychological Association, Halifax, NS.

Leiter, M. P. (1990). 'The impact of family resources, control coping, and skill utilisation on the development of burnout: a longitudinal study'. *Human Relations*, 43, 1067–83.

Leiter, M. P. (1991). 'The dream denied: professional burnout and the constraints of human service organisations'. *Canadian Psychology*, 32 (4), 547–55.

Leiter, M. P. (1992). 'Burnout as a crisis in self-efficacy: conceptual and practical implications'. *Work and Stress*, 6, 107–15.

Leiter, M. P. (1993). 'Burnout as a developmental process: consideration of models'. In: W. B. Schaufeli, C. Maslach, T. Marek (eds), *Professional Burnout: Recent Developments in Theory and Research*. Washington, DC: Taylor & Francis, 237–50.

Leiter, M. P., Maslach, C. (1988). 'The impact of interpersonal environment on burnout and organisational commitment'. *Journal of Organisational Behaviour*, 9, 297–308.

Lemkau, J. P., Rafferti, J. P., Perdy, R. R., Rudisill, J. R. (1987). 'Sex role stress and job burnout among family practice physicians'. *Journal of Vocational Behaviour*, **31**, 81–90.

Levi, L. (1973). 'Humanokologie-psychosomatische gesichtpunkte und forschungsstrategien'. *Psychosomatic Medicine*, **5**, 92–102.

Levi, L. (1974). 'Stress, distress and psychosocial stimuli'. In: A. McLean (ed.), *Occupational Stress*. Springfield, IL: Charles C. Thomas.

Lloyd, G. (1995). 'Social work responses to HIV disease'. In: L. Bennett, D. Miller, M. W. Ross (eds), *Health Workers and AIDS*. Reading: Harwood Academic Press, 259–70.

Locke, E. A. (1976). 'The nature and causes of job satisfaction'. In: M. D. Dunnette (ed.), *Handbook of Industrial and Organisational Psychology*. Chicago: Rand-McNally.

Lopez, D., Getzel, G. (1987). 'Strategies for volunteers caring for persons with AIDS'. *Social Case Work: The Journal of Contemporary Social Work*, January, 47–54.

Lovejoy, N. C. (1988). 'Family and care giver responses to HIV infection'. In: G. Gee, T. A. Moran (eds), *AIDS: Concepts in Nursing Practice*. Baltimore: Williams & Wilkins, 379–401.

Lunt, B., Yardley, J. (1988). *Home Care Teams and Hospital Support Teams for the Terminally Ill*. Southampton: Cancer Care Research Unit, Royal South Herts Hospital.

Lyall, A. (1989). 'The prevention and treatment of professional burnout'. *Loss, Grief and Care*, **3** (1–2), 27–32.

Maj, M. (1991). 'Psychological problems of families and health workers dealing with people infected with human immunodeficiency virus 1'. *Acta Psychiatrica Scandinavica*, **83**, 161–8.

Mann, J. (1995). 'Human Rights and the New Public Health'. *Health and Human Rights*, **1**(3), 229–33.

Mann, J., Tarantola, D., Netter, T. W. (1992). *AIDS in the World: A Global Report*. Cambridge, MA: Harvard University Press.

Margolis, B. L. (1974). 'Job stress: an unlisted occupational hazard'. *Journal of Occupational Medicine*, **16**, 659–61.

Marks, G., Richardson, J., Lochner, T., *et al.* (1988). 'Assumed similarity of attitudes about AIDS among gay and heterosexual physicians'. *Journal of Applied Social Psychology*, **18**, 774–86.

Martin, C. A., Julian, R. A. (1987). 'Causes of stress and burnout in physicians caring for the chronically and terminally ill'. *The Hospice Journal*, **3**, 121–46.

Maslach, C. (1993). 'Burnout: a multidimensional perspective'. In: W. B. Schaufeli, C. Maslach, T. Marek (eds), *Professional Burnout: Recent Developments in Theory and Research*. Washington, DC: Taylor & Francis, 19–32.

Maslach, C., Jackson, S. E. (1978). 'Lawyer burn-out'. *Barrister*, **5** (2), 52–4.

Maslach, C., Jackson, S. E. (1981). 'The measurement of experienced burnout'. *Journal of Occupational Behaviour*, **2**, 99–113.

Maslach, C. H., Jackson, S. E. (1982). 'Burnout in health professions: a social psychological analysis'. In: G. S. Saunders, J. Suls (eds), *Social Psychology of Illness*. London: Lawrence Erlbaum.

Maslach, C., Jackson, S. E. (1985). 'The role of sex and family variables in burnout'. *Sex Roles*, **12**, 837–51.

Maslach, C., Jackson, S. E. (1986). *The Maslach Burnout Inventory. Manual* (2nd edn). Palo Alto, CA: Consulting Psychologists Press.

Maslach, C. H., Ozer, E. (1995). 'Theoretical issues related to burnout in AIDS health workers'. In: L. Bennett, D. Miller, M. W. Ross, (eds), *Health Workers and AIDS:*

Research, Intervention and Current Issues in Burnout and Response. Reading: Harwood Academic Press, 1–14.

Maslach, C., Schaufeli, W. B. (1993). 'Historical and conceptual development of burnout'. In: W. B. Schaufeli, C. Maslach, T. Marek (eds), *Professional Burnout: Recent Developments in Theory and Research*. Washington, DC: Taylor & Francis, 1–16.

Maslanka, H. (1992). 'Social support, rewards and burnout in AIDS volunteers'. Poster presented at VIII International Conference on AIDS/III STD World Congress, Amsterdam, 18–24 July. (Unpublished)

Maslanka, H. (1995). 'HIV volunteers'. In: L. Bennett, D. Miller, M. Ross (eds), *Health Workers and AIDS*. Reading: Harwood Academic Press; 151–74.

Maslanka, H (1996). 'Burnout, social support and AIDS volunteers'. *AIDS Care*, 8(2), 195–206.

Maynard, E. D. (1985). 'The intervener: managing personal crises'. *Emotional First-Aid: A Journal of Crisis Intervention*, 2 (3), 39–46.

McCann, K., Wadsworth, E. (1992). 'The role of informal carers in supporting gay men who have HIV related illness: what do they do and what are their needs?' *AIDS Care*, 4, 25–34.

McCarthy, M. (1989). 'Burnout: what price care-giving?' *Loss, Grief and Care*, 3 (1–2), 67–71.

McElroy, A. (1982). 'Burnout – a review of the literature with application to cancer nursing'. *Cancer Nursing*, 5, 211–17.

McNabb, K., Keller, M. L. (1991). 'Nurses' risk-taking regarding HIV transmission in the workplace'. *Western Journal of Nursing Research*, 13(6), 732–45.

Meier, S. T. (1983). 'Toward a theory of burnout'. *Human Relations*, 36, 899–910.

Meier, S. T. (1984). 'The construct validity of burnout'. *Journal of Occupational Psychology*, 57, 211–19.

Miller, D. (1987). *Living with AIDS and HIV*. London: MacMillan Press.

Miller, D. (1989). 'HIV counselling: an international perspective'. Paper presented at the American Medical Association International HIV Conference: Counselling, Testing and Early Care, Montreal, 3–4 June. (Unpublished)

Miller, D. (1991). 'Occupational morbidity and burnout: lessons and warnings for HIV/AIDS carers'. *International Review of Psychiatry*, 3, 439–49.

Miller, D. (1992a). 'Staff stress in HIV health care workers (Amsterdam summary)'. *AIDS Care*, 4 (4), 429–32.

Miller, D. (1992b). 'Stress and coping of HIV/AIDS health care workers: a review and a challenge'. Poster presented to VII International Conference on AIDS in Africa, Yaounde, Cameroon, 8–11 December. (Unpublished)

Miller, D. (1993). 'HIV/AIDS health worker stress and stress prevention'. *AIDS Care*, 5(4): 517–21.

Miller, J. D. (1995a). 'Dying to Care?: Occupational Morbidity and Burnout, and Preferences for Staff Support in HIV and Oncology Health Care'. Unpublished Doctoral thesis, University of Nottingham.

Miller, D. (1995b). 'Models of management for occupational morbidity and burnout'. In: L. Bennett, D. Miller, M. W. Ross (eds), *Health Workers and AIDS: Research, Intervention and Current Issues in Burnout and Response*. Reading: Harwood Academic Press, 175–90.

Miller, D. (1995c). 'The UK Multicentre Occupational Morbidity Study (MOMS): issues of methodology, volunteer bias and preliminary findings on preferences for staff support in HIV/AIDS health staff'. In: L. Bennett, D. Miller, M. W. Ross (eds), *Health Workers and AIDS: Research, Intervention and Current Issues in Burnout and Response*. Reading: Harwood Academic Press, 213–28.

Miller, D. (1996). 'Stress and burnout in HIV/AIDS carers'. *AIDS*, 10 (Suppl. A), S213–S219.

Miller, D., Brown, B. (1988). 'Developing the role of clinical psychology in the context of AIDS'. *The Psychologist*, 2, 63–6.

Miller, D., Gillies, P. (1993). *Prevention of Occupational Morbidity in Management of HIV Infection and Disease: Interim Report on Study Phase One*. London: Department of Health.

Miller, D., Gillies, P. (1996) 'Is there life after work: experiences of HIV and oncology health staff'. *AIDS Care*, 8(2), 167–82.

Miller, D., Green, J. (1986). 'Counselling for HIV infection and AIDS'. *Clinics in Immunology and Allergy (AIDS and HIV infection)*, 6 (3), 661–83.

Miller, D., Riccio, M. (1990). 'Functional psychiatric syndromes associated with HIV1 infection and disease'. *AIDS*, 4 (5), 381–88.

Miller, D., Weber, J., Green, J. (1986). *The Management of AIDS Patients*. London: MacMillan Press.

Miller, D., Gillies, P., Elliott, C. (1994a). 'Successful staff burnout prevention: lessons from six major UK HIV/AIDS treatment sites'. Paper presented at X International Conference on AIDS/IV International Conference on STD, Yokohama, 7–12 August. (Unpublished)

Miller, D., Nott, K. H., Vedhara, K. (1994b). 'HIV and psychoimmunology: evidence promising and forthcoming'. *Journal of The Royal Society of Medicine*, 87, 687–90.

Miller, D., Gillies, P., Elliott, C. (1996). *Prevention of Occupational Morbidity and Burnout in Management of HIV Infection and Disease: Final Report*. London: Department of Health.

Miller, D., van Praag, E., Lloyd, G., Kalibala, S. (1999). 'HIV/AIDS counselling: The WHO model and its implementation'. In: D. Miller, J. Green (eds), *The Psychology of Sexual Health*. London: Blackwell Science, in press.

Miller, M. M., Potter, R. E. (1982). 'Professional burnout among speech-language pathologists'. *ASHA*, 24 (3), 177–81.

Miller R., Bor, R., Salt, H., Murray, D. (1989). 'AIDS and children: some of the issues in haemophilia care and how to address them'. *AIDS Care*, 1, 59–65.

Milne, R., Keen, S. (1988). 'Are general practitioners ready to prevent the spread of HIV?' *British Medical Journal*, 296, 533–5.

Moos, R. H., Insel, P. M. (1974). *Combined Preliminary Manual, Family Work and Group Environmental Scales*. Palo Alto, CA: Consulting Psychologists Press.

Moreland, L., Legg, S. (1991). *Managing and Funding AIDS Organisations*. London: Department of Health/Compass Partnership.

Morin, S. F., Batchelor, W. F. (1984). 'Responding to the psychological crisis of AIDS'. *Public Health Reports*, 99, 4–9.

Moser, C., Kalton, G. (1979). *Survey Methods in Social Investigation* (2nd edn). London: Heinemann Educational Books.

Munodawafa, D., Bower, D. A., Webb, A. A. (1993). 'Perceived vulnerability to HIV/AIDS in the US and Zimbabwe'. *International Nursing Review*, 40(1), 13–16.

National Association for Staff Support (NASS) (1992). *A Charter for Staff Support for Staff in the Health Care Services*. Woking: NASS.

Nesbitt, W. H., Ross, M. W., Sunderland, R. H., Shelp, E. E. (1996). 'Prediction of grief and HIV/AIDS-related burnout in volunteers'. *AIDS Care*, 8(2), 137–44.

Nicholls, S. E. (1986). 'An overview of the psychological and social reactions to AIDS'. In: J. C. Gluckman, E. Vilmer (eds), *Acquired Immundeficiency Syndrome (International Conference on AIDS, Paris 1986)*. Paris: Elsevier, 261–270.

O'Donnell, L., O'Donnell, C., Pleck, J., Snarey, J., Rose, R. (1987). 'Psychosocial responses of hospital workers to Acquired Immune Deficiency Syndrome (AIDS)'. *Journal of Applied Social Psychology*, 17, 269–85.

O'Driscoll, M. P., Schubert, T. (1988). 'Organisational climate and burnout in a New Zealand social service agency'. *Work and Stress*, 2 (3), 199–204.

Offit, A. (1994). *Virtual Love: A Novel*. New York: Simon and Schuster.

Omoto, A. M., Snyder, M. (1990). 'Basic research in action: volunteerism and society's response to AIDS'. *Personality and Social Psychology Bulletin*, 16(1), 152–65.

Osborne, C., van Praag, E., Jackson, H. (1997). 'Models of care for patients with HIV/AIDS. *AIDS*, 11 (Suppl. B), S135–S,141.

Otway, H. J., Misenta, R. (1980). 'The determinance of operator preparedness for emergency situations in nuclear power plants'. Paper presented at International Workshop on Procedural and Organisational Measures for Accident Management: Nuclear Reactors, Laxenburg, Austria, 28–31 January 1980. (Unpublished)

Paradis, L. F., Miller, B., Runnion, V. M. (1987). 'Volunteer stress and burnout: issues for administration'. *Hospice Journal*, 3, 165–83.

Parsons, C. D. F. (1995). 'Infection control in the era of HIV/AIDS'. In: L. Bennett, D. Miller, M. W. Ross (eds), *Health Workers and AIDS: Research, Intervention and Current Issues in Burnout and Response*. Reading: Harwood Academic Press, 341–60.

Pasacreta, J. V., Jacobsen, P. B. (1989). 'Addressing the need for staff support among nurses caring for the AIDS population'. *Oncology Nursing Forum*, 16, 659–63.

Patton, C. (1989). 'The AIDS industry: construction of "victims", "volunteers", and "experts"'. In: E. Porter, S. Watney (eds), *Taking Liberties: AIDS and Cultural Politics*. London: The Serpent's Tail.

Paykel, E. S. (1983). 'Methodological aspects of life events research'. *Journal of Psychosomatic Research*, 27 (5), 341–52.

Payne, R. (1984). 'Review of W. Paine's "Job stress and burnout: research theory and intervention perspectives"'. *Journal of Occupational Psychology*, 57, 175–6.

Pearlin, L. I., Semple, S., Turner, H. (1988). 'Stress of AIDS caregiving: a preliminary overview of the issues'. *Death Studies*, 12 (5–6), 501–17.

Perlman, B., Hartman, E. A. (1982). 'Burnout: summary and future research'. *Human Relations*, 35 (4), 283–305.

Piemme, J., Bolle, J. (1990). 'Coping with grief in response to caring for persons with AIDS'. *The American Journal of Occupational Therapy*, 44 (3), 266–9.

Piercy, F. P., Wetchler, J. L. (1987). 'Family work interfaces of psychotherapists'. *Journal of Psychotherapy and the Family*, 3 (2), 17–32.

Pinching, A. J. (1986). 'AIDS: dilemmas for the psychiatrist' (letter). *The Lancet*, 1 March 1986, 496–7.

Pines, A. (1982). 'Helpers' motivation and the burnout syndrome'. In T. A. Wills (ed.), *Basic Processes in Helping Relationships*. New York: Academic Press, 453–75.

Pines, A., Kafry, D. (1981). 'Tedium in the life and work of professional women as compared to men'. *Sex Roles*, 7 (10), 963–77.

Pines, A., Maslach, C. (1978). 'Characteristics of staff burnout in mental health settings'. *Hospital and Community Psychiatry*, 29, 233–7.

Pines, A., Aronson, E., Kafry, D. (1981). *Burnout: From Tedium to Personal Growth*. New York: Free Press.

Plant, M. L., Plant, M. A., Foster, J. (1992). 'Stress, alcohol, tobacco and illicit drug use amongst nurses: a Scottish study'. *Journal of Advanced Nursing*, 17, 1057–67.

Plaut, S. M. (1997) 'Boundary violations in professional–client relationships: overview and guidelines for prevention'. *Sexual and Marital Therapy*, 12(1), 77–94.

Pomerance, L., Shields, J. (1989). 'Perinatal nurses' knowledge and attitudes about AIDS'. *Journal of Obstetric, Gynaecological and Neonatal Nursing*, 18, 363–8.

Pretty, G. M. H., McCarthy, M. E., Catano, V. M. (1992). 'Psychological environments and burnout: gender considerations within the corporation'. *Journal of Organisational Behaviour*, 13, 701–11.

Price, D. M., Murphy, P. A. (1984). 'Staff burnout in the perspective of grief theory'. *Death Education*, 8, 47–58.

Procter, B. (undated). 'Supervision: a co-operative exercise in accountability'. In: M. Marken, M. Payne (eds), *Enabling and Ensuring*. Leicester National Youth Bureau and Council for Education and Training in Youth and Community Work.

Pruyser, P. W. (1984). 'Existential impact of professional exposure to life-threatening or terminal illness'. *Bulletin of the Menninger Clinic*, 48, 357–67.

Raphael B., Kelly, B., Dunne, M., Greig, R. (1990). 'Psychological distress among volunteer AIDS counsellors'. *Medical Journal of Australia*, 152, 275.

Redfern, N. (1990). 'Morbidity among anaesthetists'. *British Journal of Hospital Medicine*, 43, 377–81.

Reed, P., Wise, T. N., Mann, L. S. (1984). 'Nurses' attitudes regarding acquired immunodeficiency syndrome (AIDS)'. *Nursing Forum*, 21, 153–6.

Reynolds, S., Briner, R. B. (1994). 'Stress management at work: with whom, for whom and to what ends?' *British Journal of Guidance and Counselling*, 22 (1), 75–89.

Rogers, J. C., Dodson, S. C. (1987). 'Burnout in occupational therapists'. *The American Journal of Occupational Therapy*, 42 (12), 787–92.

Rose, R., Jenkins, C. D., Hurst, M. W. (1978). *Air Traffic Controller Health Change Study: Report to the Federal Aviation Administration*. Boston: Federal Aviation Administration.

Ross, M. W., Seeger, V. (1988). 'Determinants of reported burnout in health professionals associated with the care of patients with AIDS'. *AIDS*, 2, 395–7.

Roth, N. L. (1995). 'Structuring burnout: interactions among HIV/AIDS health workers, their clients, organisations and society'. In: L. Bennett, D. Miller, M. W. Ross, (eds), *Health Workers and AIDS: Research, Intervention and Current Issues in Burnout and Response*. Reading: Harwood Academic Press, 73–92.

Rottier, J., Kelly, W., Tomhave, W. K. (1983). 'Teacher burnout – small and rural school style'. *Education*, 104 (1), 72–9.

Rugg, D., Schulz, S. L., Fagan, R., Rhodes, F. (1989). 'Job related stress among HIV antibody test counsellors'. Paper presented at V International Conference on AIDS, Montreal, 4–9 June. (Unpublished)

Russell, D. W., Altmaier, E., Van Velzen, D. (1987). 'Job-related stress, social support, and burnout among classroom teachers'. *Journal of Applied Psychology*, 72, 269–74.

Sallis, J. F., Trevorrow, T. R., Johnson, C. C., *et al.* (1987). 'Worksite stress management: a comparison of programmes'. *Psychology and Health*, 1, 237 55.

Salovey, P., O'Leary, A., Stretton, M. S., *et al.* (1991). 'Influence of mood on judgements about health and illness'. In: J. P. Forgas (ed.), *Emotion and Social Judgement*. Oxford: Pergamon Press, 241–62.

Salt, H. (1997). Personal communication.

Savicki, R., Cooley, E. (1983). 'The relationship of work environment and client contact to burnout in mental health professionals'. Paper presented at annual meeting of the American Psychological Association, San Francisco. (Unpublished)

Schaufeli, W. B., Enzmann, D., Girault, N. (1993a). 'Measurement of burnout: a review'. In: W. B. Schaufeli, C. Maslach, T. Marek (eds), *Professional Burnout: Recent Developments in Theory and Research*. Washington, DC: Taylor & Francis, 199–215.

Schaufeli, W. B., Maslach, C., Marek T. (eds) (1993b), *Professional Burnout: Recent Developments in Theory and Research*. Washington, DC: Taylor & Francis.

Schneider, J. (1984). *Stress, Loss and Grief: Understanding their Origins and Growth Potential*. Baltimore, MD: University Park.

Schuler, R. S. (1980). 'Definition and conceptualisation of stress in organisations'. *Organisation Behaviour and Human Performance*, 25, 184–215.

Schwab, R. L., Iwanicki, E. F. (1982). 'Perceived role conflict, role ambiguity, and teacher burnout'. *Educational Administration Quarterly*, 18, 60–74.

Seeley, J., Kajura, E., Bachengana, C., *et al.* (1993). 'The extended family and support for people with AIDS in a rural population in west Uganda: a safety net with holes?' *AIDS Care*, 5, 117–22.

Selder, F. E., Paustian, A. (1989). 'Burnout: absence of vision'. *Loss, Grief and Care (Special Edition on 'Professional Burnout in Medicine and the Helping Professions')*, 3 (1–2), 1–19.

Selye, H. (1956). *The Stress of Life*. New York: McGraw-Hill.

Selye, H. (1976). *Stress in Health and Disease*. Boston: Butterworths.

Sheldon, T. A., Borowitz, M. (1993). 'Changing the measure of quality in the NHS: from purchasing activity to purchasing protocols'. *Quality in Health Care*, 2 (3), 149–50.

Sherr, L., George, H. (1989). 'Effects of HIV and AIDS work on staff involved in caring'. In: P. Bennett, J. Weinman (eds), *Proceedings of the 2nd Conference of the Health Psychology Section*. Leicester, British Psychological Society.

Shilts, R. (1987). *And The Band Played On: Politics, People, and the AIDS Epidemic*. London: Penguin.

Shinn, M., Rosario, M., Morch, H., Chestnut, D. E. (1984). 'Coping with job stress and burnout in the human services'. *Journal of Personality and Social Psychology*, 46 (4), 864–76.

Shirom, A., *et al.* (1973). 'A sketch of the policeman's working personality'. In: A. Niederhoffer, A. S. Blumberg (eds), *The Ambivalent Force*. San Francisco, CA: Rhinehart Press, 132–43.

Sigman, A. (1992). 'The state of corporate health care'. *Personnel Management*, Feb, 24–31.

Smail, D. (1993). *The Origins of Unhappiness: A New Understanding of Personal Distress*. London: HarperCollins.

Smyser, M. S., Bryce, J. B., Joseph, G. (1990). 'AIDS-related knowledge attitude and precautionary behaviours among emergency medical professionals'. *Public Health Reports*, 105(5), 496–504.

Smyth, M., Browne, F. (1992). *General Household Survey 1990*. London: HMSO.

Sontag, S. (1990). *Illness as Metaphor, and AIDS and its Metaphors*. New York: Anchor.

Sorensen, J. L., Constantini, M. F., London, J. A. (1989). 'Coping with AIDS: strategies for patients and staff in drug abuse treatment programmes'. *Journal of Psychoactive Drugs*, 21 (4), 435–41.

Spector, P. E. (1992). 'A consideration of the validity and meaning of self-report measures of job conditions'. In: C. L. Cooper, I. T. Robertson (eds), *International Review of Industrial and Organisational Psychology*. Chichester: John Wiley, 123–51.

Stevens, M. J., Pfost, K. S. (1983). 'A problem-solving approach to staff burnout in rehabilitation settings'. *Rehabilitation Counselling Bulletin*, 27 (2), 101–7.

Stewart, B., Meyerowitz, B., Jackson, L., *et al.* (1982). 'Psychological stress associated with out-patient oncology nursing'. *Cancer Nursing*, 5, 383–7.

Strassmeier, W. (1986). Early intervention and ecology. *Fruhforderung-interdisziplinar*, 5 (4), 151–62.

Sunderland, R. H., Shelp, E. E. (1993). 'Supervision solves volunteer "burn-out" problem'. Paper presented at IX International Conference on AIDS IV STD World Congress. Berlin, 6–11 June 1993. (Unpublished)

Taylor, A. J. (1991). 'Method in my madness: song or swan song'. *Bulletin of New Zealand Psychological Society*, 71, 14–19.

Taylor, K., Eakin, J., Skinner, H., *et al.* (1990). 'Physicians' perception of personal risk of HIV infection and AIDS through occupational exposure'. *Canadian Medical Association Journal*, 143(6), 493–500.

Temoshok, L., Dreher, H. (1992). *The Type C Connection: The mind-body Link to Cancer and your Health*. New York: Plume.

Theorell, T. (1974). 'Life events before and after onset of a premature myocardial infarction'. In: B. S. Dohrenwend, B. P. Dohrenwend (eds), *Stressful Life Events: Their Nature and Effects*. New York, Wiley.

Tomlinson, B. (1993). *Making London Better*. London: Department of Health Publications.

Treiber, F. A., Shaw, D., Malcolm, R. (1987). 'Acquired immunodeficiency syndrome: psychological impact on health personnel'. *Journal of Nervous and Mental Disease*, 175 (8), 496–9.

Turner, H. A., Catania, J. A., Gagnon, J. (1994). 'The prevalence of informal caregiving to persons with AIDS in the US: caregiver characteristics and their implications'. *Social Science and Medicine*, 38, 1543–52.

Ullrich, A., FitzGerald, P. (1990). 'Stress experienced by physicians and nurses in the cancer ward'. *Social Science and Medicine*, 31 (9), 1013–22.

Ursprung, A. W. (1986). 'Incidence and correlates of burnout in residential service settings'. *Rehabilitation Counselling Bulletin*, 29, 225–93.

van Dis, H., van Dongen, E. (1993). *Burnout in HIV/AIDS Health Care and Support: Impact for Professionals and Volunteers*. Amsterdam: University of Amsterdam Press.

van Servellen, G., Leake, B. (1993). 'Burn-out in hospital nurses: a comparison of acquired immunodeficiency syndrome, oncology, general medical, and intensive care unit nurse samples'. *Journal of Professional Nursing*, 9 (3), 169–77.

van Servellen, G., Lewis, C., Leake, B. (1988). 'Nurses' responses to the AIDS crisis: implications for continuing education programs'. *Journal of Continuing Education in Nursing*, 19, 4–8.

Visintini, R., Fossati, A., Fontana, S., *et al.* (1995). 'The measurement of the impact of working with HIV-patients on nurses: reliability, construct and criterion-related validity of the AIDS impact scale'. In: L. Bennett, D. Miller, M. W. Ross (eds), *Health Workers and AIDS: Research, Intervention and Current Issues in Burnout and Response*. Reading: Harwood Academic Press, 93–114.

Visintini, R., Campanini, E., Fossati, A., *et al.* (1996). 'Psychological stress in nurses' relationship with HIV-infected patients: the risk of burnout syndrome'. *AIDS Care*, 8(2), 183 91.

Wade, K., Perlman Simon, E. (1993). 'Survival bonding: a response to stress and work with AIDS'. *Social Work in Health Care*, 19 (1), 77–89.

Wall, T. D., Kemp, N. J., Jackson, P. R., Clegg, C. W. (1986). 'Outcomes of autonomous workgroups: a long term field experiment'. *Academy of Management Journal*, 29, 280–304.

Wallace, J. E., Brinkerhoff, M. (1991). 'The measurement of burnout revisited'. *Journal of Social Service Research*, **14** (1), 85–111.

Walsh, S. (1990). 'Personal and professional threat: a model of self care for clinicians'. Unpublished MSc thesis, University of Exeter.

Warr, P. B. (1987). *Work, Unemployment and Mental Health*. Oxford: Clarendon Press.

Warr, P., Jackson, P. (1985). 'Factors influencing the psychological impact of prolonged unemployment and of re-employment'. *Psychological Medicine*, **15** (4), 795–807.

Webb, S., Gouse, V., Ford, A., Lutz, B. (1993). 'Conflict in the trenches: local health officials and HIV community leaders'. Paper presented at IX International Conference on AIDS, Berlin, June 6–11 (POD 244140). (Unpublished)

Whittington, A., Wilson, S., Avery, T. (1993). *Unemployment and Health: a Literature Review*. Nottingham: Department of General Practice, and Department of Health Medicine and Epidemiology monograph.

Wilcoxon, S. A. (1989). 'Leadership behaviour and therapist burnout: a study of rural agency settings'. *Journal of Rural Community Psychology*, **10** (2), 3–14.

Williams, M. J. (1988). 'Gay men as "buddies" to persons living with AIDS and ARC'. *Smith College Studies in Social Work: Special Issue on AIDS*, **59**, 38–52.

World Health Organization (1992). *Global Programme on AIDS Progress Report 1991*, Geneva: World Health Organization.

World Health Organization (1995). *Counselling for HIV/AIDS: A Key to Caring*. Geneva: World Health Organization/Global Programme on AIDS (WHO/GPA/TCO/HCS/95. 15).

World Health Organization/UNAIDS (1997). *The Implications of Antiretroviral Treatments: Informal Consultation, April 1997*. Geneva: WHO/UNAIDS (WHO/ASD/97. 2).

Zabel, R. H., Zabel, M. K. (1982). 'Factors in burnout among teachers of exceptional children'. *Exceptional Children*, **49**, 261–3.

Index

The following abbreviations have been used in the index: MBI Maslach Burnout Inventory

Printed in the United States
by Baker & Taylor Publisher Services